SENILE DEMENTIA: A BIOMEDICAL APPROACH

Developments in Neuroscience

SENILE DEMENTIA:
A BIOMEDICAL APPROACH

Proceedings of the Conference held in St. Louis, Missouri, U.S.A. on March 22-23, 1978

Edited by

KALIDAS NANDY

Geriatric Research, Education and Clinical Center, Veterans Administration Hospital, Bedford, Massachusetts, and Department of Anatomy and Neurology, Boston University School of Medicine, Boston, Massachusetts, U.S.A.

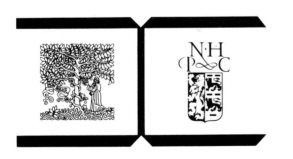

ELSEVIER/NORTH-HOLLAND BIOMEDICAL PRESS
NEW YORK • AMSTERDAM • 1978

with the exception of the contributions authored by Paul L. Haber (pp. xi—xxi), Ralph Goldman (pp. 3—17), Kalidas Nandy (pp. 19—32), Carolyn B. Smith (pp. 45—60), Clarence J. Gibbs et al. (pp. 115—130), and Irwin Feinberg (pp. 155—168), which are works of the United States Government.

Published by:

ELSEVIER NORTH-HOLLAND, INC.
52 Vanderbilt Avenue
New York, New York 10017

Sole distributors outside U.S.A. and Canada:

ELSEVIER/NORTH-HOLLAND BIOMEDICAL PRESS
335 Jan Van Galenstraat, P.O. Box 211
Amsterdam, The Netherlands

ISBN: 0-444-80028-X (series)
ISBN: 0-444-00271-5 (vol. 3)

Library of Congress Cataloging in Publication Data
Main entry under title:

Senile dementia: a biomedical approach

   (Developments in neuroscience ; v. 3)
   Bibliography: p.
   Includes index.
   1. Senile psychosis—Congresses. 2. Senile psychosis—Physiological aspects—Congresses.
I. Nandy, Kalidas II. Series. [DNLM: 1. Psychosis, Senile—Congresses. 2. Dementia, Presenile—Congresses. 3. Aging—Congresses.
4. Brain chemistry—Congresses. W1 DE998K v. 3/ WT150 B615s 1978]
RC524.S46   618.9'76'8983   78-9358

Manufactured in the United States of America

CONTENTS

CONTRIBUTORS

MELVYN J. BALL, Departments of Pathology and Clinical Neurological Sciences, University of Western Ontario, London, N6A 5C1, Ontario, Canada

STEPHEN BOBIN, Immunobiology Laboratory, Department of Pathological Neurobiology, New York State Institute for Basic Research in Mental Retardation, 1050 Forest Hill Road, Staten Island, New York 10314, USA

ROLAND BRANCONNIER, Geriatric-Psychopharmacology Unit, Boston State Hospital, 591 Morton Street, Boston, Massachusetts 02124, USA

JONATHAN CHAFFEE, Immunobiology Laboratory, Department of Pathological Neurobiology, New York State Institute for Basic Research in Mental Retardation, 1050 Forest Hill Road, Staten Island, New York 10314, USA

JONATHAN O. COLE, McLean Hospital, 115 Mill Street, Belmont, Massachusetts 02178, USA

NORMA A. COOKE, Neuropsychology Laboratory, Department of Neurology, Baylor College of Medicine, Houston, Texas 77030, USA

JOHN O. EICHLING, Edward Mallinckrodt Institute of Radiology, Washington University School of Medicine, 510 South Kingshighway, St. Louis, Missouri 63110, USA

IRWIN FEINBERG, Psychiatry Service, Veterans Administration Hospital, San Francisco, California, USA and Department of Psychiatry, University of California, San Francisco, California, USA

MOKHTAR GADO, Edward Mallinckrodt Institute of Radiology, Washington University School of Medicine, 510 South Kingshighway, St. Louis, Missouri 63110, USA

D. CARLETON GAJDUSEK, Laboratory of Central Nervous System Studies, National Institute of Neurological and Communicative Disorders and Stroke, National Institutes of Health, Bethesda, Maryland 20014, USA

JOE R. A. GAY, Neuropsychology Laboratory, Department of Neurology, Baylor College of Medicine, Houston, Texas 77030 USA

MITCHELL GERSOVITZ, Department of Nutrition and Food Science, Massachusetts Institute of Technology, Cambridge, Massachusetts, USA

CLARENCE J. GIBBS, JR., Laboratory of Central Nervous System Studies, National Institute of Neurological and Communicative Disorders and Stroke, National Institutes of Health, Bethesda, Maryland 20014, USA

RALPH GOLDMAN, Assistant Chief, Medical Director for Extended Care, Veterans Administration Central Office, Washington, D.C.

ROBERT L. GRUBB, JR., Edward Mallinckrodt Institute of Radiology, Washington University School of Medicine, 510 South Kingshighway, St. Louis, Missouri 63110, USA

PAUL A.L. HABER, Assistant Chief, Medical Director for Professional Services, Veterans Administration Central Office, Washington, D.C.

CHARLES P. HUGHES, Department of Neurology and Neurological Surgery (Neurology), Washington University School of Medicine, 660 South Euclid, St. Louis, Missouri 63110, USA

O. HUNZIKER, Sandoz Institute of Basic Medical Research, Lichtstrasse 35, CH-4002 Basel, Switzerland

P. IWANGOFF, Sandoz Institute of Basic Medical Research, Lichtstrasse 35, CH-4002 Basel, Switzerland

STEPHEN E. KARPIAK, Division of Neuroscience, New York State Psychiatric Institute, 722 West 168th Street, New York, New York 10032, USA

THOMAS L. KEMPER, Boston City Hospital, Boston, Massachusetts, USA

COLIN L. MASTERS, Laboratory of Central Nervous System Studies, National Institute of Neurological and Communicative Disorders and Stroke, National Institutes of Health, Bethesda, Maryland 20014, USA

WILLIAM MEIER-RUGE, Sandoz Institute of Basic Medical Research, Lichtstrasse 35, CH-4002 Basel, Switzerland

HENRY J. MICHALEWSKI, Andrus Gerontology Center, University of Southern California, University Park, Los Angeles, California 90007, USA

HERBERT F. MÜLLER, EEG Department, Douglas Hospital, Montreal, H4H 1R3, Canada and McGill University, Montreal, Canada

KALIDAS NANDY, Geriatric Research, Education and Clinical Center, Veterans Administration Hospital, Bedford, Massachusetts, USA and Boston University School of Medicine, Boston, Massachusetts, USA

MERVAT NASSEF, Immunobiology Laboratory, Department of Pathological Neurobiology, New York State Institute for Basic Research in Mental Retardation, 1050 Forest Hill Road, Staten Island, New York 10314, USA

THOMAS NEWCOMB, Assistant Chief, Medical Director for Research and Development, Veterans Administration Central Office, Washington, D.C.

FRANCISCO I. PEREZ, Neuropsychology Laboratory, Department of Neurology, Baylor College of Medicine, Houston, Texas 77030, USA

ERIC PFEIFFER, Department of Psychiatry, University of Colorado School of Medicine, Denver, Colorado, USA

M. LINDA POWERS, Department of Pediatrics, Harvard Medical School, Endocrine Division, Children's Hospital Medical Center, Boston, Massachusetts, USA

MARCUS E. RAICHLE, Edward Mallinckrodt Institute of Radiology, Washington University School of Medicine, 510 South Kingshighway, St. Louis, Missouri 63110, USA

MAURICE M. RAPPORT, Division of Neuroscience, New York State Psychiatric Institute, 722 West 168th Street, New York, New York 10032, USA and Department of Biochemistry, Columbia University College of Physicians and Surgeons, 722 West 168th Street, New York, New York 10032, USA

K. REICHLMEIER, Sandoz Institute of Basic Medical Research, Lichtstrasse 35, CH-4002 Basel, Switzerland

P. SANDOZ, Sandoz Institute of Basic Medical Research, Lichtstrasse 35, CH-4002 Basel, Switzerland

RONALD E. SAUL, Department of Neurology, Rancho Los Amigos Hospital, 7601 Imperial Highway, Downey, California 90242, USA

IRA SHOULSON, Department of Neurology, University of Rochester School of Medicine, 601 Elmwood Avenue, Rochester, New York 14642, USA

CAROLYN B. SMITH, Laboratory of Cerebral Metabolism, National Institute of Mental Health, Bethesda, Maryland 20014, USA

LARRY W. THOMPSON, Andrus Gerontology Center, University of Southern California, University Park, Los Angeles, California 90007, USA

DOROTHY B. VILLEE, Department of Pediatrics, Harvard Medical School, Endocrine Division, Children's Hospital Medical Center, Boston, Massachusetts, USA

VERNON YOUNG, Department of Nutrition and Food Science, Massachusetts Institute of Technology, Cambridge, Massachusetts, USA

PREFACE

The mean life expectancy has changed significantly in the past decades in the United States. The growing number of older people has already made a significant impact on the health care system as well as the socio-economic condition of the country. About 21 million people are currently over 65 years of age and this number is expected to double by the turn of the century. Based on the hospital and nursing home statistics, nearly 3 million people in this group are suffering from a varying degree of clinically detectable mental impairment and this figure may represent only the tip of the iceberg. It is expected that the number of demented patients might progressively increase as more and more people will approach the maximum lifespan.

At present there are about 30 million veterans in the United States of which about 6 million are over 65 years. With the current growth trend of the population, this number might increase to about 12 million by the end of the century. It is said 1 out of 3 American males over 65 years of age will be veterans by the year 1990. This serious and growing problem was recognized by the Veterans Administration. As a result, eight Geriatric Research, Education and Clinical Centers (GRECC) within the Extended Care Program have been established initially under the leadership of Dr. Paul A.L. Haber and subsequently under the direction of Dr. Ralph Goldman. The purpose of these centers is to develop a better understanding of the complex biomedical and socio-economic problems of the aged and to enhance the quality of life of the older veterans.

In order to discuss this devastating and dehumanizing disease, senile dementia, a symposium was organized in St. Louis jointly by South-Central Regional Medical Education Center and the Veterans Administration Central Office in March, 1978. This book is published as the proceedings of the symposium and an outstanding group of physicians and scientists participated as contributors. The first part of the book deals primarily with epidemiological, histopathological,

immunological and neurochemical aspects of the brain changes. The
more clinical aspects including neuropsychological manifestations,
sleep and EEG changes, differential diagnosis and treatment are included in the second part of the book. Special chapters on Huntington's
disease, progeria and nutritional requirements have also been added.
An introductory chapter describing the more fundamental concepts of the
biological aging process has been included for the clinicians. It is
hoped that the book will advance the knowledge of the physicians and
scientists and eventually lead to a better understanding and management
of the complex biomedical problem.

The editor is grateful to John D. Chase, M.D., Chief, Medical
Director, Veterans Administration Central Office, for permission to
publish the proceedings of the symposium. I am also indebted to Paul
A. L. Haber, M.D., Assistant Chief, Medical Director for Professional
Services, Ralph Goldman, M.D., Assistant Chief, Medical Director for
Extended Care and Thomas F. Newcomb, M.D., Assistant Chief, Medical
Director for Research and Development for their participation and sup-
port in this venture. I am expressing my deep appreciation to Francis
A. Zacharewicz, M.D., Medical Director, Mr. Vern Gomes, M.A., M.S.,
Associate Director and especially Ms. Dorothy Sassenrath, M.S., Educa-
tional Specialist of South-Central Regional Medical Education Center
for their efficient management of and strong support in organizing the
symposium. The support of Mead Johnson & Company, Sandoz, Inc.,
American Hoechst Corporation, Schering Corporation, and Ciba-Geigy
Corporation is gratefully acknowledged. Finally, the editor
expresses his sincere thanks to the publisher for the continued
cooperation and understanding in dealing with the problems in the
preparation of this volume.

K. NANDY

FOREWORD

While research related to the aging process often appears to direct
itself towards pushing back the inevitable time of death, that is the
seeking of immortality, that objective should remain secondary to its
predecessor -- that the quality of life be optimal. This requires
that an individual remain functional, mentally and physically, that
he or she have a meaningful place in society, that a sufficient degree
of mobility be retained to permit continued social interaction, and
that each remain an individual person -- unique in some special way.
With our occasional preoccupation with the extension of life, we
sometimes neglect attention to these qualities of life. Dementia
strikes at the heart of them particularly. Although an afflicted in_
dividual's life may not be greatly shortened, the presence of this
disability attacks all of the aspects contributing to quality.
Whereas a locomotor disability might interfere with physical function
and mobility, or loss of hearing might require special adaptation to
remain employed, the individual afflicted with dementia has few op-
tions for adaptation and witnesses his own destruction as an individual. In many respects, the attachment of the word "senile" in
creation of the phrase "senile dementia" immediately fixes one's
thought processes towards the inevitability of aging and mental
deterioration. As the Proceedings of this conference will demonstrate, there are many avenues of approach to a solution of the problem we now call senile dementia. Some of these indeed have their
roots in a study of the aging process whereas others do not. At the
present time, when many of our correlations must be descriptive, we
should be especially cautious not to associate cause and effect with
these correlations. Different perspectives might be obtained when
one compares persons with dementia to others of the same age as distinct from studying the problem of dementia by starting with the

normal aged.

This conference brings together investigators from a variety of disciplinary origins. Each sees the problem somewhat differently and indeed each may be seeing a different problem. For the present, however, it is important for these individuals to hear each other and for the reader of these Proceedings to look for the individualities as independent from the commonalities. Integration into a common explanation must await further work and will probably lead to the conquest of at least a portion of what is now called senile dementia.

Thomas F. Newcomb, M.D.

INTRODUCTION

BIOMEDICAL ASPECTS OF AGING:
A REVIEW OF THEORY AND PHILOSOPHICAL PRINCIPLES

PAUL A. L. HABER

In undertaking to write an introductory review to a consideration of Biomedical Aspects of Senile Dementia it seems appropriate to review the biomedical aspects of aging in general. It may be most profitable to orient those considerations towards a review of the current theories of aging in general. There are many compilations of theories of aging but it would be useful to create one that relates particularly to the concerns about senile dementia and the review of theories of aging which contribute most significantly to our understanding of the aging of the brain. If aging in man is at all different from aging of other species, it may be because of the higher degree of organismal organization, quite probably not more evident in any tissues than in those of the central nervous system. It is difficult at this point in our studies to determine absolutely whether this further extension of differentiation and organization (so much a part of what separates man from his fellow creatures) renders human beings more or less susceptible to the degredations of the aging process. While it is clear that the more highly integrated an organ system becomes, the more vulnerable it will be to perturbations of any sort, in the case of the brain it might be argued that the higher the degree of organization becomes, the more potent will be the organism's coping ability.

The timeliness of these considerations must be apparent to anyone who is concerned with the delivery of health care. In these days when the probability of some form of National Health Insurance coverage grows ever larger, a great deal of national consciousness has focused on the cost of health care delivery in the United States. It is now estimated that the total expenditures for health care both through direct and indirect reimbursements and delivery modes approaches the staggering sum of $160 billion dollars, which approximates 8.5% of the Gross National Product. There has been a great public outcry protesting the rate of increase of health care expenditures. Knowles[1] has shown that the rate of growth has been threefold in the ten year period between 1965 and 1975. Tibbits[2] has noted that there are over 1.2 million nursing home beds in the United States with expenditures to support them of seven and a half billion dollars annually. Carver[3] has stated that the number of elderly with mental conditions in such institutions is about 79%: Thirty-four percent having a diagnosis of advanced senility, twenty-eight percent having senility without psychosis, and seventeen percent having some other mental condition. Chien[4] has estimated that the number of mentally ill elderly in such nursing homes may be between 60 and 80 percent of the total population. But the problem is not confined to nursing homes alone. Whanger[5] has pointed out that ten percent of admissions to state mental hospitals and about a third of in-hospital population are aged sixty-five or more. Most of these have some form of chronic brain disease. Finally, it is known that of all short-stay hospital discharges there are 1.55 per 100 discharges due to chronic brain syndrome according to Health, Education & Welfare[6] figures. The conclusion that forces itself upon the observer is that senile brain disease and the dementias which accompany or are part of the syndrome have enormous economic impact upon the health care delivery system of the United States.

The emergence of senile dementia as a major cause of concern is a phenomenon of our time. The major reason for this to be true is the fact that there are so many older people living in our society. It is likely that the problems associated with aging have not been a cause of grave concern to any society because no society ever had to cope with large numbers of aging individuals. Hayflick[7] and others have indicated that the existence of large numbers of aged individuals is a biological luxury which has not been exercised by any species or society in the past. Whether because of the advances of modern medicine, or because of cultural advances, the life expectancy (though not the life span) of adult individuals has increased greatly. Ordinarily the bioecology of any species requires that individuals reach the age of reproduction and early child rearing. It does not require their continued existence into old age, however, in order to assure the propagation of the species. So that the emergence of senile dementia is a condition which now affects the economic well-being of the whole society. If some way could be found to ameliorate the ravages of the senile dementias to the affected population, the whole society would undoubtedly profit economically and socially as well.

The sad fact is that while Medicare and Medicaid have undoubtedly wrought great progress in the care and treatment of aging Americans, in the public mind, at least, those social programs created to help provide medical treatment for the aging are associated with the idea of demented patients inhabiting nursing homes. And it is precisely the behavior pattern of patients with senile brain disease that makes it so difficult to maintain patients at home or in other less costly surroundings than nursing homes. If some way could be found to delay or prevent senile brain disease, the resultant benefit might make it possible to reduce the nursing home permanent population by half.

There is a conflict today voiced widely in circles concerned with research into aging which pits advocates of research leading to a longer life against those who would concentrate instead on trying to ameliorate those conditions which tend to degrade the quality of life in the aged person. Briefly put, the dilemma runs to whether we ought to concentrate on the length or quantity of life as against the quality of life. But research into the cause of senile dementia must surely be given high priority regardless of which camp wins, because it is clear that both the length and the nature of living must be favorably altered if the process of senile dementia can be prevented.

Certainly one of the most venerable theories of aging is that of "Cross-linking". This theory as originally conceived obtained most particularly to supporting tissues, but it has been extended now to cover other systems, especially DNA. This theory holds that cross-linking agents such as a variety of aldehydes, metals (such as copper, aluminum and manganese), organic acids (such as fumaric and succinic acid) and certain amino acids, occur naturally in body fluids and that they tend to attach themselves at right angles to the long axis of parallel chains of the substrate substances. This cross attachment causes disruption in the functioning of the main elements. Cross-linking of parallel strands of collagen begins in the precursor substance, tropocollagen. As collagen ages, the degree of cross-linking increases. This process can be demonstrated by inhibition of the normal shortening of aging tendon tissue when thermal stress is applied, or the failure to exhibit normal swelling when exposed to some solution. This progress of cross-linking in collagen causes a decrease in elasticity which has long been observed in aging animals. The degree of cross-linking is specific for animal species and is related to the pace of aging. Thus the amount of cross-linking in a two and a half year old rat tail (an aged rat) is much greater than collagen in a two and a half year old human infant, but quite comparable to the amount of cross-linking in an aged human of seventy-five years. Concurrent with the loss of elasticity there is also a certain brittleness which has been compared to the excessive tanning of leather. There is some relationship between the degree of cross-linking and the presence of free radicals and the effects of oxidation and peroxidation.

In the case of elastin[8] cross-linking is a potent factor in explaining the aging process but its dynamics are not as well worked out as in the case of collagen. The amino acids, desmosine and isodesmosine are implicated in the cross-linking process here. It is also known that this cross-linking does increase during normal maturation, but may be constant in the otherwise intact aging animal. The theories of aging that indict disruption of the supporting rather than parenchymal tis-

sues seem to be more directly involved in an explanation of the damage
wrought by aging in that the parallel strand structure of supporting
tissues is readily seen as susceptible to cross-linking. The mechanical nature of this theory seems to fit closely with a structural change
familiar to many chemists working with polymers.

A second theory of aging has to do with the production of free
radicals which are highly reactive molecular groupings produced in the
course of oxygenation of a large number of complex organic substances.
These free radicals have been implicated in the aging of such everyday
substances as rubber and plastics. In biological tissues they have
been thought by some to cause degradation of membranes,
mucopolysacchares, elastin, collagen and of other connective tissue
components. But most intriguing is the possible interaction of free
radicals with DNA. This interaction between DNA and the free radicals
causes the formation of intermediate substances which are highly unstable. They cause DNA alterations which are passed on to RNA and
bring about the formation of malsynthesized proteins. Inhibitors of
free radicals such as Vitamin E have recently been thought to be useful
in minimizing the degradative effects of free radicals and have earned
a vogue in popular methods of "preventing" aging. The proponents of
the free radical theory of aging have not fully worked out the process
imputed by them to effect aging, but the free radicals are thought to
interfere with oxygenation and peroxidation mechanisms.

One particularly appealing aspect of the free radical theory has
been the effect on unsaturated fatty acids which appear to be among the
most vulnerable substances to be attacked by free radicals. Harman has
called attention to this phenomenon[9] particularly to the effect of perturbation of membrane mechanics. The smooth functioning of membranes
depends to a large extent on uninterrupted electron transfer in the
normal oxidation chain which, if interrupted by the action of free radicals, renders the membranes' function imperfect. This has the effect

of aging the cell and reducing its vitality.

In considering the free radical theory of aging one passes logically to another theory - that of radiation. Following the atom-bomb blasts of the Second World War it became widely known that the effects of ionizing radiation in many ways mimicked the effects of aging. Indeed, in some quarters, it was thought that radiation itself was the cause of aging. Although radiation does produce harmful effects on the cell in a variety of ways, the one that seems most likely to account for its effect is through the production of free radicals. The tremendous effect of free radicals on cellular dynamics is evidenced by the knowledge that if but one molecule within a cell out of every million molecules is destroyed the cell would not survive. Coupled with the age-old observation that the exposed portions of the body (the throat, face, hands) show the classic skin changes of aging such as thickening, wrinkling and loss of elasticity is the disquieting knowledge that we are constantly exposed to background radiation of the order of 0.1 rad per year and one cannot dismiss the effects of radiation on aging. It has been proposed that finding some way in which to totally shield animals or humans from radiation might prove an interesting counter to the normal effects of aging. Certainly experimentations on that thesis would seem to yield useful information.

Still another theory of aging has to do with the rate of energy expenditure. It has been postulated that the total amount of energy available to a given individual is peculiar to the species and that the rate of expenditure is inversely proportional to the life span. A faster rate of consumption is exhibited by short-lived animals while animals with greater species longevity are characterized by a slower rate of energy disposition. This phenomenon is also related to the size of the species particularly among warm-blooded animals since smaller species exhibit higher metabolic rates than do larger ones. The need for smaller animals to metabolize faster than larger ones is related to the rate of heat production versus heat loss and this in turn derives from the fact that animals of small size have a disproportionately larger part of their mass devoted to surface area in the integument than do larger ones.

Some illustrative data help confirm the above facts. Thus, the mouse has an average weight of 0.021 kg. Its BMR is 3.6 cal/day for a total of 171 kcal/kg/day and its average lifespan is between two and a half and three years. On the other hand the pig which weighs 128 kg, has a metabolic rate of 2443 kcal/day or 19.1 kcal/kg/day and its lifespan is 30 years.[10] That the theory has its limits is attested to by the fact that heavier mammals such as the rhinoceros, elephant, hippopotamus although weighing many times more than man do not show proportionate differences in metabolic rate or lifespans. Data of a different kind tend to support the idea that at least among some lower forms of life, longevity appears to be increased when the ambient temperature is lowered for significant periods of time. This appears to be particularly true if the young or adolescent animal is exposed to lower than usual temperatures and if the animal is simultaneously kept on a diet which is restrictive in caloric intake.

The accumulation of waste products in the cell has been the basis for yet another theory of aging. In this theory it has been postulated that degradation products of cellular metabolism tend to accumulate with age and that the resultant cell mass tends to occupy more and more space in the aging cell and thus mechanically interferes with the normal movement of metabolites within the cell and impinges on the living space of the cellular organelles. Lipofuscin for example is a pigment which is the byproduct of cellular metabolism and is composed of complete fatty acid derivatives. Cephalin, sphingomyelin, cholesterol esters, and lecithin have been found to form part of the composition of lipofuscin. The origins of lipofuscin have been postulated to be remnants of membranes or of mitochondria, but whatever its origin it is now generally accepted that the accumulation of lipofuscin increases with age. It has been found in increased quantities within certain tissues such as nervous tissue, bone, and myocardium.

Although lipofuscin has been implicated in this theory of the accumulation of waste products, other substances have been investigated as well. Calcium and magnesium in particular have been thought to increase in concentration with increased age. Indeed the entire role of trace elements has been investigated with some success. In the case of trace elements it is felt that deficiency as well as excess can cause cellular mischief. A host of metallic ions such as zinc, iron, copper, and chromium are found to be necessary in minute quantities for many enzymatic processes to function. A recent seminar at the VA Center in Bay Pines, Florida has called attention to the role of trace elements in aging.[11]

Altered endocrine function as a basis for aging has long been observed in virtually every gland. Thus, decreased function has been documented in the aged state in thyroid, gonad, pituitary, pancreas, and adrenal gland to name but some of the target, endocrine systems. Some have found it useful to parallel the prototype of the aged individual with the classic case of hypothyroidism - slow speech, cracked voice, obtunded sensorium, cold extremities, constipation, querulous personality and indeed there was a fad in medical practice (now thankfully defunct) to prescribe thyroid hormone almost routinely for older patients. Another endocrine function well studied in aging has been the rold of pancreatic secretion of insulin and the altered effects of insulin on glucose metabolism in the aged animal. Here we now know that the usual profile of glucose metabolism demonstrated in humans by the normal glucose tolerance test is not at all a valid statement in the aged human where responses to glucose loading may show higher peaks and longer elevations of blood glucose levels than would be compatible with normal states in the younger individual. Other endocrines are less clearly understood. This is particularly true of growth hormone where puzzling changes are known to exist. The total amount of growth hormone has not been shown to decrease with aging yet the presence of muscle wasting, so widely seen in the aged animal, would seem to indicate either a shortage of or loss of efficacy of growth hormone. One particularly interesting finding is that single injection of androgen to the neonate invokes premature aging by altering the hypothalamus.[12]

The immunologic theory of aging has attracted many advocates in recent years. There are two sorts of immunologic activity associated with aging. There is, of course, a decline in immunocompetence both of the cellular mediated and the humoral mediated types. It has been estimated that an individual at age 80 has one tenth the immunocompetency of the 20 year old human. This renders the individual much more susceptible to infections and accounts for the generally observed phenomenon that aged individuals suffer higher mortality with many kinds of respiratory infections than do younger counterparts. But on the other hand the disturbances associated with altered immunocompetence also lead to a phenomenon of autoimmunity and the production of altered proteins and a host of adverse reactions to their production and presence in the body. Makinodan[13] has called attention to the loss of immunocompetence with aging, to the difficulty of stimulating immunologic response in the aging animal, and finally to the increase of age-associated malignancy in older animals with a consequent increase in the number of aberrant cells. That not all of this series of phenomena is understood is attested to by the observation that some older animals exhibit an anamnestic response when challenged by antigens to which they were exposed in youth.

We are indebted to Professor B. Strehler[14] for his analysis of yet another group of aging theories. The first of these is the Brody-Failla Theory which maintains that the mortality rate is inversely proportional to vitality, a hypothetical physiological property which

decreased with time as a first-order decay process. The second theory
is the Simms-Jones Theory which holds that the lessening of vitality
with aging is really due to the accumulation of stresses experienced
during aging. The third theory, the Sacher Theory, postulates a "mean
physiological state" which decreases in linear fashion with aging. As
random events perturb the equilibrium of the aging animal, it is
forced beyond a certain inherent limiting value with the result that
death occurs. The final theory is the Strehler-Mildvan Theory which
differs from the Sacher Theory in that the random events which will
eventually cause the animal's death occur not in a Gaussian distribution (Sacher's postulate) but in a Maxwell-Boltzman fashion.

Finally Strehler[15] has evolved his own theory, that of codon restriction which deals with the programming of development and aging.
He cites four postulates dealing with cell-specific codon languages,
programmed changes in these languages during aging, facilitation or
expansion of the languages, and fourth a postulate for language con-
traction. He uses these postulates to construct a theory of aging
which is applicable not alone to explain the aging of an animal system, but in the case of man to hypothesize specific function of the
central nervous system, particluarly the creation and storage of memory. The reader is referred to his classic text for further explanation.

It is fitting that the discussion of theories of aging in this
brief recapitulation should end with a reference to memory. Probably
as much as any function, the senile dementias are heralded by a loss
of memory function. The papers comprising this collection of reflec-
tions on the aging brain and senile dementia will hopefully lead to
new research, new clinical trials, new approaches to the problems of
the old central nervous system of the human.

BIBLIOGRAPHY

1. Knowles, J. H., "Doing Better and Feeling Worse"; Health in the United States, p.g., Daedalus, Journal of the American Academy of Arts and Sciences. Winter 1977.

2. Tibbits, C., "Introduction" p. 4, Ethical Considerations in Long Term Care, edited by Winston, Wm. and Wilson, A. Eckerd College Gerontology Center, 1977.

3. Carver, E. J. Geropsychiatric Treatment, Where, Why, How, Drug Issues in Geropsychiatry p. 67, Williams and Wilkins, Baltimore, 1974.

4. Chien, C. P. "Psychiatric Treatment for Geriatric Patients: Pub or Drug". American J. Psychiatry, 127, 1070, 1971.

5. Whanger, A. D., "Management of the Elderly in State Hospitals" Drug Issues in Geropsychiatry, p. 103, Williams and Wilkins, Baltimore, 1974.

6. Health Insurance Statistics, U.S. Dept. HEW, DHEW Publication No. 75-11702, March 14, 1975.

7. Hayflick, L., "The limited in vitro lifespan of human diploid cell strains", Exp. Cell Res. 37;614, 1964.

8. Kohn, R., Principles of Mammalian Aging, p. 40, Prentice Hall, Englewood Cliffs, N.J., 1971.

9. Harman, D., The Free Radical Theory of Aging: The Effect of Aging on Serum Mercaptan, evels, J. of Gerontology, 15:38, 1960.

10. Kleiber, M., The Fire of Life. pp. 181-205, New York, 1961.

11. Dawton, A., Introductory Remarks, Trace Elements in Aging, p. 5, The Biomedical Role of Trace Elements in Aging, edited by Hsu, J. et. al., Eckerd College Gerontology Center, 1976.

12. Leathem, J., "Endocrine Changes With Aging". pp. 177-193 Epide miology of Aging. DHEW Publication No. (NIH) 75-711, 1972.

13. Makinodan, T., "Aging and the Immune System A Brief Summary of Current Knowledge". pp. 161-176. Epidemiology of Aging. DHEW Publication No. (NIH) 75-711, 1972.

14. Strehler, B., Time Cells, and Aging. p. 113-116, Academic Press, New York, 1977.

15. Strehler, B. Op Cit pp 291 et seq.

SECTION I

PHYSIOPATHOLOGY

THE SOCIAL IMPACT OF THE ORGANIC DEMENTIAS OF THE AGED

RALPH GOLDMAN, M.D.
VA Central Office

Senile dementia has been a catch-all diagnosis, poorly defined. Yet,
it points to a problem, increasingly recognized, of great social importance.
There are now more than one million individuals, almost all over the age
of sixty-five years, who are in nursing homes. Two-thirds of these residents are stated to have intellectual impairment. The vast majority of
first admissions to mental institutions for patients over the cited age
are for organic brain disease, obviously also admitted because of evidence
of intellectual deterioration. Uncounted are those who, because of a
protective environment, are able to continue in their own homes or communities. This is truly a problem of vast dimensions, tragic in its implications, and immense in the social requirements that it creates.

	White Men		White Women		Black Men		Black Women	
To Age	1900	1972	1900	1972	1900	1972	1900	1972
65	39	67	44	82	19	50	22	68
75	21	41	25	64	9	28	11	46
85	5	14	7	32	2	11	4	24

Table 1. Survival Percentages 1/

1/ Vital Statistics of the U.S., Vol. II, 1973.

It is ironic that society should strive for a state of public
health which would allow the majority of its members to reach old age,
yet be so demoralized by a corollary outcome when the goal is achieved.
When less than five percent of the population reached the age of sixty-
five, the problems of old age were of little social concern. Now that
over two-thirds of the population will reach that age, their problems
must be the primary concern of the health and social welfare services,
as well as of the public as a whole. Table 1 shows the proportionate
increase in these population components in the short period since the
beginning of this century.

For purposes of the present discussion, dementia will refer to
the loss of intellectual capacity, regardless of the cause. The precise
evaluation of intellectual capacity continues to be controversial,
however, the fact of impairment, with confusion, disorientation, lack

3

of insight and inability to reason, is so overt at the time of clinical
presentation that its presence is rarely in doubt. The relatively small
decrements which may or may not be present as a feature of modal aging
are not the present subject of concern. Since senile dementia is a term
generally reserved for a specific entity, my discussion will be expanded
to include all causes of dementia in the aged. When not otherwise quali-
fied, senile dementia will refer only to dementia which has Alzheimer-
like qualities and is without apparent cause.

As a means of approaching the problem, I will examine the following
questions:
1. What are the causes of dementia in the aged?
2. What is the significance of acute brain syndrome?
3. What is the frequency of dementia in this age group?
4. To what extent is dementia treatable?
5. What are the social implications of dementia in the aged?
6. What specific problems does dementia create for the VA?

The causes of dementia

It is not my intent to get involved in the technicalities of diagnosis, but only to develop some relevant points. It is common to either
avoid the diagnosis of dementia entirely, focusing only on the major
medical problem, to hide the diagnosis under a vague generality, such
as "cerebral arteriosclerosis", or to fuse all patients into the undifferentiated entity of senile dementia, senility, or organic brain
syndrome. While the statistical likelihood that an organic cause
associated with aging may be high, such an undifferentiated approach
leads both to diagnostic errors and neglect. Many reports are available of attempts at greater precision. In one recent example Seltzer
and Sherwin[1] reviewed 80 patients in a VA facility, with, however, an
average age of only 66 years, thus, a relatively young group, and found
31 percent with a primary psychiatric diagnosis of senile dementia, 19
percent with alcoholic dementia, 14 percent with Korsahoff's syndrome,
11 percent with schizophrenia, and the remaining 25 percent scattered
through a number of diagnoses. These included no patients with apparently reversible forms of dementia, although three had no apparent

abnormality of the mental state when later reviewed and in three the diagnosis was undetermined.

In another recent study from Australia, Smith, Kiloh, Ratnovale and Grant[2] reviewed 100 patients who had been referred for dementia. Twelve of these were under 45 years of age, 22 were over 65 years, and the remaining 66 were between 45 and 65 years. The average age of the 49 men was 54.5 years, while that of the 51 women was 58.5 years. Dementia was confirmed in 81 patients, and in all the 22 patients over the age of 65 years. Of the 19 patients without dementia, eight had drug intoxication and eleven had pseudodementia due to depression (4), schizophrenia (5), hypomania (1), and hyperthyroidism (1).

The 81 patients with confirmed dementia consisted of 16 patients with a variety of identifiable causes, of which eight had potentially reversible dementia, 17 had probable alcoholism, 12 had arteriosclerosis, and 36 had presumed senile dementia. The cases with identifiable causes included low pressure hydrocephalus (7), head injury (4), Huntington's chorea (2), and one each of Kuf's syndrome, epilepsy, and hypothyroidism. The only patients over age 65 with potentially reversible dementia were two with low-pressure hydrocephalus.

One of the most comprehensive studies of organic brain syndrome of the elderly was made by the psychiatric screening unit of the San Francisco General Hospital. The study included all patients referred to this unit who were over 60 years and were admitted for the first time[3,4,5]. The results are shown in Table 2.

"Chronic brain syndrome" included both senile dementia and arteriosclerosis. The group with "other organic brain disease" included 46 with evidence of change due to alcoholism alone. Another 25 alcoholics were included in the senile or arteriosclerotic brain disease categories as well. This study was particularly important because of the data presented which also reviewed the characteristic course and outcome for each of the entities.

Table 2. Psychiatric Diagnoses in the Elderly
San Francisco General Hospital - 1959

	Patients	Percent
Chronic brain syndrome	150	28
Acute brain syndrome	71	13
Mixed (acute & chronic) brain syndrome	177	33
Psychogenic disorder only	58	11
Other organic brain disorder	69	13
Undiagnosed	9	2
Total	534	100

A number of other studies of the distribution of underlying etiologies for organic dementia in the aged are available, and all show a similar distribution[6,7]. Several include cases under the age of 65 years, and the diagnostic variety in these reports appears to be greater than when only older patients are surveyed.

The current classification of organic brain syndromes of the American Psychiatric Association (DSM II)[8] appears to be reasonably adequate for the purpose:

II. Organic Brain Syndromes (OBS)
A. Psychoses
    290 Senile and presenile dementia
    291 Alcoholic psychosis
    292 Psychosis associated with intracranial infection
    293 Psychosis associated with other cerebral conditions
        (includes vascular lesions, epilepsy, neoplasm, degeneration, trauma)
    294 Psychosis associated with other physical conditions
        (includes endocrine, metabolic, and nutritional disorders, systemic infection, drug or poison intoxication other than alcohol)
B. Nonpsychotic OBS
    309 Inclusive

Acute Brain Syndrome

Acute brain syndrome is characterized by its reversibility. In the classic study of acute brain syndrome by Simon and Cahan[4], the average duration of symptoms before hospitalization was seven days, as compared to fifteen days for a mixed acute and chronic brain syndrome group and 34 months for patients with uncomplicated chronic brain syndrome. Fluctuating confusion and memory loss were the most prominent symptoms. Drug and alcohol ingestion, cardiac failure, malnutrition, and cerebral vascular accidents were the predisposing factors in over three-fourths of the combined cases of acute and mixed acute and chronic brain syndrome. It should be noted that only 29 percent of 248 patients with acute brain syndrome did not also have evidence of a complicating chronic brain syndrome.

While no data were found to provide an age specific incidence of acute brain syndrome, several reports have appeared which suggest that the incidence increases with age, with or without evidence of chronic brain syndrome. Doty[9] followed the general hospital course of 1,044 patients ranging in age from 12 to 84 years. Delerium occurred in 4 percent of those under age 40 years and 14.5 percent of those over that age. In a recent study of the cognitive integrity of patients, also in a general hospital, Jacobs and his associates[10] found that the average age of those showing deficits was 73 years, whereas the total group averaged 65 years. Since periods of delerium are not uncommon during acute illness, particularly in the aged, they are usually considered to be symptoms which are not diagnostically indexed for later access and characterization.

In view of the concern regarding pseudodementia, the characteristics of acute brain syndrome in the aged should be more precisely documented. The apparent increased vulnerability of the aged and the presence of a frequently demonstrable underlying chronic brain syndrome suggests the possibility of an age-related loss of reserve, which reaches a threshhold value under the stress of conditions often associated with a relative cerebral hypoxia.

I remember one patient who had retained all of his rather remarkable intellectual and technical skills until the age of 86. During an acute myocardial infarction he became confused and delerious, but recovered almost entirely within six weeks. It was hard to visualize that under the same stress he would have undergone the same reaction thirty or forty years earlier.

Table 3. Age-Specific Incidence of Dementia
in Nursing Home Residents 1/

Age	Percent of Population in Nursing Homes 2/		Percent of NH-Patients with Dementia		Percent of Pop. in NH with Dementia	
	Men	Women	Men	Women	Men	Women
65-74	1.13	1.28	48	48	0.54	0.61
75-84	4.08	7.05	62	63	2.53	4.44
85+	18.04	27.44	68	70	12.27	19.21

1/ National Nursing Home Survey 1973-1974.
2/ Extrapolated from (1) and census data, Department of Commerce
Series P-25, No. 519, April, 1974.

The Frequency of Dementia in the Aged

Data regarding the frequency of dementia in the aged are essential to
resource planning. The patient who is confused, forgetful, and in-capable of
performing essential functions requires extensive personal assistance regardless of the diagnosis. The problem is to determine the actual number of such
patients at risk.

The National Nursing Home Survey of 1973-1974 [11] provides one approach to
the data. This survey indicated the number of residents, by age, and from census
data it was possible to determine the age specific rate of nursing home utilization.
From the survey it was also possible to obtain a crude value for intellectual
impairment. The data are summarized in Table 3. It should be recognized that on
one hand this represents the casual evaluation of nursing home staff, and includes
all levels of impairment. On the other hand, it does not include those patients
still in the community or in other more formal institutions.

Kay [12] has extensively reviewed the literature, including his own studies,
to determine incidence. The data trends are similar, and indicate that there is
actually a comparable incidence to that indicated by the indirect evidence just
presented (Table 4). The data are all quite consistent in showing a geometric
increase in frequency with age. As widely scattered areas as Japan, Demark,
England and the United States have similar trends, and of particular note is the
abrupt rise in frequency after age eighty (Table 5).

An important study was performed by Larsson, Sjogren, and Jacobsen in 1963 [13].
These investigators studied only senile dementia and reviewed all of the cases in
Stockholm over a period of several years. They found not only did the cumulative
incidence increase with age, but that the risk to first degree relatives was in-

creased more than fourfold. Table 6 indicates this trend.

Table 4. Prevalence of Chronic Brain Syndromes at Ages 65 and Over 1/

Author	Country	% Severe	% Mild
Greenberg	USA	6.8	
Primrose	Scotland	4.5	
Nielsen	Denmark	3.1	15.1
Kay (1961)	England	5.6	5.7
Parsons	England	4.4	10.0
Kaneho	Japan	7.2	
Hagnell	Sweden	9.1	7.0
Akesson	Sweden	1.0	
Kay (1970)	England	6.2	2.6

1/ From Kay, 1972.

Table 5. Prevalence of Chronic Brain Syndrome by Age 1/

	Japan	England	Denmark
60-69	2.3	2.3*	0
70-79	5.9	3.9	1.9
80 +	19.8	22.0	13.2
All ages	4.4	6.2	3.1

* 65-69

1/ From Kay, 1972.

Table 6. Cumulative Risk of Senile Dementia 1/

Age	General Population	First Degree Relatives
60	–	0.2
70	0.4	2.0
75	1.2	5.7
80	2.5	11.3
85	3.8	16.9
90	5.2	23.0

1/ From Larsson, Sjogren, and Jacobson, 1963.

Both the data of Kay[12] and that of Simon[3] indicate a great increase in mortality in patients with dementia regardless of type. Severe chronic dementia requiring institutionalization was associated with an approximate annual mortality of 40 percent in Kay's series, and 36 percent in that of Simon.

Three important issues emerge from these observations. First, the exact fraction of the population over age 65 requiring services because of dementia is not precisely known, but is probably at least five percent. Second, the risk increases geometrically with age. In view of the recent relatively more rapid increase in the over-eighty population than any other segment, it may be anticipated that there will be an acceleration in need. Valid estimates require not only knowledge of the number of individuals over age 65, but the relative size of the age cohorts within that age group in order to prepare useful projections. Finally, senility, even when unassociated with any specific disease, has a high mortality. The facilities required are determined by the duration of disability as well as the incidence.

The Treatment of Dementia

The approach to the treatment of dementia can be divided into two distinct categories: 1) The cure, or reversal, of the dementing process, and 2) The optimum
maintenance of those patients with what is clearly irreversible destruction of brain
tissue. It would be inappropriate, nor is it my intent, to explore treatment in
detail, but only to outline my view of the general problems and possible strategies
to be adopted.

The foregoing review has examined superficially some of the variables in the
diagnosis of dementia. It is clear that in each case a specific diagnosis must be
made. What is less unclear is the extent to which pseudodementias and reversible
dementias are now being missed. Acute dementia will resolve relatively quickly.
Since the early mortality is high, and related to the precipitating cause, early
medical diagnosis is imperative. A group more likely to be masked is that of the
pseudodementias, particularly those with depression and those due to drug excess.
Patients with occult anemia, hypothyroidism, CNS syphilis, head injury, pellagra,
normal pressure hydrocephalus, and brain tumors should be recognized. With a routinely high index of suspicion and modern diagnostic aids the exclusion of these
conditions should be neither difficult nor expensive, especially when balanced against
the alternative of prolonged institutionalization.

Since members of the public are concerned about the therapeutic nihilism regarding dementia, they are extremely receptive to reports of the frequency of missed diagnoses. There is clearly a difference between the number of cases of various categories that present for diagnosis, the number for whom diagnosis is too late for
effective treatment, and the number who are never correctly diagnosed. Such data are
necessary, and limits of acceptable uncertainty should be set. The availability of
this information should do much to improve public confidence, as well as our own
standards. The reviews available seem to indicate that after elimination of patients
with depression and chronic drug toxicity, an upper limit of fifteen percent of potentially treatable cases of organic dementia could be expected.

Once the irreversibility and extent of the organic damage has been established,
social policy and medical potentials must play an increasingly interactive role. Can

the patient's function be significantly improved, can it be stablized at the best possible level and further decline arrested or delayed, or is no regimen effective? The burden of proof now lies with those who make the claim that input above that which is necessary for humane management produces any significant effect. This is a question which must be asked and re-asked as therapeutic regimens change. Social policy depends upon the answer. The extreme negative view is expressed by Rossman[14] and Wershow[15]. Ultimately, are we more obliged to give penicillin to an unresponsive patient with chronic organic brain disease who develops pneumonia than we are to maintain the respirator on a patient with the criteria of brain death? The best information should be available and policy evolved through informed public consensus.

Beyond this question is that of long-term care after adequate diagnosis and stabilization. Should it be institutional or non-institutional? Since the medical aspects can be managed in either locale, the problem evolves into the question of achieving the balance between effectiveness, cost, and acceptability.

The Social Implications of Dementia

There is probably no condition which creates more anxiety than the fear of mental incompetence in oneself or one's family. Granting even that the patient becomes unaware of the disability, the emotional, physical, and economic burdens on the family may often be totally disruptive.

It is no wonder that the acceptance of dementia as a major public problem is met by massive public denial. I'm sure that we all have had the experience of being told that dementia is the result of social neglect, or some other social or environmental factor, and that both cause and effect are capable of reversal. The theme of a widely distributed teaching film, "Peege", strongly implies this concept. The attitude is reinforced by frequent news and magazine articles.

I have previously reviewed the magnitude of the problem, citing the large number of individuals who are demented, in institutions, or require assistive and protective services. It is essential, however, to also see the problem in perspective. Wershow[16] recently reviewed the last year in the lives of a consecutive series of individuals over the age of seventy-five years who died in Birmingham, Alabama. Sixty percent were ambulatory one week before death and 80 percent had been ambulatory two months earlier. Although the criteria were vague, less than five percent were reported to have had mental disturbances for a prolonged period, except for white women who had 10 to 15 percent impairment. Since women live so much longer than men, the incidence is greater, but the age-specific rates are similar. The five percent frequency of chronic mental disturbance is comparable to the other data presented, and should be reassuring. There was a forty to fifty percent incidence of confusion during the last week of life.

Although the individual risk is low, five percent of more than twenty million individuals is itself a population of over one million. It is for this group that our planning must be directed.

The assumption must be made that an adequate diagnosis will be made in each case and that acute hospital facilities will be available and properly utilized when needed. The major problem is the appropriate placement for the long-term management of those patients for whom current therapy is incapable of restoring adequate competence to eliminate the need of constant supervision and attendance. The twin goals should be the optimal situation and the minimum social cost. Two general alternatives are possible, institutional placement, usually a nursing home, or the equivalent, and community placement, usually with the patient's family or a family surrogate. Another possibility is a combination solution in which the patient lives at home, but can be placed in a day care center or in a nursing home for brief periods in order to allow the caretaker to function and to gain periods of respite.

The common wisdom proclaims that both goals are best achieved by keeping the patient out of an institution. An example will illustrate some of the problems. An 89-year old man can no longer care for himself, and because he wanders, cannot be left alone. His daughter-in-law, a clinical laboratory supervisor, gives up her job to care for him. Apparently a good solution. Yet, the family loses her income, the government loses a significant amount of income tax, society loses her skilled productivity, and she gives up a 40-hour a week job for a 168-hour a week responsibility.

Such a solution may have been valid when the temporal demand upon a woman's labor was unlimited and its value trivial because she was not considered to be in the work force. It is doubtful that that such logic would find much current acceptance by those who would bear its burden. In addition, it can be argued that it is not cost effective, and that the resultant isolation of the patient from his age peers might actually reduce the amount of social interaction and activity. Yet, there is evidence that where families exist, most patients are maintained in the home as long as is possible.

It should be noted that 78.2 percent of the men and 91.5 percent of the women in nursing homes have no spouse. Age and disability appear to be manageable as long as there is a competent companion. Nineteen percent of the individuals in nursing homes have never married. When infertile marriages and family separations are added, an even larger segment of this population must have no children who could provide an alternate home.

One solution of relative promise is the personal care home, in which a family undertakes to care for several residents. Although this method has been used for psychiatric patients, its potential for geriatric patients has not been equally well explored. At present the costs are reasonable, but it is possible that with insistence on standards and organization of the operators into interest groups that these costs would also rise.

The availability of home health aids and other services may make retention of the patient in the home more practical. However, since a good nursing home can function with only 0.7 staff (on a 40-hour week basis) per patient, the economic balance might make this alternative seem less attractive.

It is clear that the care of these patients will be an increasing and vexing problem. It behooves us to examine the alternatives carefully, and to develop a variety of solutions to meet the diverse individual needs. We must recognize and accept the fact that we have an obligation, and that it will be impossible to maintain the standards that we demand without paying the appropriate price.

Problems of the Veterans Administration

The problems of the Veterans Administration in regard to dementia are comparable to those of the community at large, but with several somewhat unique features. The most important is that the veteran population corresponds to America's wars. There are now nearly thirty million living veterans. Only 750,000 World War I veterans remain, but the thirteen million members of the largest group, the World War II veterans, now have an average age of 58 years. In 1970 there were only 2,000,000 veterans over the age of 65 years, by 1995 there will be a peak number of 8,000,000. The number of very old veterans, over the age of 85, will not reach its maximum until the early years of the twenty first century. Using the Larsson, Sjogren, and Jacobson estimates for senile dementia alone, the number will increase from 31,500 in 1980 to 96,000 in 2000. The demand upon the VA for the care of these patients must be anticipated.

Second, since the VA is one of the few public sources of extended care for individuals ineligible for Medicaid, the VA cares for a larger than usual fraction of veterans in this category. As a result, the VA also provides support for many younger patients with dementia. None of the current legislative proposals includes plans for expansion of long term care facilities.

Third, the veteran patient who utilizes the VA is more likely to be without a family or substantial personal resources. Therefore, the option of placing the patient in his own home with family caretakers is limited.

Fourth, the veteran patient is also very likely to be an alcoholic, with many of the problems, including dementia, which may result. All four of these problems intensify the present and future role of the VA.

For convenience, the placement of these patients can be classified into institutional and non-institutional settings. The former include hospitals, nursing homes, and domiciliaries; the latter include the patient's home, personal care (foster) homes, boarding houses, halfway houses and the like. The VA program encompasses all of these alternatives.

The length of hospital stay is determined by the need for care and the ability to outplace the patient. Patients with dementia are usually placed in nursing homes. The VA supports three programs, VA Nursing Home Care Units, State Veterans Homes, and Community Nursing Homes. All of the 90 VA Nursing Home Units are physically adjacent to VA Hospitals. In concept these Units care for the more complex patients who require recurrent hospitalization. They can also serve as sites for training personnel. The State Veterans Home Nursing Care Units are sponsored by the states, but receive partial per diem remuneration from the VA. The VA also has a grant program for State nursing home and domiciliary construction. The community nursing homes care for the veterans on a contract basis. Their major advantage is that they can provide care in the veterans' home communities. The greatest potential for expansion lies in this sector.

The VA and the State Veterans Homes both maintain domiciliary programs. However, domiciliary residents are required to be able to care for themselves, and the domiciliaries are not structured to care for patients with significant mental impairment.

It is important that nursing homes be suitable to the purpose and that only appropriate patients be retained. To the maximum extent possible the VA goal is to deinstitutionalize its patients by placing them back into their own homes or in personal care homes. In order to facilitate this movement the VA is expanding its network of support services. These include outpatient clinics, hospital-based home care for patients incapable of movement and to instruct families in appropriate procedures, aid and attendance fees where needed as a supplement to pensions, the encouragement of the development of senior citizens centers at Veterans' Service Organization Posts to reinforce socialization, and the planned exploration of geriatric day care centers to relieve caretakers and to provide medical supervision and assistance.

Recognizing the need for further research into the problems of dementia, four of the VA Geriatric Research, Education, and Clinical Centers are focussing on fundemental problems in this area. These include the Boston Outpatient Clinic-Bedford Hospital, Minneapolis, Seattle-American Lake, and Sepulveda (California) GRECC's. This conference is an outgrowth of that commitment.

Finally, recognizing that there has been an inadequate academic and professional interst in aging, the VA has established a Geriatric Fellowship which will commence in July, 1978. Although this fellowship is designed to prepare physicians for the full range of geriatric problems, the importance of dementia to a geriatric practice will assure an increased focus on this area.

Conclusion

Given the fact that nerve cells are post-mitotic, and not capable of replacement after destruction, it should not be surprising that organic deficits accumulate with age. It should be similarly unsurprising that a society dedicated to human survival and an increasing average age should also accumulate individuals with intellectual deficits who would not be capable of survival in a less protective environment. It is really a philosophical issue whether, for the individual, death with or without an intact intellect is the less tragic. What is important is that life achieve its maximum potential and that society have the resources to achieve this end. First, it is necessary to be certain that all individuals with reversible dementia be recognized and treated. Second, society must accept that there will then be a large residual population of individuals for whom organic damage will be so severe that environmental modification, while necessary for humanitarian reasons, will have little effect on the level of intellectual function. Third, research must be intensified to recognize and treat identifiable causes of dementia before irreversible damage is produced, and to slow its progress, should senile dementia be, in fact, a normal process. Fourth, accepting the problems of organic dementia, once it has occurred, systems must be developed which maximize the well-being of the patients, yet are within our social resources. Above all, we must be honest. No problems can be solved by denial or wishful thinking. Professional, scientific, and public awareness must be heightened, and action based on the best available data.

BIBLIOGRAPHY

1. Seltzer, B. and Sherwin, I. (1978) "Organic Brain Syndromes",
    An Empirical Study and Critical Review, Am. J. Psychiatry, 135,
    13-21.

2. Smith, J.S., et. al. (1976) The Investigation of Dementia, The
    Results in 100 Consecutive Admissions, Med. J. Australia, 2,
    403-405.

3. Epstein, L.J. and Simon, A. (1967) Organic Brain Syndrome in the
    Elderly. Geriatrics, 22,145-150.

4. Simon, A., and Cahan, R.B. (1963) The Acute Brain Syndrome in
    Geriatric Patients. Psychiatric Research Reports 16, 8-21.

5. Simon, A., et. al. (1968) Alcoholism in the Geriatric Mentally Ill.
    Geriatrics, 23, 125-131.

6. Freemon, F.R. (1976) Evaluation of Patients With Progressive
    Intellectual Deterioration. Arch Neurol., 33, 658-659.

7. Marsden, C.D. and Harrison, M.J.G. (1972) Outcome of Investiga-
    tion of Patients with Presenile Dementia. Br. Med. J., 2, 249-252.

8. American Psychiatric Association. (1968) Diagnostic and Statistical
    Manual of Mental Disorders (DSM II). Washington, D.C.

9. Doty, E.J. (1946) The Incidence and Treatment of Delerious
    Reactions in Later Life. Geriatrics. 1, 21.

10. Jacobs, J.W., et. al. (1977) Screening for Organic Medical Syndromes
    in the Medically Ill. Ann. Int. Med. 80, 40-46.

11. United States 1973-74: National Nursing Home Survey (1977). U.S.
    Government Printing Office, Washington, D.C.

12. Kay, D.W.K. (1972) Epidemiological Aspects of Organic Brain
    Disease in the Aged. In: Aging and the Brain, Gaitz, C.M., ed.,
    Plenum. New York.

13. Larsson, T., et. al. (1963) Senile Dementia. Acta Psychiat.
    Scand. 39, Suppl. 167.

14. Rossman, I. (1973) Alternatives to Institutional Care. Bulletin
    of the New York Academy of Medicine, Second Series, 49, 1084-1092.

15. Wershow, H.J. Comment: (1977) Reality Orientation for Gerontologists:
    Some Thoughts About Senility. The Gerontologist. 17, 297-302.

16. Wershow, H.J. The Last Year of Life of Those Aged Seventy-Five
    and Over. To be published.

MORPHOLOGICAL CHANGES IN THE AGING BRAIN

KALIDAS NANDY

Geriatric Research, Education and Clinical Center, Veterans Administration Hospital, Bedford, Massachusetts and Boston University School of Medicine, Boston, Mass.

INTRODUCTION

Gerontologists have described aging as the changes in the structure and functions following reproductive maturity resulting in decreased ability to overcome environmental challenges and increased probability of death with time[1]. These changes are also considered to be intrinsic, universal within a species, progressive and deleterious to the organism as a whole[2]. The functional units of CNS are the neurons which are postmitotic in nature and are, therefore, likely to show effects of aging of the organism. The brain is also considered to be an important organ controlling not only directly by providing the electrical impulses to the contractile tissues, but also indirectly by influencing other systems through various neuroendocrine mediators. In the higher animals, particularly the mammals, the size of the brain and also the brain weight-body weight ratio has been considered to be related to the lifespan of the animals, although the precise nature of the relationship is not understood[3]. A certain degree of deterioration of brain functions is commonly associated with aging.. A severe degree of impairment of cognitive and other functions are found in older individuals in the clinical syndrome known as senile dementia. (Table 1)

TABLE 1

The major changes in the brain associated with aging and senile dementia are:

GROSS CHANGES

1. Reduction of brain weight
2. Reduction of brain volume
3. Increase in the ventricular size
4. Increase in the size of the sulci

MICROSCOPIC CHANGES

1. Loss of neurons
2. Deposition lipofuscin age pigment
3. Loss of dendritic spines
4. Amyloid changes
5. Senile (neuritic) plaques
6. Formation of neurofibrillary tangles

There are numerous studies on the changes in the mammalian brain associated with aging of the individuals as well as in the patients with senile dementia. The changes such as loss of neurons, loss of dendritic spines, intracytoplasmic deposition of lipofuscin pigment and frequent development of amyloid lesions are consistently found in the brain of aging mammals[4-13]. On the other hand, formation senile (neuritic) plaques in neuronal parikarya and the intracytoplasmic development of neurofibrillary tangles are more characteristic of senile and presenile dementia and are rather infrequent in the brain of normal old people[14-17].

In this chapter the discussion will be focussed on the lipofuscin pigment formation which is one of the most consistent cytological changes in the brain of aging mammals. The pigment in the nerve cells of vertebrates was probably first reported by Hannover[18], although the term lipofuscin was first introduced in the literature by Borst[19]. The pigment has been variously named as chromolipid, ceroid, lipochrome, age pigment, wear and tear pigment, cytolipochrome, hemofuscin, etc. by different investigators[20-26].

DISTRIBUTION AND PROPERTIES

Lipofuscin pigment is easily demonstrated in tissue sections by histochemical, fluorescence and ultrastructural methods using both frozen and paraffin sections. Since some lipid components of the pigment might be removed by the use of lipid solvents used during paraffin embedding, frozen sections fixed in 1% cold formalin have been used.

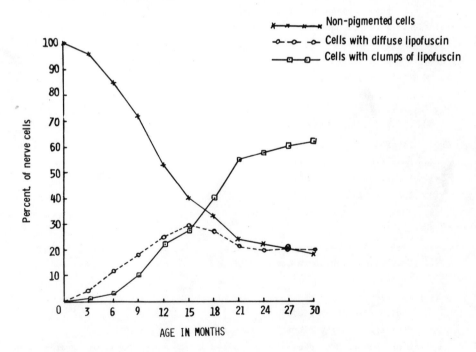

Fig. 1. Lipofuscin distribution in pyramidal cells of cerebral cortex (layer III) in mice of different ages.

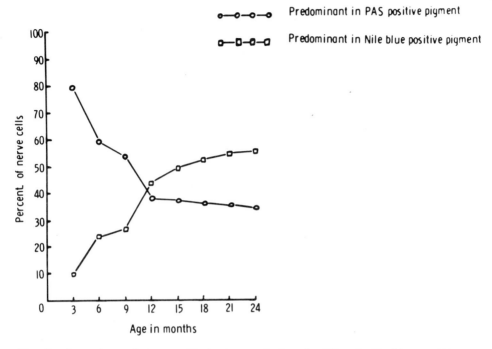

Fig. 2. Percentage of nerve cells having predominantly PAS and nile blue positive material in the cerebral cortex of mice of different ages.

The neurons in the CNS of rodents exhibited a variable pattern of pigmentation in their cytoplasm. The pigment was not generally detected in the neurons in the first two months of age. While the pigment was rather diffuse in its distribution in the neurons in younger mice (3-5 months), it appeared to surround the nucleus (perinuclear) and form clumps near the axon hillock (unipolar) or near axon hillock and principle dendrites (bipolar) in older animals. The percentages of nerve cells showing heavy (clumpy), moderate (diffuse)and no pigmentation among the Purkinje cells of cerebellum and pyramidal cells of cerebral cortex were studied in mice of different ages. The number of nonpigmented cells steadily decreased with age from 100% in the newborn to 20% at 24 months. The cells showing diffuse and clumpy (perinuclear and polar) distribution of lipofuscin appeared to increase with age from zero to 20 and 60% respectively (Figure 1). The percentages of neurons showing predominantly PAS and Nile blue positive lipofuscin among the pigmented pyramidal cells of cerebral cortex and Purkinje cells of cerebellum were also studied[5]. While the cells containing PAS positive materials gradually decreased from 80 to 30%, the cells containing predominantly Nile blue positive materials steadily increased from zero to 70% by the age of 24 months (Figure 2).

Lipofuscin pigment in the neurons exhibited a variation in the staining properties in young and old mice. It appeared that Sudan black B and PAS positive pigments were predominant in younger mice (3-5 months) and showed a similar distribution. On the other hand, the pigment in the neurons of older mice (12 months or more) were more easily stained by Nile blue and ferric-ferricyanide methods. A difference in the fluorescence properties was also noted in these two types of pigment. Upon activation at a wave length of 3650 A^o, the pigment in younger mice gave mostly a greenish-yellow autofluorescence with an emission spectrum of 2400-4200 A^o and a peak of 3400 A^o. The autofluorescence of the lipofuscin in older animals was mostly orange-yellow with an emission spectrum of 3000-4000 A^o and a peak at 3800 A^o [5].

A variable effect of the chemicals on the staining and fluorescence properties of the lipofuscin pigment was also noted. Chemicals such as HCl, NaOH, DMSO, diastase, hyaluronidase and ribonuclease had no effect on the staining properties of lipofuscin, and disruption of the tissues took place when the concentration was substantially increased. On the other hand, when the sections were treated with trypsin and lipase, a reduction in the PAS and Sudan black B positive materials occurred. A similar reduction of the material was also noted when the sections were treated with chemicals such as chloroform:methanol (2:1), ether, pyridine and acetone, although Nile blue positive pigment was also partially removed[5].

The staining properties of the pigment in mice fed on vitamin E deficient diet were somewhat different from those found in control animals. A variable stainability of the pigment was noted in these mice. These could be stained, although less uniformly, by PAS, Sudan black B, Nile blue and carbol fuchsin methods and were not stained by ferric-ferricyanide method. The autofluorescence of this pigment included both green-yellow and orange-yellow types. The pigment also appeared to be rather resistant to treatment with the enzymes and lipid solvents[5].

The activity of acid phosphatase, β-glucuronidase, simple esterase, succinate dehydrogenase and cytochrome oxidase was noted in the neurons of old mice, particularly in the areas of lipofuscin deposition. A moderate reaction was observed in the pigmented areas in the younger animals and the intensity increased markedly in heavily pigmented cells in older animals. On the other hand, the activity of specific cholinesterase, adenosinetriphosphatase and thiamine pyrophosphatase was substantially reduced in the neurons of old animals and their distribution did not appear to be related to lipofuscin deposition.

It appears that lipofuscin formation is a continuous process starting as early as two months in mice and increasing progressively as a function of age. The pigment seems to have early and late stages during its development. The early stages predominant in younger animals, was more easily stained with Sudan black B and PAS, and had a greenish-yellow autofluorescence. The later form more frequently encountered in older animals was easily stainable by Nile blue and ferric-ferricyanide methods, and had a golden-yellow autofluorescence. The early form of

TABLE 2

THE PROPERTIES OF LIPOFUSCIN PIGMENT

	Early type	Late type
Distribution:	Scattered granules	Perinuclear or polar clumps
Staining properties:	More easily stained by PAS and Sudan black B	Commonly stained by Nile blue, ferric-ferricyanide methods
Autofluorescence:	Greenish-yellow with an emission spectrum of 2300-4200 A^O and a peak at 3200 A^O	Orange-yellow with emission spectrum of 3000-4000 A^O and a peak at 3800 A^O
Extraction by lipid solvents:	Marked	Less marked
Digestion by lipase and trypsin:	Partially digestible	Nil
Enzyme activity:	Moderate activity of acid phosphatase, β-glucuronidase, simple esterase, succinic dehydrogenase, cytochrome	Strong activity of the enzymes
Ultrastructure:	Fine granules associated with lysosomes and vacuoles	Large masses of the pigment materials surrounded by lysosomal membranes containing vacuoles of varying sizes

the pigment could be partially digested by lipase and trypsin, and markedly dissolved in lipid solvents, while the mature form was more resistant to such treatment[5] (Table 2).

BIOCHEMICAL STUDIES ON LIPOFUSCIN

Lipofuscin pigment has been isolated from the brains of animals by the method modified from that described by Siakotos, et.al[27]. Ten animals from different age groups were studied in each experiment and the study was repeated twice to judge the reproducibility of the results.

Ten animals, each from six different age groups (4-6 weeks, 3-4, 6-8, 12-14, 18-20, 24-26 months) were pooled at random. Their brains, including cerebrum, cerebellum, and brainstem, were dissected out. The materials from each age group were blended in a sucrose solution (0.14M sucrose, 0.05M Tribase, 0.01M KCl EDTA, PH 8.0) for 30 seconds in a Waring blender in the proportion of 1 gm of brain to 10 ml of the solution.

The preparations were placed in silicone coated tubes and centrifuged in an ultracentrifuge (Beckman $L_5$65) at 140,000g for one hour, yielding pellet and supernatant fractions. The supernatant fluid containing the brownish pigment layer near the top were pipetted out and mixed with NaCl to make 10% solution in weight volume. After the salt was dissolved, the mixture was centrifuged similarly for one hour at 140,000g. The top brownish band was aspirated out and mixed with equal volume of distilled water and centrifuged again. The centrifuge tube containing the layers of lipofuscin were sliced in a tube slicer and were collected by a pipette from the upper part of the sliced tube. The materials were then studied by fluorescence, histochemical and electron microscopic methods to check the purity of the samples.

Since the brain lipofuscin preparation, particularly in low concentration, does not form pellets which can be handled with ease, all preparations were manipulated as suspensions. Hence, volumetric procedures were employed rather than pelleting or sedimentation. Acid phosphatase in the isolated lipofuscin were quantitated by the hydrolysis of p-nitrophenyl phosphate followed by spectrophotometric determination of the free nitrophenol at 420 mμ [28,29]. All enzyme assay were carried out under identical conditions and the spectrophotometer was checked frequently for consistent results. Since other sources of the enzyme were eliminated by the isolation procedure, the high specific activity of acid phosphatase in brain lipofuscin, 5,000 nM/mg of protein/hour, were used to quantitate the yield of brain lipofuscin per unit of fresh tissue[30]. In other words, hydrolysis of 500 nM of paranitrophenol phosphate per hour is equal to 1/10 mg of lipofuscin protein. This approach permitted a quantitation of small differences in lipofuscin concentration in the different samples. The correction factor for total amount of lipofuscin relative to a milligram of lipofuscin protein will be calculated from a large amount of pure lipofuscin separated from additional brain samples.

This study indicated that the methods of isolation are sensitive and can be used routinely to quantitate lipofuscin content in brain samples in small quantity. The results of the study are consistent and the difference in lipofuscin protein contents in samples from different age groups is significant (Figure 3).

TABLE 3

THE QUANTITY OF LIPOFUSCIN

The numbers represent the micrograms of lipofuscin protein per gram of wet brain tissue.

Age of Mice	4-6 wks.	3-4 mos.	6-8 mos.	12-14 mos.	18-20 mos.	24-26 mos.
Sample 1	0.005	0.85	2.34	3.62	5.25	8.42
Sample 2	0.032	1.25	1.92	3.94	6.47	7.81
Sample 3	0.041	1.04	2.04	3.56	5.90	8.08
Sample 4	0.025	0.56	2.15	4.12	6.28	8.64
Mean	0.025	0.925	2.11	3.81	5.97	8.24
	±.015	±.293	±.178	±.265	±.538	±.366

Samples for electron microscopy were treated with Dowex 50 to remove sodium ions retained from the density gradients employed for isolation. The deionized and neutralized preparation were fixed in 2% osmic acid buffered with 0.1M collidine buffer at pH 7.5-7.6 for 16 hours in the cold. The material was centrifuged for 10-30 minutes in a clinical centrifuge and pellets at the bottom were dehydrated through a graded series of ethanol (35%, 50%, 70%, 95%, and 100% alcohol for five

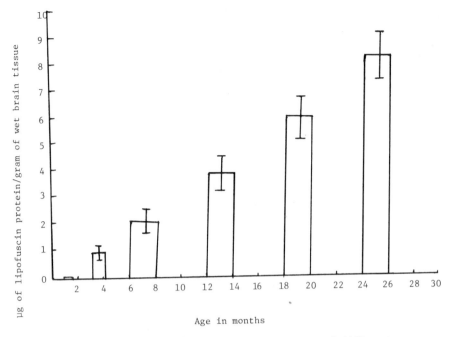

Figure 3 Lipofuscin content in brain samples from mice of different ages.

minutes each. This was then treated with Spurr low viscosity medium, embedded in
pure medium and polymerized for 8-12 hours. Thin sections (600-900 A^o thick) were
cut in an ultramicrotome and were examined in RCA-3G after counterstaining with 1%
uranly acetate in 70% EDTH followed by lead citrate for ten minutes. The major
indicator of purity of lipofuscin was the absence of other sub-cellular particulates.
The study indicated that the isolated lipofuscin fractions are pure with no contamination with myelin, lysosomes or microsomes in any of the preparations. A progressive increase of electron dense lipid bodies and lipofuscin particulates was
consistently noted as a function of age.

    The study carried out by isolating lipofuscin pigment from mouse brains of
different ages yielded measurable quanties of lipofuscin by spectrophotometric
measurements of acid phosphatase as the marker enzyme. Since this approach did not
provide sufficient pigment in some samples, quantitation was carried out by
measuring the activity of acid phosphatase in brain lipofuscin[30]. Three major
subcellular sources of acid phosphatase in the brain are lysosome, lipofuscin and
soluble protein fractions. The procedure followed in isolating lipofuscin resolved
in a lipofuscin preparation with a density of approximately one[33]. Since the
density of brain lysosomes is intermediate between that of brain nerve-endings and
mitochondrial fractions, the isolation procedures of brain lipofuscin completely
removed all traces of lysosomes having no pigment deposition. The use of Nacl

solutions in the isolation procedure removed all traces of soluble proteins[27].
Acid phosphatase appeared to be an integral part of brain lysosomes and isolated
pigment with a very high specific activity in both. The study also showed that
there is a progressive increase in the brain lipofuscin with age in these animals
and a significant difference was observed in the different age groups (Table 3).
The electron microscopic and fluorescence studies revealed a more or less pure
samples of lipofuscin by the isolation procedures. Several important questions, may
be raised by these studies. Although all precautions were taken to prevent loss of
pigment during the isolation procedures, the possibility of loss of some materials
during fractionation and collection of the materials cannot be ruled out. Another
nagging question is the possibility of the variation of acid phosphatase activity in
the pigment from mice of different ages. A comparative biochemical and histochemical
study of acid phosphatase activities in the brain samples from mice of different ages
might provide some answer to this question.

LIPOFUSCIN FORMATION IN VITRO

Lipofuscin pigment formation has been studied in two uncloned lines (T59 and H8)
and one adrenergic clone (NBA2) of mouse C1300 neuroblastoma cells in culture.
Neuroblastoma cells are derived from neural crest tissue and under appropriate
experimental conditions, can express properties of mature nerve cells[34]. Inhibition
of cell division leads to the formation of neurite-like processes, generation of
electrical properties similar to those of differentiated neurons and increases in
neuronal enzymes. The cells were grown in a monolayer in Falcon plastic flask or on
glass coverslips in Ham's chemically defined synthetic medium (GIBCO Ham's F-12).

Lipofuscin pigment has been demonstrated for the first time in mouse neuroblastoma cells in culture using standard histochemical, fluorescence and electron
microscopic procedures[35,36]. It was observed that the staining properties, enzyme
histochemistry, fluorescence and ultrastructural characteristics of the pigment in
neuroblastoma cells are similar to the corresponding properties of neurons in
animals[37]. The percentage of the cells containing pigment increased with time when
the cells were maintained in culture. This is particularly true when the cultures
are at confluent density and a larger proportion of the cells ceased to divide.
Pigment formation was also enhanced in cultures in which cell division was inhibited
by the addition of papaverine, prostaglandin E_1 or media containing 1% serum.
Additionally, resumption of the cell division by omission of these agents in the
media was accompanied by a reduction in the number of cells containing pigment.

LIPOFUSCIN IN PATHOLOGICAL CONDITIONS

Lipofuscin pigment in excessive amounts in the neurons of CNS have been reported
in a number of pathological conditions of the brain with shortened lifespan. An
early formation lipofuscin pigment in abnormally high quantities has been observed
in the neurons of patients with Progeria and Werner's syndrome[38]. Similar observa-

tions were made in a group of mutant mice who appeared to have a condition of premature aging[39]. The animals usually died within eight weeks of age and lipofuscin pigment in quantities comparable to that in neurons of 12 month old mice was found in neurons with hyperchromatic nuclei. In another pathological condition, Batten-Vogt syndrome, also known as neuronal ceroid-lipofuscinosis, an excessive amount of lipofuscin-like pigment in the neurons has been described[40]. Subsequently, Siakotos, et.al.[30], succeeded in isolating pigment from English Setters with a genetically determined neuronal ceroid-lipofuscinosis, in which the homozygous animals exhibit clinical and morphological picture similar to the Spielmeyer-Sjogren type. The pigment was described as ceroid and the chemical analysis of the isolated pigment revealed some difference from the typical lipofuscin[30]. The two pigments, lipofuscin and ceroid, have been distinguished on the basis of their cation composition, enzymatic and lipid contents. It was noted that ceroid contained a higher concentration of acidic lipid polymer, iron, calcium and copper[30]. It has been hypothesized that the peroxidation of unsaturated fatty acids resulted in the accumulation of pigments in the residual bodies with a progressive death in the bulk of the affected nerve cells and gross brain atrophy[41]. Histochemical study of this pigment material revealed that the stored material is more easily extractible in the unfixed state with acidified or alkalized chloroform-methanol mixtures than lipofuscin[42].

GENESIS AND SIGNIFICANCE OF LIPOFUSCIN

Despite numerous reports on the lipofuscin pigment in the literature on its various aspects, information on two most fundamental questions, namely its mode of origin and physiopathologic significance, are surprisingly lacking. The investigators seem to differ widely in their views on the genesis of the pigment. The pigment appear to be derived from one or more of the organelles within the cell. The more accepted notion has been in favor of the lysosomal origin of the pigment. The stong acid phosphatase activity and the striking ultrastructural similarity between the two are the major evidences for this hypothesis[5,23,43]. Biochemical isolation of the pigment from the brain samples followed by electron microscopy provide further evidence in support of this hypothesis[30].

The arguments have also been made in favor of the possible origin of the pigment from the mitochondria[44,45].The areas of pigment formation in the neurons of the mesencephalic nucleus of the trigeminal nerve have been correlated with high concentration of the mitochondria[46]. It has been suggested that the pigment formation may be preceded by an increased concentration and clumping of mitochondria resulting in the disturbance of normal metabolic activity. This latter condition might lead to the accumulation of insoluble fatty acids which are introduced in the pigment formation[47,48]. These authors have further extended the work in the lipofuscin formation in tissue culture with similar observations.

The possible origin of the pigment from Golgi apparatus and endoplasmic reticulum have also been explored. The evidence in favor of the origin of lipofuscin from Golgi apparatus mainly came from the Sudanophilic and osmiophilic properties of both the organelle and the pigment[49,50]. Although there is no direct evidence of the association of the pigment with the endoplasmic reticulum, the location of the pigment in the striations of the cardiac muscle[51] and decreased level of sytoplasmic RNA in the neurons of aged human brain have been considered in favor of this argument [52]. It is difficult at this time to make any precise statement on the origin of this pigment. The available evidences in the literature tend to indicate that the origin of the pigment may take place from a variety of intracellular organelles and cell membranes which have undergone wear and tear and deterioration during aging. The final breakdown of the materials probably takes place in the lysosomes where these are segregated in an attempt to metabolize and probably reutilize the materials.

There are numerous reports in the literature to indicate that lipofuscin is found in the nondividing cells, which are more likely to show the effects of aging [5,23,46,53,54,55]. Recent studies in our laboratory using neuroblastoma cells in culture have provided further evidences along this line. These tumor cells are capable of dividing indefinitely in tissue culture, but exhibit properties of normal neurons if division is arrested by chemicals such as papaverine, cyclic AMP or prostaglandin E_1. However, when these agents were omitted in the culture media, the cells resumed their division. It has been observed that the differentiated neuroblastoma cells show aging like normal neurons in the animals and develop lipofuscin pigment. On the other hand, omission of the differentiating agents in the media was associated with the resumption of cell division and marked reduction in the pigment formation[35]. The repeatation of the experiment provided further confirmation on the positive correlation between cell differentiation and lipofuscin formation. Several intriguing questions still remain to be answered. Why do nondividing cells accumulate the pigment unlike the mitotic cells? Why does lipofuscin pigment accumulate in the neurons of older animals but not in the young? It may, however, be speculated that the cells in the young animals may have the special ability to metabolize or reutilize the products of intracellular wear and tear, which might be lost during the aging process. For example, a change or loss certain lysosomal enzymes might take place during the lifetime of animals and this might account for the accumulation in the old neurons of partially digested or undigested cellular residue or "garbage" as lipofuscin pigment. Further studies along these lines might appear promising.

The understanding on the functional significance of the pigment in the neurons is even more lacking. While some investigators think that the pigment might be harmful to the cells, others are in favor of its beneficial effects. This confusion may be partly due to the lack of direct evidences on the functions of the cells with and without the pigment. Ideally, studies should be carried out on the functional properties of the cells before and after the formation of pigment as well as following the removal of the pigment by drugs. The studies by Nandy[43], and Nandy and Lal[56], showed a significant improvement of learning and memory in mice following centrophenoxine treatment, which was also associated with a reduction in lipofuscin in the neurons of cerebral cortex and hippocampus. On the other hand, Lal et.al.[57], demonstrated that rats subjected to vitamin E deficient diet showed a deterioration of the learning and memory and an increase in the lipofuscin pigment in the neurons of the cerebral cortex and hippocampus. It may, therefore, be argued that a relation between lipofuscin formation and neuronal function might exist. Although there is no direct evidence to indicate that lipofuscin is harmful or toxic to the cells, it appears reasonable to assume that the process of wear and tear, underlying pigmentogenesis might still be detrimental to the cellular functions. Lipofuscin may, therefore, represent the ashes after the fire rather than a causative factor. On the other hand, the accumulation of large amounts of the pigment occupying a substantial part of the cell soma might also be detrimental to smooth functional operations within the cells.

SUMMARY

This paper outlines the major changes associated with aging and Senile dementia and deals in detail about the lipofuscin pigment. The pigment is commonly visualized by its histochemical, fluorescence and ultrastructural characteristics. Various studies indicate that the pigment formation is a continuous process starting in 2-3 months in mice and thereafter increasing progressively as a function of age. Lipofuscin appears to develop in early and late stages, which differ in their histochemical, fluorescence and ultrastructural properties. The early stage, predominant in younger mice, is more easily stained by PAS and Sudan black B methods and has a greenish-yellow fluorescence. The late stage, on the other hand, is frequently encountered in older animals. This is more easily stainable with Nile blue and ferric-ferricyanide methods, and has an orange-yellow fluorescence. The mature form is also more resistant to treatment with enzyme and lipid solvents. The pigment in the brain has been isolated and quantitated by differential centrifugation followed by spectrophotometric measurement of acid phosphatase. A progressive increase of the pigment with age was also seen by this method. Lipofuscin formation has also been studied in neuroblastoma cells in culture. The pigment formation was enhanced in the cultures when the cell division was inhibited by certain agents, and was reduced when those agents were omitted. This study also confirmed the earlier notion that lipofuscin is a feature of the differentiated cells. There are evidences in support of the origin of lipofuscin from lysosomes, mitochondria and other organelles, although deposition appears to be related to lysosomes. Although there is no direct evidence in support of the harmful effects of the pigment, it has been suggested that the age-associated wear and tear within the cells underlying pigment formation could still be detrimental to the cells.

29

ACKNOWLEDGEMENTS

The works presented here were supported by the U. S. Public Health Grants HD-04188, NS-11964 and the Veterans Administration Research Funds. The author acknowledges technical assistance of Miss Nancy Roy and the typing assistance of Mrs. Arline Barrett.

REFERENCES

1. Strehler, B.L. ed (1960) "The Biology of Aging" Am. Inst. Biol. Sci., Washington, D.C.

2. Strehler, B.L. (1967) "Environmental Factors in Aging and Mortality" Environmental Research 1, 46-88.

3. Sacher, G. (1977) "Life Table Modification and Life Prolongation" in Handbook of the Biology of Aging C.E. Finch and L. Hayflick (eds.) Van Nostrand Rheinhold Company, New York, pp. 582-638.

4. Nandy, K. (1977) "Immune Reactions in Aging Brain and Senile Dementia" in The Aging Brain and Senile Dementia K. Nandy and I. Sherwin (eds.) Plenum Press, New York, pp. 181-196.

5. Nandy, K. (1971) Acta Neuropath 19:25-32.

6. Nandy, K. (1968) J. Geront. 23, 82-92.

7. Brody, H. (1955) J. Comp. Neurol., 102, 511-556.

8. Brody, H. (1960) J. Geront., 16:258-261.

9. Brizzee, K. R., Kaack, B. and Klara, P. (1975) "Lipofuscin: Intra-and Extra neuronal Accumulation and Regional Distribution" in Neurobiology of Aging, J. M. Ordy and K. R. Brizzee (eds.) Plenum Press, New York, pp. 463-484.

10. Reichel, W., Hollander, J., Clark, J. H., Strehler, B. L. (1968) J. Geront. 23, 71-78.

11. Corsellis, J.A.N. (1976) "Some Observations on the Purkinje Cell Population and on Brain Volume in Human Aging" in Neurobiology of Aging R. D. Terry and S. Gershon (eds.), Raven Press, New York, pp. 205-209.

12. Feldman, M. L. (1977) "Dendritic Changes in Aging Rat Brain: Pyramidal Cell Dendritic Length and Ultrastructure" in The Aging Brain and Senile Dementia, K. Nandy and I. Sherwin (eds.), Plenum Press, New York, pp. 23-28.

13. Scheibel, M. E. and Scheibel, A. B. (1977) "Differential Changes with Aging in Old and New Cortices" in The Aging Brain and Senile Dementia K. Nandy and I. Sherwin (eds.), Plenum Press, New York, pp. 39-58.

14. Wisniewski, H. M. and Terry, R. D. (1976) "Neuropathology of the Aging Brain" in Neurobiology of Aging, R. D. Terry and S. Gershon (eds.), Raven Press, New York, pp. 265-280.

15. Igbal, K., Wisniewski, H. M., Grunde-Igbal, Inge and Terry, R. D. "Neurofibril-lary Pathology: An Update" in The Aging Brain and Senile Dementia, K. Nandy and I. Sherwin (eds.) Plenum Press, New York, pp. 209-228.

16. Selkoe, D. J. and Shelanski, M. L. (1977) "The Fibrous Proteins of Brain: A Primer for Gerontologists" in The Aging Brain and Senile Dementia, K. Nandy and I. Sherwin (eds.), Plenum Press, New York, pp. 247-264.

17. Tomlinson, B. E. and Henderson, G. (1976) "Some Quantitative Cerebral Findings in Normal and Demented Old People" in Neurobiology of Aging, R. D. Terry and S. Gershon (eds.), Raven Press, New York, pp. 183-204.

18. Hannover, A. (1842) Videnskapsselsk. Naturvidensk. Math. Afh., Copenhagen, 10.

19. Borst, M. (1922) Pathogische Histologie, Vogel, Leipzig, 210.

20. Pearse, A. G. E. (1964) Histochemistry: Theoretical and Applied, Little, Brown & Co., Boston, pp. 661-675.

21. Bondareff, W. (1957) J. Geront., 12, 364-369.

22. Gatenby, J. B. (1953) J. Roy. Micr. Soc., 73, 61-81.

23. Samorajski, T., Keefe, J. R., Ordy, J. M. (1964) J. Geront., 19, 262-276.

24. Sulkin, N. M. (1953) J. Geront., 8, 435-448.

25. Bourne, G. H. (1973) "Lipofuscin" in Neurobiological Aspects of Maturation and Aging, D. H. Ford (ed.), Elsevier, Amsterdam, pp. 187-201.

26. Sekhon, S. S. and Maxwell, D. S. (1974) J. Neurocytol., 3, 59-72.

27. Siakotos, A. N., Watanabe, I., Siato, A. and Flesicher, S. (1970) Biochem. Med., 4, 361-375.

28. DeDuve, C., Pressman, B. C., Gianetto, R., Wattiaux, R. Applemans, F. (1955) Biochem. J., 60, 604-617.

29. DeDuve, C., Wattiaux, R. and Baudhuin, P. (1962) Adv. Enzymol, 24, 291-298.

30. Siakotos, A. N., Goebel, H. H., Patel, V., Watanabe, I. and Zeman, W. (1972) "The Morphogenesis and Biochemical Characteristics of Ceroid Isolated from Cases of Neuronal Ceroid-Lipofuscinosis" in Sphingolipid, Sphingolipidosis and Allied Disorders, B. W. Volk and S. M. Aronson (eds.), Plenum Press, New York, Vol. 19, pp. 53-61.

31. Rouser, G., Kritchevsky, C., Siakotos, A. N., Yamanoto, A. N., (1970) "Lipid Composition of the Brain and its Subcellular Structures" in Neuropathology: Method and Diagnosis, C. G. Tedeschi (ed.), Little, Brown and Co., Boston, pp. 691-753.

32. Siakotos, A. N. and Rouser, G. (1965) J. Am. Oil Chem. Soc., 42, 913-919.

33. Sellinger, D. Z., Rucker, D. L. and Belbian Verseter, R. D. (1964) J. Neurochem. 11, 271-280.

34. Minna, J. D. (1973) "Genetic Analysis of the Mammalian Nervous System Using Somatic Cell Culture Techniques" in Tissue Culture of the Nervous System, G. Sato (ed.), Plenum Press, New York, pp. 161-185.

35. Nandy, K. and Schneider, H. (1976) "Lipofuscin Pigment Formation in Neuroblastoma Cells in Culture" in Neurobiology of Aging, R. Terry and S. Gershon (ed.), Raven Press, New York, pp. 245-264.

36. Nandy, K. and Schneider, H. (1978) Gerontology 24 (Suppl 1), pp. 66-70

37. Schneider, H. and Nandy, K. (1977) J. Geront., 32, 132-139.

38. Reichel, W. and Garcia-Bunuel, R. (1970) Am. J. Clin. Path., 53, 243.

39. O'Steen, K. W. and Nandy, K. (1970) Am. J. Anat., 128, 359-365.

40. Zemen, W. (1971) "The Neuronal Ceroid Lipofuscinosis-Batten-Vogt Syndrome: A. Model for Human Aging?" in Adv. in Geront. Res., B. L. Strehler (ed.), Academic Press, New York, Vol. 3, pp. 147-169.

41. Semen, W. (1974) J. Neuropath. Exp. Neurol., 33, 1-12.

42. Elleder, M. (1977) Acta Neuropath., 38, 117-122.

43. Nandy, K. (1978) J. Am. Geriat. Soc., 26 (No. 2), 74-81.

44. Hess, A. (1955) Anat. Rec., 123, 399-424.

45. Roizin, L. (1964) J. Neuropathol. Exp. Neurol., 23, 209-252.

46. Hasan, M. and Glees, P. (1972) Gerontologia, 18, 217-236.

47. Gopinath, G. and Glees, P. (1974) Acta Anat., 89, 14-20.

48. Glees, P. and Gopinath, G. (1973) Z. Zellforsch, 141, 285-298.

49. Bondareff, W. (1964) "Histopathology of the Aging Nervous System" in Advances in Gerontological Research, Academic Press, New York, Vol. 1, pp. 1-22.

50. Dalton, A. J. (1957) Symp. Soc. Exp. Biol., 10, 148-154.

51. Strehler, B. L. (1964) "On the Histochemistry and Ultrastructure of Age Pigment" in Advances in Gerontological Research, B. L. Strehler (ed.), Academic Press, New York, Vol. 1, pp. 343-384.

52. Mann, D. M. A. and Yates, P. O. (1974) Brain, 97, 481-488.

53. Brody, H. and Vijayashanker, N. (1977) "Anatomical Changes in the Nervous System" in Handbook of the Biology of Aging, C. E. Finch and L. Hayflick (eds.), Van Nostrand Rheinhold Company, New York, Vol. 1, pp. 241-261.

54. Samorajski, T., Ordy, J. M. and Keefe, J. R. (1965) J. Cell Biol., 26, 779-261.

55. Brody, H. (1960) J. Geront., 15, 258-261.

56. Nandy, K. and Lal, H. (1978) "Neuronal Lipofuscin and Learning Deficits in Aging Mammals" in Neuropsycho-pharmacologicum, E. Domino (ed.), Pergamon Press, New York, pp. 1633-1645.

57. Lal, H., Pogacar, S., Daly, P. R. and Puri, S. K. (1973) "Behavioral and Neuropathological Manifestations of Nutritionally Induced Central Nervous System Aging in the Rat" in Neurobiological Aspects of Maturation and Aging, D. Ford (ed.), Elsevier, New York, pp. 129-140.

ALTERATIONS OF MORPHOLOGICAL AND NEUROCHEMICAL PARAMETERS OF THE
BRAIN DUE TO NORMAL AGING

W. MEIER-RUGE, O. HUNZIKER, P. IWANGOFF, K. REICHLMEIER and P. SANDOZ

Sandoz Institute of Basic Medical Research, Lichtstrasse 35, CH-4002
Basel (Switzerland)

ABSTRACT

Age-dependent changes of morphometric and neurochemical parameters
are studied in autopsic human brains free of metabolic, neurologic or
psychiatric diseases.

A morphometric investigation of the main part of the inferior olivary
nucleus shows a significant, 19.7 % nerve cell loss between the ages of
20 and 80 years.

The capillary network of the brain cortex develops an age-related increase in the mean capillary diameter, an increase in capillary length
per unit brain volume and a decrease in the mean capillary distance.
These findings demonstrate that decreased cerebral blood flow in the elderly is possibly the result of an adaptation to changed anatomical parameters and not a sign of insufficiency.

Neurochemical investigations of 13 glycolytic enzymes of brain cortex
and putamen demonstrate a change in activity in only two cases : soluble
hexokinase activity increases and that of phosphofructokinase decreases
with age. The alterations in these key enzymes are regarded as being
rate-limiting for ATP synthesis. On this presupposition, the conclusion
is drawn that, a therapeutic increase in glucose uptake by the brain
seems not to be reasonable.

Carbonic anhydrase decreases significantly in the aging brain. It is
likely that this particular alteration is of importance for an instability of the CO_2 regulation of cerebral blood flow. The age-induced decrease in acetylcholinesterase was significant only in the putamen, a
finding which may be relevant to extrapyramidal symptoms in the aged.
Further, an age-induced decrease in cAMP stimulated protein kinase was
observed.

INTRODUCTION

Aging is an event of normal life with progressive impairment of adaptation due to inadequate responses to environmental stimuli.

This characterizes aging as a slowly developing process of deviation from normal life.

With reference to the brain, it is surprising how low the incidence of age-related brain diseases is.

Slater and Roth[1] estimated the following prevalence rates of mental disorders in the elderly (over 65, living at home or permanently in a nursing home or a geriatric hospital) :

- Manic-depressive disorders, paraphrenia and   3.49 %
  unspecific severe brain syndromes

- Senile dementia (incl. arteriosclerotic   4.56 %
             dementia)

- Senile psychosis   8.05 %

- Minor symptoms of senility   83.90 %

Many of these mental aging diseases seem to be linked to a hereditary disposition.

Broe et al.[2] reported in a normal population of the elderly in Glasgow (Scotland) a 5.8 % morbidity rate for senile dementia and observed minor symptoms of aging in 83.6 % of the elderly who were investigated. This shows that a large proportion of the complaints from the elderly are due to minor symptoms of aging, which have, however, a number of serious consequences for the daily life of the aging individual, since aging reduces the functional redundancy of the different organs, in particular the brain, the kidney, the heart etc..

Currently limited knowledge of normal brain aging forced us to study the morphological and neurochemical characteristics of this process. A knowledge of these parameters is a prerequisite for the development of a pathogenic concept of senile dementia and other aging diseases of the brain.

MATERIAL AND METHODS

All studies were accomplished with human brain tissue obtained at autopsy. All cases were free of metabolic, neurologic or psychiatric diseases and prior to death none of the cases had been undergoing psychiatric treatment. The post-mortem delay was 4 to 24 hours.

a) Morphometric procedure

The post-mortem changes in stereological parameters of cerebral capillaries were investigated by Hunziker and Schweizer[3] and the randomized sampling procedures for selecting sections were described by Sandoz[4].

Investigations of the nerve cell number from the human inferior olive is described elsewhere[5].

The optic electronic image analysis procedure for measuring the architecture of cerebral capillaries in aging human brains was described by Hunziker[6,7].

The study on capillaries was performed with 8 brains. The cases were divided into tow groups : young (19-49 years), and aged normotonic (66-72 years). Brain cortex from the frontal, parietal (anterior and posterior central gyrus), superior and inferior temporal gyrus and occipital areas was investigated. The capillaries were selectively stained with alkaline phosphatase reaction. The selectivity of the staining was verified by a three-dimensional reconstruction of the brain capillary network[8].

b) Neurochemical methods

The neurochemical investigations were carried out with 48 human brains obtained at autopsy. The calendar ages of the individuals were from 19 to 92 years.

Brain tissue examined was cortex of the frontal pole and putamen. The tissue was frozen in dry ice and stored at -80°C.

The glycolytic enzymes were investigated as described by Bergmeyer[9] and by Bücher et al.[10].

The following enzymes were studied : hexokinase, phosphoglucose isomerase, fructose-6-phosphate kinase, fructose-1,6-diphosphate aldolase, triose-phosphate isomerase, glyceraldehyde-3-phosphate dehydrogenase, 3-phosphoglycerate kinase, phosphoglycerate mutase, enolase, pyruvate kinase, lactate dehydrogenase, glucose-6-phosphate dehydrogenase, and glycerol-3-phosphate dehydrogenase.

ATPases were determined by the method of Bonting et al.[11]. The details of the modification used are described elsewhere[12].

Protein kinase was studied as described by Reichlmeier[31]. The other two enzymes analysed systematically were carbonic anhydrase and acetylcholinesterase[44,45].

The influence of the cause of death and the duration of agony was investigated by Iwangoff et al.[13]. It was shown that the duration of agony is of greater significance than the time interval between death and autopsy.

RESULTS

The morphometric investigation of the main part of the human inferior olivary nucleus demonstrated that the number of neurons decreases
significantly (p < 0.02) as function of age (Figure 1).

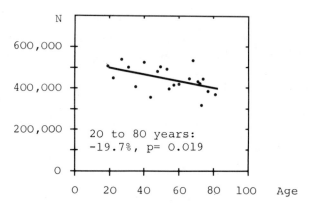

Fig. 1. Age-related decrease in the number of nerve cells (N) in
the main part of the inferior olivary nucleus[5]

Between the ages of 20 and 40 years a linear regression of the number
of nerve cells can be observed, reaching -19.7 % at 80 years.

In contrast, the total volume of the olivary nucleus decreased by only 6.7 % which was, however, not statistically significant.

The investigation of the stereological parameters in the brain cortex of a young and an elderly group demonstrated that, in individuals
with normal blood pressure, the mean capillary diameter increases significantly with age. The mean capillary distance decrease and the capillary lengths per unit volume of brain cortex increase (Figure 2).

Neurochemical studies of the enzymes of the glycolytic pathway demonstrate that most of these enzymes are changed in their activity not
at all or only slightly by the aging process; this is true e.g. for
phosphoglucose isomerase, aldolase, triose-phosphate isomerase, glycer-
aldehyde-3-phosphate dehydrogenase, 3-phosphoglycerate kinase, enolase,
pyruvate kinase, lactate dehydrogenase glucose-6-phosphate dehydrogenase (brain cortex) and glycerol-3-phosphate dehydrogenase.

In contrast to these findings, the two key enzymes hexokinase and
phosphofructokinase are significantly changed. The soluble hexokinase
increases and fructose-6-phosphate kinase decreases significantly with
age (Figure 3). Na^+/K^+-ATPase (cortex; $y = 3.41 - 0.003$ x, $R^2 = 0.004$)

precentral gyrus of human brain cortex

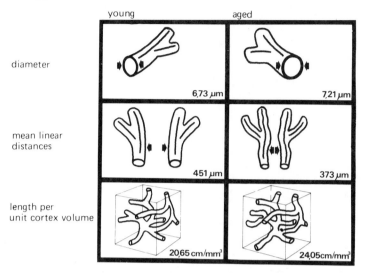

young   aged

diameter   6,73 μm   7,21 μm

mean linear distances   451 μm   373 μm

length per unit cortex volume   20,65 cm/mm³   24,05 cm/mm³

Fig. 2. Comparison of capillary parameters in the brain cortex of young and old humans[21].

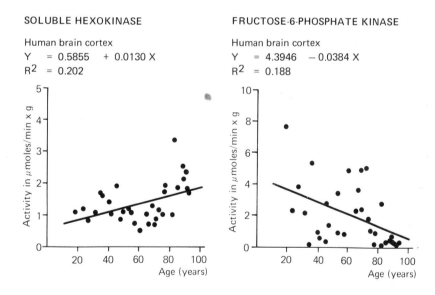

SOLUBLE HEXOKINASE

Human brain cortex
$Y = 0.5855 + 0.0130 X$
$R^2 = 0.202$

FRUCTOSE-6-PHOSPHATE KINASE

Human brain cortex
$Y = 4.3946 - 0.0384 X$
$R^2 = 0.188$

Fig. 3. Age-dependent changes of the glycolytic key enzymes hexokinase and phosphofructokinase which are rate limiting in the glycolytic pathway [13,22].

and Mg^{++}-ATPase (cortex; $y = 9.45 - 0.01 \, x$, $R^2 = 0.009$) is only negligibly reduced.

However, carbonic anhydrase shows a significant ($p = 2\alpha < 0.01$) decrease in its activity (Figure 4). Acetylcholinesterase (brain cortex; $y = 1.36 - 0.001 \, x$, $R^2 = 0.002$) decreases only in the putamen ($y = 63.84 - 0.31 \, x$, $R^2 = 0.171$, $p = 2\alpha < 0.01$) in old age. Protein kinase stimulation by cAMP declines progressively with increasing age (Figure 5), the decrease being more pronounced in the brain cortex ($y = 92.42 - 0.45 \, x$, $R^2 = 0.186$) than in putamen ($y = 65.85 - 0.19 \, x$, $R^2 = 0.032$). Phosphoglycerate mutase decreases significantly with age ($p = 2\alpha < 0.05$) in the brain cortex ($y = 73.12 - 0.31 \, x$, $R^2 = 0.124$; putamen $y = 77.40 - 0.21 \, x$, $R^2 = 0.029$). Glucose-6-phosphate dehydrogenase increases only in the putamen ($y = 0.55 + 0.004 \, x$, $R^2 = 0.174$).

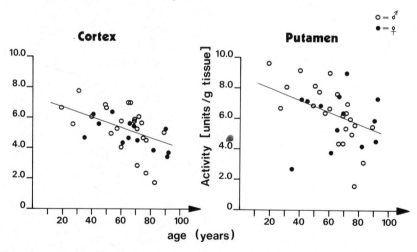

Fig. 4. Age-induced decrease of carbonic anhydrase in the human brain cortex and putamen [32].

DISCUSSION

The old concept that aging is accompanied by a progressive nerve cell loss [14] is seriously in need of correction.

We know today that only a moderate loss, of the order of 20 to 25 %, of the neuronal cells in the brain cortex occurs with age [15-18].

Activation of cAMP-Protein Kinase in Human Brain

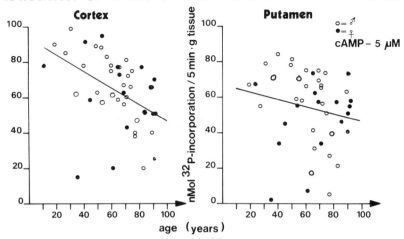

Fig. 5. Reduction of cAMP stimulation of protein kinase with increasing age [32].

The morphometric determination of the number of nerve cells in the main olivary nucleus in man is today controversial.

Monagle and Brody[19] observed no significant alterations of the nerve cell number. We found a 20 % decrease in the nerve cells between the ages of 20 and 80 years [5]. A 20 % cell loss may possibly be responsible for a slight subclinical sensomotor impairment, but not for a severe psychomotor abnormality.

The old theory that senile mental decline is the result of an age-related decrease in cerebral blood flow [20], was examined by means of a morphometric investigation of the capillary network of the brain cortex. The morphometric parameters of the capillaries were examined by an optic electronic image analysis system [6,7]. The results demonstrate (Figure 2) that the ratio of capillary vessels to brain tissue shifts in favour of the blood supplying capillary network [21].

The age-related increase in capillary diameter, the increase in the capillary length per unit brain cortex volume and an about 17 % decrease in the mean capillary distance demonstrate that a 10 - 15 % decrease in brain blood flow in the elderly is completely compensated by the altered parameters of the capillary network. So the decreased cerebral blood flow in the aged [20] may be an adaptative phenomenom and not a symptom of insufficient blood supply.

Neurochemical alterations in the aging brain can be better correlated with cognitive disorders, and a knowledge of neurochemical changes in the brain metabolism in the course of physiologic aging may also be of fundamental importance in the interpretation of pathogenic aspects of aging diseases of the brain such as senile dementia etc..

Our neurochemical studies demonstrate (Figures 3 - 5), that the aging process is accompanied by changes in some enzyme activities of the energy metabolism. It is surprising that in the glycolytic pathway most enzymes remain unchanged and only the key enzymes hexokinase and phosphofructokinase show an alteration [22]. The decrease of fructose-6-phosphate kinase may impair the glucose splitting capacity of the glycolytic pathway and explain the reduced cerebral glucose consumption in aged subjects [23]. Since glycolysis is the first metabolic step in glucose degradation before entering into the citric acid cycle and the respiratory chain, all energy formation, which results in the synthesis of the energy carrier ATP, depends upon the metabolic turnover capacity of the glycolytic pathway. This seems to be significant because the total energy formation in the brain depends almost exclusively upon the glycolytic capacity.

In view of these findings it does not seem reasonable to increase therapeutically the glucose uptake by the brain except in the case of a drug which improves the glucose turnover at the rate limiting steps hexokinase and fructose-6-phosphate kinase (Figure 6).

The reduction in ATP synthesis capacity due to an age-induced limitation of the glucose turnover rate is of particular interest, because the ATPases are only slightly changed with age, possibly resulting in exhaustion of the limited ATP stores under conditions of an accerelated ATP turnover.

Further studies will be needed to prove, whether or not the increase of soluble hexokinase is the result of a membrane alteration with a consequent decrease of membrane-bound hexokinase.

An age-dependent decrease in carbonic anhydrase may be relevant to an impairment of CO_2 exchange under conditions of increased metabolic turnover, these findings indicate that, with increasing age, CO_2 regulation of cerebral blood flow becomes labile, and is combined with a tendency to instability of brain blood flow autoregulation.

Investigations of acetylcholinesterase in the human brain demonstrate only a slight change in enzyme activity in the brain cortex. In the putamen, however, there is a significant decrease of acetylcho-

Glycolytic Pathway

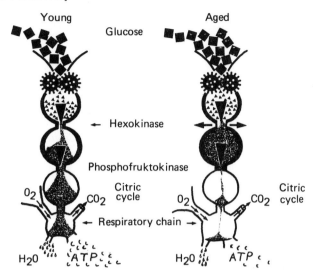

Fig. 6. Schematic representation of the limitations of the glycolytic pathway by an age-induced alteration of hexokinase and
phosphofructokinase activity and the subsequent reduction of the
capacity of ATP synthesis (right) in comparison with the normal
situation (left).

linesterase activity. The putamen, which is one of the striatal nuclei
of the brain, belongs to the extrapyramidal system regulating involunt-
ary movements in gait, statics, balance, etc.. These neurochemical
findings confirm earlier observations in aging rats [24-26].

The   decrease in acetylcholinesterase activity in the putamen and
consequent decline of metabolic turnover seem to be at least in part
consistent with an age-related reduction in the electrical activity in
the brain, which is characterized by a continuous shift of the dominant
alpha-frequency to lower frequencies [27-30].

A decrease in cAMP stimulated protein kinase with age (Figure 5) was
observed in animal and human brain [31,32].

Greengard[33] postulates that a decrease in cAMP stimulated protein
kinase has effects on the phosphorylation of membrane proteins.
This is expected - among other things - to be of functional consequence
in the phosphorylation of the synaptosomal membranes which could result
in a disturbance of short term memory.

It is surprising that our knowledge of physiological brain aging is
today extremely limited, though 85 % of people over 65 suffer from a

series of psychogeriatric abnormalities such as disturbed cognitive function, affective lability, decreased vigilance, etc.. Most papers deal with different forms of pathological aging - senile dementia and Alzheimer's disease [34-37], Huntington's chorea [37-40] and Parkinson's disease [41,42] - despite the fact that these diseases (10 - 15 %) are relatively rare. These studies demonstrate mainly characteristic disturbances of transmitter turnover. Because, however, pathological aging of the brain is not the result of an accelerated physiological aging process, there exists the danger that a false therapeutic principle could subsequently be developed from such findings.

The few investigations of physiological brain aging show a decrease in transmitter enzymes such as DOPA decarboxylase, glutamic decarboxylase and tyrosine hydroxylase [42,43]. In this connection, the present data may be a further contribution in this particular area of science.

Our results have shown that aging is, generally speaking, characterized by a decreased adaptability to adverse environmental stimuli. Better insights into the normal aging process will probably help to elucidate the pathogenesis of senile dementia.

CONCLUSION

The results demonstrate that physiological aging of the human brain is accompanied by a moderate loss of neuronal cells, which is far below the level that would cause neurological deficit symptoms.

Morphometric investigations of the density of the capillary network show that the ratio of capillary to brain cortex volume increases. It is possible that a decrease in cerebral blood flow in the elderly is completely compensated by an unchanged blood supply to a smaller brain cortex volume.

Neurochemical examination of the enzymes of the glycolytic pathway demonstrates that the key enzymes hexokinase and phosphofructokinase, which are rate limiting in the glucose turnover of the brain, become significantly changed with age. This finding confirms the observation of a decreased glucose uptake in aged individuals. In the light of these results a therapeutic increase of glucose uptake of the brain obviously makes sense only, if these key enzymes can be normalized.

ACKNOWLEDGEMENTS

The authors are grateful to Professor H.U. Zollinger (Institute of Pathology, University of Basel), Professor J. Ulrich (Department of Neuropathology, Institute of Pathology, Basel) and Professor W. Wegmann (Pathological Institute of the Kantonsspital of Basel-Land, Liestal) for kindly providing us with the autopsic material.

REFERENCES

1. Slater, E. and Roth, M. (1977) Clinical Psychiatry, Baillière Tindall, London, pp. 533 - 544.

2. Broe, G.A., Akhtar, A.J., Andrews, G.R., Caird, F.J. Gilmore, A. J.J. and McLennan, W.J. (1976) J. Neurol Neurosurg. Psychiatr. 39, 362 - 366.

3. Hunziker, O. and Schweizer, A. (1977) Beitr. Pathol. 161, 244 - 255.

4. Sandoz, P.A. (1977) Microscopica Acta, Suppl. 1, 201 - 202.

5. Sandoz, P. and Meier-Ruge, W. (1977) IRCS Medical Science 5, 376.

6. Hunziker, O., Frey, H. and Schulz, U. (1974) Brain Res. 65, 1 - 11.

7. Hunziker, O. Bangerter, D., Leimgruber, W., Schieweck, CH., Vinzenz, S. and Wiederhold, K.-H. (1974) Microscopica Acta 75, 452 - 458.

8. Wiederhold, K.-H., Bielser, W., Schulz, U., Veteau, M.-J. and Hunziker, O. (1976) Microvascular Research 11, 175 - 180.

9. Bergmeyer, H.U. (1970) Methoden der enzymatischen Analyse, Verlag Chemie, Weinheim.

10. Bücher, TH., Luh, W. and Pette, D. (1964) in Handbuch der physiologischen und pathologisch-chemischen Anaylse, Hoppe-Seyler / Thierfelder eds. Vol. VIA, Springer-Verlag, Berlin - Heidelberg - New York.

11. Botting, S.L., Simons, K.A. and Hawkins, N.M. (1961) Arch. Biochem. Biophys. 95, 416 - 423.

12. Meier-Ruge, W., Enz, A., Gygax, P., Hunziker, O., Iwangoff, P. and Reichlmeier, K. (1975) in Genesis and Treatment of Psychologic Disorders in the Elderly, Aging Vol. 2, Gershon, S. and Raskin, A. eds., Raven Press, New York, pp. 379 - 387.

13. Iwangoff, P., Armbruster, R., Enz, A. and Sandoz, P. (1978) IRCS Medical Science 6, 83.

14. Brody, H. (1955) J. Comp. Neurol. 102, 511 - 516.

15. Brody, H. (1973) in Development and Aging in the Nervous System, Rockstein, M. and Sussman, M.L. eds., Academic Press, New York, pp. 121 - 133.

16. Brody, H. (1976) in Neurobiology of Aging, Aging Vol. 3, Terry, R. D. and Gershon, S. eds., Raven Press, New York, pp. 177 - 181.

17. Shefer, V.F. (1973) Neurosci. Behav. Physiol. 6, 319 - 324.

18. Tomlinson, B.E. and Henderson, G. (1976) in Neurobiology of Aging, Aging Vol. 3, Terry, R.D. and Gershon, S. eds., Raven Press, New York, pp. 183 - 204.

19. Monagle, R.D. and Brody, H. (1974) J. Comp. Neurol. 155, 61 - 66.

20. Kety, S.S. (1956) Res. Publ. Assoc. Res. Nerv. Ment. Dis. 35, 31 - 45.

21. Hunziker, O., Abdel'Al, S., Frey, H., Veteau, M.-J. and Meier-Ruge, W. (1978) Gerontology 24, 27 - 31.

22. Iwangoff, P., Armbruster, R. and Enz, A. (1977) Sixth Internat. Meeting of the Internat. Soc. for Neurochem. Copenhagen, Denmark, Abstr. 17.

23. Sokoloff, L. (1975) in Genesis and Treatment of Psychologic Disorders in the Elderly, Aging Vol. 2, Gershon, S. and Raskin, A. eds., Raven Press, New York, pp. 45 - 54.

24. Samorajski, T. and Ordy, J.M. (1972) in Aging and the Brain, Gaitz, C.M. ed., Plenum Press, New York, pp. 41 - 61.

25. Samorajski, T. and Rolsten, C. (1973) Progr. Brain Res. 40, 253 - 265.

26. Meier-Ruge, W., Reichlmeier, K. and Iwangoff, P. (1976) in Neurobiology of Aging, Aging Vol. 3, Terry, R.D. and Gershon, S. eds., Raven Press, New York, pp. 379 - 387.

27. Obrist, W.D. (1954) Electroenceph. Clin. Neurophysiol. 6, 235 - 244.

28. Busse, E.W., Obrist, W.D. and Wang, H.S. (1965) J. Gerontol. 20, 315 - 320.

29. Wang, S.H. and Busse, E.W. (1974) in Normal Aging II, Erdman Palmore ed., Duke-University-Press, Durham / N.C., pp. 160 - 167.

30. Roubicek, J. (1977) J. Am. Geriatr. Soc. 25, 145 - 152.

31. Reichlmeier, K.D. (1976) J. Neurochem. 27, 1249 - 1251.

32. Reichlmeier, K.D., Schlecht, H.-P. and Ermini, M. (1976) 29th Ann. Meeting Gerontol. Soc. New York, Abstr. 39.

33. Greengard, P. (1976) Nature (London) 260, 101 - 108.

34. Bowen, D.M., Smith, C.B., White, P. and Davison, A.N. (1976) Brain Res. 99, pt. 3, 459 - 496.

35. Bowen, D.M., Smith, C.B., White, P. and Davison, A.N. (1976) in Neurobiology of Aging, Aging Vol. 3, Terry, R.D. and Gershon, S. eds., Raven Press, New York, pp. 361 - 378.

36. Gottfries, C.G., Roos, B.E. and Winblad, B. (1976) Akt. geront. 6, 429 - 435.

37. Perry, T.L., Hansen, S. and Kloster, M. (1975) New Engl. J. Med. 288, 337 - 342.

38. Bird, E.D., Mackay, A.V.P., Rayner, C.N. and Iversen, L.L. (1973) Lancet 1, 1090 - 1092.

39. Bird, E.D., Gales, J.S. and Spokes, E.G. (1977) J. Neurochem. 29, 539 - 545.

40. McGeer, P.L. and McGeer, E.G. (1976) J. Neurochem. 26, 65 - 76.

41. Ehringer, H. and Hornykiewicz, O. (1960) Klin. Wschr. 36, 1236 - 1239.

42. McGeer, E. and McGeer, P.L. (1976) in Neurobiology of Aging, Aging Vol. 3, Terry, R.D. and Gershon, S. eds., Raven Press, New York, pp. 389 - 403.

43. McGeer, P.L., McGeer, E.G. and Suzuki, J.S. (1977) Arch. Neurol. 34, 33 - 35.

44. Ellman, G.L., Courtney, K.D., Andres, V. and Featherstone, R.N. (1961) J. Biochem. Pharmacol. 7, 88 - 95.

45. Armstrong, J.M., Myers, D.V., Verpoorte, J.A. and Edsall, J.T. (1966) J. Biol. Chem. 241, 5137 - 5149.

STUDIES ON BIOCHEMICAL CHANGES IN AGING BRAIN

CAROLYN B. SMITH

Laboratory of Cerebral Metabolism, National Institute of Mental Health, Bethesda,
Maryland 20014

ABSTRACT

Biochemical indices of brain structure and function have been assessed in young,
middle-aged and aged rats and in tissue from human subjects, both normal elderly
and demented. The results demonstrate that in the whole temporal lobes of patients
with 'senile-type' dementia there was at least a 50% loss of neuronal constituents
compared with age-matched normal controls. In the mentally normal subjects, age-
related losses occurred in 4 of the 8 indices of neural cells. Preliminary results
from a study of the local cerebral glucose utilization in aged rats indicate that
in the course of normal aging regionally selective decreases in glucose metabolism
may occur. These changes may reflect a decrease in functional activity, a loss of
neurons or neuronal processes and/or an essential metabolic defect.

INTRODUCTION

Losses of neurons[1,2] and dendritic spines[3,4] have been described as essential
features of the neuropathology of both senile dementia and normal aging. Considering
the limitations in current quantitative morphological methods[5], in this current study
biochemical techniques have been applied in order to assess cellular and subcellular
changes in the brain. The application of biochemical techniques provides the added
advantage of an assessment of the functional as well as the structural integrity of
brain structures. This study involves the analysis of biochemical changes in brain
tissue from aged humans, both controls and patients with 'senile-type' dementia, and
young, middle-aged and aged rats.

METHODS

Human studies

Temporal lobes from 25 human brains obtained at random, post-mortem, were examined. The interval between death and refrigeration was usually within 0.75 to 3.0 h
and brains were excised within 24 h of death. One hemisphere of each brain was
removed for histopathology (Dr. J.A.N. Corsellis).

The entire temporal lobe (tissue ventral to the lateral cerebral fissure extended to meet the occipital lobe) from one hemisphere was taken for biochemical analysis.
The lobe was homogenized in 0.32 M sucrose, 1 mM Tris-HCl, pH 6.7, using a VirTis
tissue homogenizer followed by one pass in a Potter-Elvenhjem type homogenizer. The

homogenate was apportioned for the various biochemical analyses. The mitochondrial light fraction, the water-shocked myelin fraction of a crude nuclear plus mitochondrial suspension, was prepared by differential and density-gradient centrifugation[6]. The levels of total protein in both this fraction and the whole homogenate were determined[7]. Extracts of homogenate were prepared for either lipid analyses or for gel electrophoresis of water soluble proteins[8]. Ganglioside N-acetyl neuraminic acid (ganglioside NANA) was estimated[8] in the Folch extract, and galactolipid galactose was determined[9] following hydrolysis of lower layer lipids[10]. Neuronins S-5 and S-6 were determined by quantitative gel electrophoresis[11]. Nucleic acids were extracted from the homogenate and separated[12], and RNA and DNA were determined[13-16]. The glutamic acid decarboxylase (GAD) activity was determined immediately after tissue homogenization using a slight modification[6] of the CO_2-trapping method[17]. The activities of acetylcholinesterase (AChE), adenosine 2'3'-cyclic nucleotide 3'-phosphohydrolase (CNP), succinate dehydrogenase (SDH), β-glucuronidase (β-Glu), β-galactosidase (β-Gal) and carbonic anhydrase were all determined using well-established procedures[18-23]. Most of these enzyme activities were determined on homogenates which had been stored at -20° C for one week or less. The activities of CNP and SDH, however, were measured after longer storage periods. The CNP activity was unaffected by the period of storage, whereas the SDH activity decreased with increasing storage time. The SDH activities were corrected for this loss[6].

Animal studies. Local cerebral glucose utilization was determined using the autoradiographic 2-deoxy-D-[14C]-glucose method[24] in male Sprague-Dawley rats at 3 different ages (105-140d, 480-540d and 750-810d). Rats were supplied by the National Institute on Aging. Glucose utilization was measured in 31 brain regions. After surgical preparation, under light halothane anesthesia, animals were allowed to recover for 4-6h. The 2-deoxy-D-[14C]-glucose was injected into the fully conscious, partially immobilized rats. Mean arterial blood pressure (120 ± 8 mmHg), rectal temperature (37 ± 1° C), hematocrit (51 ± 3 %), and arterial blood pH (7.46 ± 0.05), pO_2 (89 ± 3 Torr) and pCO_2 (33 ± 3 Torr) were measured in order to assess the physiological state of the animals. Rats with values differing from normal by more than 2 standard deviations were excluded from the studies.

RESULTS

Human studies

Diagnostic groups. The 25 human brains obtained for this study were divided into three diagnostic groups. The control group included cases with no clinical or histological evidence of brain pathology. These specimens were subdivided into patients who had died suddenly (8 cases) and those who had had a lingering mode of death and post-mortem evidence of multiple defects in the systems which control the blood and oxygen supply to the brain (6 cases). Several of these cases had histological abnormalities (other than 'senile-type' morphological changes). The 6 cases of 'senile-type' dementia were all clinically and histologically confirmed. Two cases were classified as senile dementia and 4 cases as mixed senile and vascular dementia. The remaining 5 cases were patients with various other neurological disorders; the results obtained from these patients will not be presented in this paper. A summary of the age, sex, and the interval from death to assay for each group is given in Table 1.

TABLE 1

SUMMARIZED HISTORY OF CASES STUDIED

Diagnostic Group	No.	Age (y) (range) mean ± S.D.	Sex F/M	Interval from Death to Assay (h) mean ± S.D.
Middle-aged & elderly controls (sudden death)	8	76 ± 17 (50–100)	0.6	22 ± 5
Middle-aged & elderly controls (signs of 'O_2 deprivation')	6	57 ± 16 (34–83)	1.0	17 ± 8
Elderly controls (sudden death)	6	83 ± 11 (70–100)	1.0	22 ± 6
Organic 'senile-type' dementia*	6	85 ± 5 (79–91)	0.6	22 ± 6

* 2 cases of senile dementia and 4 cases of mixed senile and vascular dementia.

Age-related changes in whole temporal lobe. Portions of the homogenates from the temporal lobes were analyzed for the levels of 15 chemical constituents. These were: proteins (total protein, mitochondrial light fraction protein, neuronin S-5, and neuronin S-6), nucleic acids (RNA and DNA), enzymes (GAD, AChE, CNP, β-Gal, β-Glu, SDH, and carbonic anhydrase), and lipids (ganglioside NANA and total galacto-lipid). The amount of each of these constituents was expressed *per temporal lobe*. The values obtained for lobes from male patients were made comparable to female values by multiplying by a factor of 0.83 (the ratio of the mean temporal lobe weight of the 3 female normal controls to that of the other 5 males).

The effect of age (50–100y) was investigated by carrying out linear regression analysis on the sex-corrected values for each parameter and the temporal lobe weight. Apart from GAD activity (fig. 1a), no other parameter changed significantly with age. The correlations with age, however, approached significance ($p < 0.1$) for AChE, RNA/ DNA and CNP (fig. 1b,c,d, respectively). The weight of the temporal lobe also showed a slight negative correlation with age (lobe wt. in g = 107−0.076 x age, $p < 0.1$).

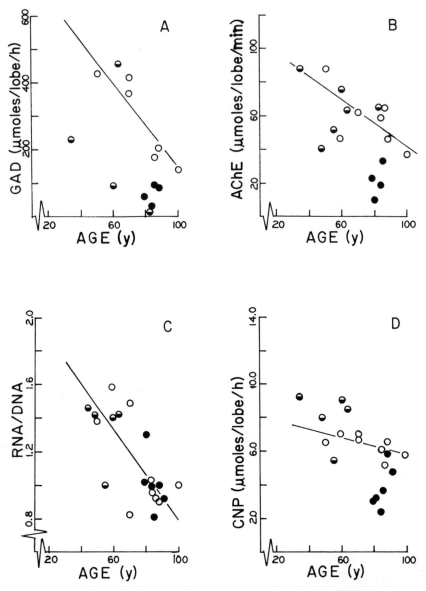

Fig. 1. Correlation of biochemical constituents in temporal lobe with age. Results from patients with 'senile-type' dementia (●) are shown in comparison with normal controls (○) and controls with signs of 'oxygen deprivation' (◑). The regression lines were calculated from the normal control values: GAD activity (μmoles/lobe/h) = 804−6.66 x age (y), p < 0.01; AChE activity (μmoles/lobe/min) = 109−0.67 x age (y), p < 0.1; RNA/DNA = 2.07−0.012 x age (y), p < 0.1; CNP activity (μmoles/lobe/h) = 8.19−0.024 x age (y), p < 0.1.

Changes due to the agonal state. Of the 7 cases of 'senile-type' dementia, 5 died of bronchopneumonia and 1 of renal failure. The normal control cases, however, all died suddenly. [The causes of death were cardiac arrests (2), bronchitis (2), aortic aneurysm (1), hemopericardium (1), post-operative hemmorage (1) and pulmonary edema (1).] In order to assess the effect of the agonal state on the 15 biochemical parameters, 6 control patients with a lingering mode of death were grouped together. [The causes of death were bronchopneumonia (2), chronic bronchitis (1), hemmorage (1), cancer (1) and carbon monoxide poisoning (1).] As shown in Table 1 this group plus the group of 8 normal controls were well-matched with respect to age, sex and pre-assay history. The biochemical results obtained from these two groups were compared by Student's t-test (Table 2). In the controls with signs of pre-mortem

TABLE 2

LEVELS OF BIOCHEMICAL CONSTITUENTS IN WHOLE TEMPORAL LOBES FROM NORMAL CONTROLS AND CONTROLS WITH SIGNS OF 'OXYGEN DEPRIVATION'

Parameter	Normal Controls	Controls with Signs of 'Oxygen Deprivation'
Carbonic anhydrase (units x 10^{-3}/h)	276 ± 86	337 ± 72
DNA (mg)	66.2 ± 16.2	82.0 ± 8.8
Galactolipid galactose (mg)	414 ± 81	N.D.
β-galactosidase (μmoles/h)	388 ± 57	416 ± 99
$\frac{\text{β-galactosidase}}{\text{β-glucuronidase}}$	19.7 ± 5.9	22.4 ± 8.2
Ganglioside NANA (μmoles)	257 ± 33	304 ± 52
β-glucuronidase (μmoles/h)	21.2 ± 5.6	20.4 ± 6.2
Mitochondrial light fraction protein (g)	2.06 ± 0.24	2.66 ± 0.64
Neuronin S-5 (mg)	7.9 ± 3.4	10.5 ± 3.2
Neuronin S-6 (mg)	14.7 ± 6.5	2.9 ± 4.9*†
RNA (mg)	72.6 ± 16.2	108.0 ± 27.0*
Succinate dehydrogenase (μmoles/h)	29.3 ± 2.4	26.7 ± 4.7
Total protein (g)	8.01 ± 1.27	8.77 ± 3.82

The values are the means ± standard deviations in 8 normal control specimens and 6 cases with signs of 'oxygen deprivation'. (Mitochondrial light fraction protein was determined in 5 normal control specimens. The value for Neuronin S-6 in the controls with signs of 'oxygen deprivation' is the mean of 5 specimens.)
† Mean value excluding that obtained from patient C.A., which was 32.2 mg. The mean ± S.D. for all 6 cases was 7.8 ± 12.7.
* $p < 0.01$.

'oxygen deprivation' the level of RNA was significantly higher than in the normal
controls. This difference is probably the result of post-mortem autolysis as 5 of
the 6 cases with signs of 'oxygen deprivation' were hospital deaths whereas only 2
of the 8 normal controls died in the hospital. The time from death to refrigeration
of the body is usually less than one hour in the hospital and more than several hours
otherwise. The level of neuronin S-6 was significantly lower in the cases with signs
of 'oxygen deprivation' if one value (32.2 mg/temporal lobe) obtained from the patient with CO poisoning was omitted. The other neuronin S-6 levels in this group
were < 7 (3 cases), 3.5 and 11.2 mg/temporal lobe.

The biochemical parameters which showed age-related changes were plotted (half-
shaded circles) in fig. 1. Apart from the GAD activities the levels of all of the
parameters appeared to be within the control range. The AChE activity may have been
lower than normal in 2 of the cases.

Comparison of the controls with the cases of 'senile-type' dementia. As shown
in Table 1, the cases of 'senile-type' dementia and the elderly controls were well-
matched with respect to age and pre-assay history. Table 3 summarizes the comparison
of the biochemical results for these two groups.

Indices of neurons, glia and atrophy. It is noteworthy that in the lobes from
patients with dementia almost all of the potential indices of nerve cells were significantly reduced whereas the tentative indices of glial cells were within the normal
range (i.e., statistically nonsignificant changes). As judged by the wet weight of
the temporal lobe, there was a significant degree of atrophy (about 22%). There was
a similar although nonsignificant loss of total protein. The mean reduction in the
6 biochemical indices of neurons which were reduced was 45% (range 37-60%).

Indices of cellularity. Neither of the potential indices of cellularity (DNA
and β-Gal/β-Glu) showed significant changes. This may seem surprising as the results
for the potential indices of neurons and glia indicated that in the demented patients
almost half of the nerve cells had been lost while the number of glial cells had not
significantly increased. However, no index of microglial cells was measured. Furthermore, the nucleic acid levels in the normal controls may be confounded by post-
mortem effects (see section on Changes due to agonal state).

Indices of cerebral 'hypoxia'. The large and significant decrease in neuronin
S-6 levels in the lobes from demented patients confirms other results[39] which show
that these patients have evidence of 'cerebral hypoxia'. The degree of change is
similar to that found in the comparison of the normal controls with the controls with
signs of 'oxygen deprivation'. Similarly the GAD activity was markedly reduced in
the demented patients. This index of the GABAergic system is also affected by pre-
death 'oxygen deprivation' (fig. 1a).

50

TABLE 3

BIOCHEMICAL INDICES OF STRUCTURAL AND FUNCTIONAL INTEGRITY OF NEURAL ELEMENTS IN 'SENILE-TYPE' DEMENTIA

Biochemical Indices[a]	Level in 'Senile-Type' Dementia (percent of Normal Elderly Controls)[b]
Cerebral hypoxia (neuronin S-6)	17***
Myelinated axons (mitochondrial light fraction protein)	55*
Nerve cell membrane (ganglioside NANA)	56***
Neuronal perikarya (β-galactosidase)	62**
Traumatized mitochondria (succinate dehydrogenase)	63***
Fresh weight of the temporal lobe	78*
Lobe weight (% of brain weight)	83**
Cellularity (β-Gal/β-Glu)	76
Neurons (neuronin S-5)	64
Total protein	76
Cellularity (DNA)	87
Ribosomes and cytoplasm (RNA)	88
Myelinated axons and microsomes (galactolipid)	81
Glia (β-glucuronidase)	73
Glia (carbonic anhydrase)	89
GABA system (GAD)†	34*
Parts distal to the parikarya (AChE)†	40***
Myelinated axons (CNP)†	63***
Relative number of neurons (RNA/DNA)†	100

The number of specimens examined were for most of the indices 6 cases of 'senile-type' dementia and 6 normal elderly controls. For neuronin S-6, 5 controls and 5 cases of dementia were compared. For the mitochondrial light fraction protein, 4 controls and 5 cases of dementia were compared. Five cases of dementia were examined for ganglioside NANA and galactolipid levels.

[a] Selected references: 11, 25-38.

[b] Calculated from data expressed as mass or enzyme activity per temporal lobe. The original data were corrected for the weight differences in temporal lobes between the sexes.

* $p < 0.05$; ** $p < 0.02$; *** $p < 0.01$.

† These biochemical constituents tend to be age-dependent (see fig. 1).

Animal studies

The biochemical results obtained from the human temporal lobes indicate that the patients with 'senile-type' dementia suffered severe terminal cerebral 'hypoxia'. This could be associated with the reduced cerebral blood flow characteristic of this disease[40] in concert with the terminal bronchopneumonia. It could also be associated with an underlying metabolic defect. [The significant reduction in SDH activity in the temporal lobes from demented paitents (Table 3) may also reflect such a defect.] The results of the human aging study at the NIMH[41] demonstrated a 23% reduction in the cerebral glucose consumption in the normal elderly and a further 22% reduction in patients with senile psychoses.

A study has been undertaken[42] at the NIMH on the local cerebral glucose utilization of normal aging rats. While the study is still in progress, the results obtained thus far are summarized in Table 4. The results suggest that there may be a regionally selective vulnerability of the rat brain to aging. The most vulnerable structures appear to be the caudate-putamen and perhaps the parietal cortex. Typical autoradiographs at the level of the parietal cortex from the 3 age groups are shown in fig. 2. Some narrowing of the cortical ribbon and loss of definition in cortical layer IV may be detected in the 2 older groups. A surprising finding is the significant *increase* in glucose consumption of the dentate gyrus in the aged rats. The globus pallidus shows a similar pattern, i.e. an increased glucose consumption in the aged animals when compared to the middle-aged animals.

DISCUSSION

Human studies

In an attempt to establish which neural elements are most affected in the organic 'senile-type' dementias, 15 biochemical constituents in the temporal lobe have been compared in control and demented cases. The analyses were carried out on homogenates of the *whole* temporal lobe and the results were expressed *per lobe*. It was anticipated that this procedure would reduce any errors due to either edema, water loss or differences in sampling. The temporal lobe was chosen for study since it is particularly affected in senile dementia[43], and changes in this region of control subjects may reflect the functional deficits that are associated with normal aging[44].

Post-mortem autolysis. Previous studies on both human and animal tissue have demonstrated the relative post-mortem stability of most of these 15 biochemical constituents for up to 3 h at 37° C[6]. Thus, provided that corpses are refrigerated after death and the interval between death and autopsy is not *greater* in the diseased compared with the control brains, data obtained for almost all the constituents should be meaningful. An estimate of the interval between death and refrigeration in the cases in this study was made based on whether death occurred

52

TABLE 4

EFFECTS OF AGING ON LOCAL CEREBRAL GLUCOSE UTILIZATION IN THE NORMAL CONSCIOUS SPRAGUE-DAWLEY RAT

Structure	Local Cerebral Glucose Utilization§ (μmoles/100g/min)		
	Young (3) (105–140d)	Middle-Aged (4) (480–540d)	Aged (3) (750–810d)
Gray Matter			
Visual Cortex	108 ± 4	87 ± 6	103 ± 8
Auditory Cortex	123 ± 6	118 ± 6	134 ± 12
Parietal Cortex	108 ± 6	84 ± 4†	105 ± 7
Sensory-Motor Cortex	114 ± 3	94 ± 4	114 ± 10
Olfactory Cortex	88 ± 7	100 ± 6	116 ± 17
Frontal Cortex	92 ± 9	85 ± 2	99 ± 11
Lateral Geniculate Body	90 ± 5	78 ± 4	93 ± 7
Medial Geniculate Body	117 ± 8	103 ± 4	113 ± 10
Thalamus: Lateral Nucleus	108 ± 10	84 ± 7	106 ± 7
Thalamus: Ventral Nucleus	92 ± 5	78 ± 2	98 ± 11
Hypothalamus	42 ± 4	49 ± 2	52 ± 1
Mamillary Body	108 ± 5	103 ± 4	118 ± 15
Hippocampus: Ammon's Horn	74 ± 6	61 ± 5	78 ± 5
Hippocampus: Dentate Gyrus	57 ± 3	59 ± 4	78 ± 3**
Amygdala	52 ± 1	46 ± 3	49 ± 3
Septal Nucleus	46 ± 2	41 ± 6	50 ± 1
Caudate-Putamen	108 ± 4	84 ± 4*	91 ± 6
Nucleus Accumbens	76 ± 8	62 ± 3	76 ± 3
Globus-Pallidus	52 ± 2	46 ± 2	56 ± 3††
Substantia Nigra	62 ± 7	52 ± 2	62 ± 4
Vestibular Nucleus	112 ± 13	103 ± 4	108 ± 3
Cochlear Nucleus	90 ± 11	119 ± 2	116 ± 11
Superior Olivary Nucleus	119 ± 9	116 ± 5	113 ± 10
Lateral Lemniscus	100 ± 9	99 ± 4	95 ± 3
Inferior Colliculus	158 ± 20	148 ± 4	158 ± 14
Superior Colliculus	102 ± 12	75 ± 4	79 ± 4
Pontine Gray Matter	61 ± 7	51 ± 1	55 ± 2
Cerebellar Cortex	59 ± 11	52 ± 2	57 ± 2
Cerebellar Nuclei	99 ± 12	89 ± 2	103 ± 8
White Matter			
Corpus Callosum	34 ± 4	29 ± .5	30 ± 3
Internal Capsule	32 ± 2	21 ± 3	25 ± 1

§ The values are the means ± standard errors obtained in the number of animals indicated in parentheses.

* Statistically significantly different from the young animals, $p < 0.05$.

** Statistically significantly different from both the young and the middle-aged animals, $p < 0.01$.

† Statistically significantly different from both the young and the aged animals, $p < 0.05$.

†† Statistically significantly different from the middle-aged animals, $p < 0.05$.

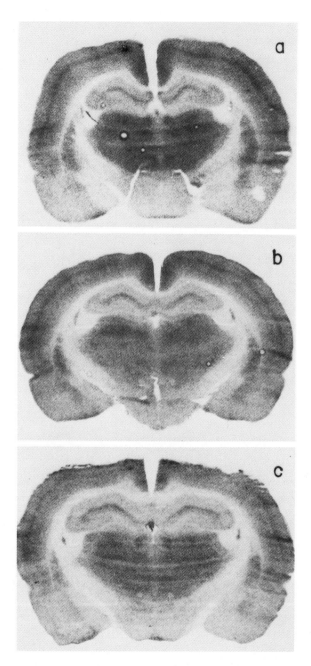

Fig. 2. Autoradiographs of coronal brain sections from rats injected with 2-deoxy-D-[14C]-glucose. The three sections are representative autoradiographs at the level of the parietal cortex from the three age groups studied: a, 105–140d; b, 480–540d; and c, 750–810d.

at home or in the hospital. All of the cases of 'senile-type' dementia died at Runwell Hospital where a special effort was made to refrigerate the body within 1 h. Five of the 6 cases with signs of 'oxygen deprivation' and only 2 of the 8 normal controls died in the hospital. Thus the mean interval from death to refrigeration was highest in the normal controls.

Agonal state. In contrast, it has been established[6] that the state of the patient during the period immediately preceeding death is the crucial factor that must be considered in studies on post-mortem tissue. In these studies the concentration of the soluble protein, neuronin S-6, was measured as an index of terminal cerebral 'hypoxia'[25]. The concentration of this protein in brain has been shown to correlate with the severity of disease in the systems that regulate the blood and oxygen supply to the brain and the selective vulnerability of the brain to hypoxemia[25] (see Table 2). Furthermore, in an experimental model of cerebral ischemia in baboons this protein was selectively and markedly depleted[45]. Terminal cerebral 'hypoxia' also appeared to affect the activity of GAD[25] (fig. la).

Aging. With the small number of normal controls examined and the possibly confounding affects of differences in agonal state and post-mortem handling, it is not surprising that statistically significant correlations with age were few. Only the activity of GAD showed a significant linear correlation with age (fig. la) while the activity of AChE only tended ($p < 0.1$) to decrease with age (fig. lb). Other age-dependent decreases have been demonstrated in the metabolism of catecholamines and the activities of neurotransmitter-related enzymes[46-48]. These biochemical changes are of interest for the work of Cragg[5] suggests that there may be a reduction in synaptic density with increasing age. Degenerating neurites, some of which have been identified as pre-synaptic terminals, are features of the senile plaques found in aging human brain[49]. Thus, the available evidence indicates that there is at least a decrease in synaptic function in senescence.

The tendency for the ratio of RNA to DNA (fig. lc) to decrease with age in the temporal lobes is in agreement with the findings of Chaconas and Finch[50] on the striata of senescent mice. This phenomenon may reflect a decrease in the relative number of neurons. Alternatively, there may be a decrease in the RNA content of neurons for it has been reported[51,52] that the RNA content of isolated neurons falls with increasing age.

The decrease in CNP activity with increasing age (fig. ld) may reflect a loss of myelin. This is in agreement with the work of Ansari and Loch[53] for they found that the yield of myelin basic protein was reduced in the frontal lobes of aged patients. Although neither of the other potential indices of myelin (galactolipid galactose and mitochondrial light fraction protein) changed significantly with increasing age, this may have been due to the greater variability in the data and the difficulties associated with subcellular fractionation of post-mortem tissue.

A loss of myelin would not be unexpected, for both primary and secondary (Wallerian) myelin degeneration have been noted in aging brain[49].

As judged by the morphological data[54,55] and the biochemical results described above, the question of whether widespread cortical neuronal loss occurs in non-demented aged humans remains unanswered. It is possible that the deterioration of mental performances associated with aging may be a function of the "quality of neuropil...rather than solely of the total number of neurones...or senile plaques"[56].

'Senile-type' dementia. All of the cases of senile organic dementia (2 of senile dementia and 4 of mixed vascular and senile dementia) were compared with the normal elderly controls (Table 3, fig. 1). The reductions in the concentration of neuronin S-6 and the activity of GAD in the dementias were probably due to the terminal 'hypoxic' state of these patients. Of the biochemical indices not affected by hypoxia, reduced ganglioside NANA concentration and lower AChE, CNP and β-Gal activities suggest that about one-half of the nerve cells have been lost from the temporal lobe. This is in remarkably close agreement with the results of cell counts on the neocortex of 3 cases of Alzheimer's disease[57] in which a 57% loss of neurons was found.

From an analysis of all of the data in this study[6,39] it can be concluded that CNP, AChE and β-Gal activities and the concentration of ganglioside NANA can provide relatively reliable estimates of quantitative cellular changes. β-Gal and AChE activities were measured, respectively, as potential indices of perikarya and the portion of the nerve cell most distal from the cell body, while the other two markers probably reflect axonal and possibly also dendritic (i.e. ganglioside NANA) densities. Therefore, the mean value of the changes in these 4 variables should give a reliable estimate of neuronal loss. Furthermore, since the wet weight of the lobe might be confounded by differences in water content the total protein content per lobe is probably the most reliable index of gross atrophy. It was tentatively concluded that it is probably valid to use the data for the RNA and DNA content but only for the semi-quantitative comparison of one dement lobe with another. Although it is unclear whether or not the potential markers of glia (carbonic anhydrase and β-Glu activities) are reliable [6] there was no other way available for assessing the number of glial cells. An attempt has been made to assess the degree of cellular changes in the individual cases using these 9 biochemical indices (Table 5). The amount of each of these variables per lobe was expressed as the percent reduction from age-matched normal control values.

Of the six lobes from the cases of organic 'senile-type' dementia all show biochemical evidence of neuronal loss ranging from about 25 to almost 60% (Table 5). In one case (Ca) the ganglioside NANA content and β-Glu activity was atypical, and it is unclear whether or not this specimen should be grouped with the other brains. In all the other lobes the ganglioside NANA content was reduced by a mean of 44% (range 31-58%). Based on the content of ganglioside NANA and the activities

TABLE 5

CELLULAR CHANGES IN TEMPORAL LOBES FROM INDIVIDUAL CASES OF 'SENILE-TYPE' DEMENTIA

| | Percent Reduction* | | | | | |
| | Senile Dementia | | Mixed Vascular and Senile Dementia | | | |
	Cl	Ar	Th	Pa	Ca	Wb
Potential indices of neurons						
Perikarya (β-Gal)	46	78	51	35	14	+7
Myelinated axons (CNP)	52	47	61	35	2	17
Nerve cell membrane (ganglioside NANA)	31	51	42	38	+107	58
Parts distal to perikarya (AChE)	60	82	64	ND	34	ND
All indices of neurons (mean)	47	58[a]	55	36	27[b]	25
Potential indices of						
Glia (β-Glu and carbonic anhydrase)	28	27	43	17	30[c]	+47[c]
Cellularity (DNA)	50	40	6	3	+25	+9
Ribosomes and cytoplasm (RNA)	38	36	10	30	+13	3
Temporal lobe atrophy (total protein)	40	49	40	50	+8	1
Morphological data						
'Senile' changes (scale 0-3)	1.0	2.0	2.5	1.5	1.5	1.5
Neuronal loss (scale 0-3)	2.0	2.0	3.0	1.0	1.0	2.0
Myelin loss (scale 0-3)	1.0	2.0	2.0	1.0	2.0	2.0

*Compared with normal elderly controls.
[a]Excluding value for β-Gal.
[b]Excluding value for ganglioside NANA.
[c]β-Glu activity may be abnormal.

of CNP, β-Gal and AChE, the most severly affected temporal lobe among the cases of vascular dementia had 55% fewer neurons than was appropriate for the age of the patient (Th, Table 5). The morphological changes and clinical history confirm that this patient was the most severely affected case of mixed senile and vascular demen-tia. In comparison with this case the senile dement lobes had both relatively fewer senile plaques and, by histological criteria, less neuronal loss. The biochemical results, however, suggest that the lobe from one of the non-vascular cases (patient Ar) had lost as many neurons. Similarly, the lobe from the other case of senile dementia (patient Cl) had relatively less marked morphological changes than the next most severely affected vascular case (patient Pa). Despite this, the biochemical results indicate that the lobe from the non-vascular dement had lost more neurons than the lobe from the vascular case. By comparison to results for mixed senile and vascular dementia the biochemical changes in senile dementia appear more extensive than predictable from the histopathology. In non-vascular senile dementia alterations in the metabolism of neurons may well precede slowly progressive changes in morphology, whereas in 'multi-infarction' the biochemistry may be explained solely on the basis of the resultant atrophy of ischemic neurons and tracts. This could indicate a basic difference in the pathogenesis of the two conditions.

Animal studies

The results of the NIMH study on human aging[41] also suggest that in patients with senile psychoses as well as normal elderly controls there is a significant decrease in cerebral glucose consumption. Recently a method has been developed[24] for the quantitative determination of the rates of glucose utilization simultaneously in all the component structural and functional units of the brain. Local cerebral glucose utilization has been found to be closely correlated with local functional activity and to serve to identify regions in the brain with altered functional activity[58]. This method is currently being applied to a study of the effects of normal aging in albino rats[42]. The preliminary results (Table 4) indicate that there are no regions with dramatic decreases in the aged animals although the caudate-putamen may show some decline in both of the older groups of animals. It will soon be possible to carry out similar studies in man[59] and thus provide a greater insight into the nature of the aging process in the human brain.

ACKNOWLEDGEMENTS

The studies on human brain were carried out in the Miriam Marks Department of Neurochemistry, The Institute of Neurology, University of London, London, England. I gratefully acknowledge all those who participated in those studies: D.M. Bowen, P. White, R.H.A. Flack, A.N. Davison, L.H. Carrasco and J.A.N. Corsellis. I also thank Suzanne Cook for preparing the typescript and J.D. Brown for the photography.

REFERENCES

1. Brody, H. (1955) J. Comp. Neurol., 102, 511-556.
2. Corsellis, J.A.N. (1962) Mental Illness and the Ageing Brain, Oxford University Press, New York.
3. Scheibel, M.E., Lindsay, R.D., Tomiyasu, U. and Scheibel, A. (1975) Exp. Neurol., 47, 392-403.
4. Mehraein, P., Yamada, M. and Tarnowska-Dzidnszko, E. (1975) Adv. Neurol., 12, 453-458.
5. Cragg, B.G. (1975) Brain, 98, 81-90.
6. Bowen, D.M., Smith, C.B., White, P., Goodhardt, M.J., Spillane, J.A., Flack, R.H.A. and Davison, A.N. (1977) Brain, 100, 397-426.
7. Lowry, O.H., Rosebrough, N.J., Farr, A.L. and Randall, R.J. (1951) J. biol. Chem., 193, 269-275.

8. Bowen, D.M., Smith, C.B. and Davison, A.N. (1973) Brain, 96, 849-856.

9. Svennerholm, L. (1956) J. Neurochem., 1, 42-53.

10. Radin, N.S., Brown, J.R. and Lavin, F.B. (1956) J. biol. Chem., 219, 977-984.

11. Smith, C.B. and Bowen, D.M. (1976) J. Neurochem., 27, 1521-1528.

12. Schmidt, G. and Thannhauser, S.J. (1945) J. biol. Chem., 161, 83-89.

13. Hurlbert, R.B., Schmitz, H., Brumm, A.F. and Potter, V.R. (1954) J. biol. Chem., 209, 23-29.

14. Burton, K. (1956) Biochem. J., 62, 315-323.

15. Croft, D.N. and Lubran, M. (1965) Biochem. J., 95, 612-620.

16. Giles, K.W. and Myers, A. (1965) Nature, 206, 93.

17. Bayoumi, R.A., Kirwan, J.R. and Smith, W.R.D. (1972) J. Neurochem., 19, 569-576.

18. Ellman, G.I., Courtney, K.D., Andrew, F. and Featherstone, R.M. (1961) Biochem. Pharmacol., 7, 88-95.

19. Drummond, G.I., Iyer, N.T. and Keith, J. (1962) J. biol. Chem., 237, 3535-3539.

20. Hotta, S.S., Laatsch, R.H. and Myron, P.V. (1963) J. Neurochem., 10, 841-847.

21. Cuzner, M.L. and Davison, A.N. (1973) J. neurol. Sci., 19, 29-36.

22. Hajra, A.K., Bowen, D.M., Kishimoto, Y. and Radin, N.S. (1966) J. Lipid Res., 7, 379-386.

23. Rickli, E.E., Ghazanfar, S.A.A., Gibbons, B.H. and Edsall, J.T. (1964) J. biol. Chem., 239, 1065-1078.

24. Sokoloff, L., Reivich, M., Kennedy, C., Des Rosiers, M.H., Patlak, C.S., Pettigrew, K.D., Sakurada, O. and Shinohara, M. (1977) J. Neurochem., 28, 897-916.

25. Bowen, D.M., Smith, C.B., White, P. and Davison, A.N. (1976) Brain, 99, 459-496.

26. Morell, P., Greenfield, S., Costantine-Ceccarini, E. and Wisniewski, H.M. (1972) J. Neurochem., 19, 2545-2554.

27. Lowden, J.A. and Wolfe, L.S. (1964) Can. J. Biochem., 42, 1587-1703.

28. Sinha, A.K. and Rose, S.P.R. (1972) Brain Res., 39, 181-196.

29. Hajos, F. and Kerpel-Fronius, S. (1969) Exp. Brain Res., 8, 66-78.

30. Bowen, D.M., Flack, R.H.A., Martin, R.O., Smith, C.B., White, P. and Davison, A.N. (1974) J. Neurochem., 22, 1099-1107.

31. Mahler, H.R., Moore, W.J., and Thompson, R.J. (1966) J. biol. Chem., 241, 1283-1289.

32. Zamenhof, S., Bursztyn, H., Rich, K. and Zamenhof, P.J. (1964) J. Neurochem., 11, 505-509.

33. Norton, W.T. and Poduslo, S.E. (1973) J. Neurochem., 21, 759-773.

34. Giacobini, E. (1961) Science, N.Y., 134, 1524-1525.

35. McLaughlin, B.J., Wood, J.G., Saito, K., Barber, R., Vaughn, J.E., Roberts, E. and Wu, J-Y. (1974) Brain Res., 76, 377-391.

36. De Robertis, E., Iraldi, A., Arnaiz, G. and Salganicoff, L. (1962) J. Neurochem., 9, 23-35.

37. Kurihara, T. and Tsukada, Y. (1967) J. Neurochem, 14, 1167-1174.

38. Hess, H.H. and Thalheimer, C. (1971) J. Neurochem., 18, 1281-1290.

39. Bowen, D.M., Smith, C.B., White, P., Flack, R.H.A., Carrasco, L.H., Gedye, J.L. and Davison, A.N. (1977) Brain, 100, 427-453.

40. Ingvar, D.H. and Gustafson, L. (1970) Acta neurol. scand., 46, Suppl. 43, 42-73.

41. Birren, J.E., Butler, R. N., Greenhouse, S.W., Sokoloff, L. and Yarrow, M.R., editors (1963) Human Aging: A Biological and Behavioral Study, U.S. Government Printing Office, Washington, D.C.

42. Smith, C.B., Rapoport, S.I., Fredericks, W.R. and Sokoloff, L. unpublished.

43. Tomlinson, B.E., Blessed, G. and Roth, M. (1970) J. neurol. Sci., 11, 205-242.

44. Heron, A. and Chowne, S. (1967) Age and Function, Churchill, London.

45. Bowen, D.M., Goodhardt, M.J., Strong, A.J., Smith, C.B., White, P., Branston, N.M., Symon, L. and Davison, A.N. (1976) Brain Res., 117, 503-507.

46. McGeer, E.G. and McGeer, P.L. (1976) in Neurobiology of Aging, Aging, Vol. 3, Gershon, S. and Terry, R.D. eds., Raven Press, New York, pp. 389-403.

47. Finch, C.A. (1973) Brain Res., 52, 261-276.

48. Walker, J.B. and Walker, J.P. (1973) Brain Res., 54, 391-396.

49. Wisniewski, H.M. and Terry, R.D. (1973) Prog. Brain Res., 40, 167-186.

50. Chaconas, G. and Finch, C.E. (1973) J. Neurochem., 21, 1469-1473.

51. Hyden, H. (1962) in Neurochemistry, Elliot, K.A.C., Page, I.H. and Quastel, J.H., eds., Charles C. Thomas, Springfield, Ill., pp. 331-375.

52. Ringborg, U. (1966) Brain Res., 2, 296-298.

53. Ansari, K.A. and Loch, J. (1975) Neurology, 25, 1045-1050.

54. Bowen, D.M. and Davison, A.N. (1976) in Biochemistry and Neurological Disease, Davison, A.N., ed., Blackwell Scientific Publications, Oxford, pp. 2-50.

55. Brody, H. (1976) in The Neurobiology of Aging, Terry, R.D. and Gershon, S., eds., Raven Press, New York, pp. 177-182.

56. Scheibel, M.E. and Scheibel, A.B. (1975) Structural Changes in the Aging Brain in Clinical, Morphologic and Neurochemical Aspects in the Aging Central Nervous System, Brody, H., Harman, D. and Ory, J.M. eds., Raven Press, New York, pp. 11-38.

57. Colon, E.J. (1973) Acta neuropath. (Berl.), 23, 281-290.

58. Sokoloff, L. (1977) J. Neurochem., 29, 13-26.

59. Reivich, M., Kuhl, D., Wolf, A., Greenberg, J., Phelps, M., Ido, T., Casella, V., Fowler, J., Gallagher, B., Hoffman, E., Alavi, A. and Sokoloff, L. (1977) in Cerebral Function, Metabolism, and Circulation, Ingvar, D. and Lassen, N., eds., Munksgaard, Copenhagen, pp. 190-191.

CYTOTOXIC AUTOANTIBODY TO THE BRAIN

JONATHAN CHAFFEE, MERVAT NASSEF AND STEPHEN BOBIN

New York State Institute for Basic Research in Mental Retardation, 1050 Forest Hill

Road, Staten Island, N.Y. 10314

ABSTRACT

A technique is presented for measuring the levels of cytotoxic anti-brain auto-

antibodies in human sera. Unexpectedly high levels of this antibody activity can

be detected in the sera of some apparently normal individuals, while others have

little or no measurable activity. Preliminary results show that more persons of

age 20-25 have levels of anti-brain antibody above overall average than do persons

either older or younger. The technique is sensitive enough to test the specificity

of these antibodies; in all the sera tested so far, the activity is absorbed by

both brain and thymus, and by some other tissues in varying degrees. These studies

of the incidence of autoantibodies in normal people will provide a baseline for

the investigation of anti-brain autoantibodies in conjunction with neurological

disease.

INTRODUCTION

Circulating antibodies directed against antigenic components of the brain might

attack the brain, affecting its function transiently, or permanently, by altering

brain structure. This hypothesis has received circumstantial support in recent

years. In the first place, antibodies capable of binding to brain antigens have

been detected in human sera[1] and in the sera of aging mice[2,3,4]. Serum antibodies

can make their way from circulation into the brain, although they are somewhat

retarded by the blood brain barrier under normal circumstances[5]. When this

barrier is compromised, they move very rapidly[6]. Antibodies put into tissue

culture model systems affect the function of brain cells, interfering with

synaptic transmission[7] or may cause destruction of structural elements, such as

myelin[8]. Anti-brain antibodies introduced experimentally into the brain may

61

selectively affect the behavior of animals[9,10]. In humans, reports have appeared
of increased levels of circulating anti-brain antibody appearing in conjunction
with sustained functional aberration, such as chronic schizophrenia[11,12], in Huntington's disease[13], or in conjunction with dementia in systemic lupus erythematosis[14,15].
In ataxia telangiectasia, a heritable degenerative brain disease, antibodies to brain
have been measured[16]. The involvement of the immune system in multiple sclerosis is
obvious; immune cells invade the brain,[17] and elevated levels of immunoglobulin can
be measured in the cerebral spinal fluid.[18] The target antigenic specificity of this
immunoglobulin has been difficult to establish;[19] however, serum antibodies specific
for myelin have been reported[20] and circulating humoral factors cytotoxic for lympho-
cytes themselves[21]. Taken together, this evidence emphasizes the pertinence of investigating the involvement of circulating anti-brain antibodies in neurologic
disease.

This paper presents an assay system designed to screen for anti-brain antibodies
in human serum. It is rapid and reproducibly quantitative. The assay measures cytotoxic antibodies directed against brain cell surface antigens, reasoning that in the
brain, components displayed on the surfaces of cells will be most open to attack. The
assay utilizes methods previously developed for characterizing the cell surface antigens of brain cells[22,23]. Using suspensions of cells derived from normal brain or
from brain tumors, a sensitive two stage cytotoxic test allowed measurement of the
potency of experimental antisera generated against brain components. Pre-absorption
of cytotoxic activity with portions of brain and different tissues delineated the
distribution of the antigenic targets of these antibodies[24]. A series of antigens
were identified on the surface of mouse brain cells[25,26,27,28,29,30,31]. Many of
these were shared with the brains of other species, including human brain[30,31].
Surprisingly, many of the antigens of brain cell surface were also shared with cells
of other tissues, such as kidney or sperm[30,31]. Hyperimmune antisera to these antigens have been used to partially purify cell types from suspensions of brain cells[32],
to localize the antigens in tissue sections[33], and to tag the antigens for biochemical characterization[34].

This assay system was sensitive enough to detect naturally occurring mouse antibodies to one major cell surface antigen, the NS-6 antigen [4]. This suggested that the technique could be modified to study anti-brain antibody occurring in human sera and might allow the primary auto antigenic targets to be identified. It also emphasized the "normal" occurrence of anti-brain autoantibody. Preparatory to the study of sera from patients with neurologic disease, an investigation was begun of the incidence and levels of anti-brain autoantibodies in apparently normal people in relationship to age. This report presents the technique, and some preliminary data on sera from normal people.

MATERIALS AND METHODS

Normal Serum. Tests on human sera utilized remainders of samples drawn for clinical testing with non-heparinized vacutainers (Becton Dickinson, East Rutherford, N.J.). Serum was withdrawn from clotted samples, clarified by centrifugation, and samples were stored frozen at -70° C. Samples were made available through the Community Blood Center of Greater New York. Others were obtained through the cooperation of the Veteran's Administration Extended Care Unit at St. Albans, Queens, N.Y., from patients with non-neurologic diagnoses not using drugs known to influence the immune system. Anonymity of donors is maintained. Prior to testing, sera were heat inactivated at 56° C for 20 min to destroy complement activity.

Target Cells. Target cells for cytotoxicity tests are prepared from MUNTAD (Mouse Undifferentiated Neural Tumor, ADeno virus induced) maintained in subcutaneous passage in C3H/fBi mice. Cells of this new tumor resemble subventricular cells of normal mouse brain[35]. Cells are suspended from tumor in Earles Balanced Salt Solution (EBSS) (GIBCO, Grand Island, N.Y.) by repeated passage through the flame-narrowed tip of a disposable Pasteur pipette. The suspended cells are washed free of clumps and subcellular debris by centrifugation 10 min at 70 g. The cell pellet is resuspended in saline containing 2 mci/ml ^{51}Cr (New England Nuclear, Boston, Mass.) at a volume/volume ratio of 2.5:1, cells to sodium chromate, and incubated for 45 min at 37° C. The cells are washed once by centrifugation at 70 g, then dead cells are lysed by further incubation for 7 min at 37° C with 0.25% Trypsin (Worthington TRL , Worthington Biochemical Corp., Freehold, N.J.) and 0.025% DNase (Worthington DP) in EBSS. Debris and unabsorbed ^{51}Cr are removed by 2 further EBSS washes at 70 g, and the cells are resuspended at a concentration of 4×10^6/ml in medium 199 + 2% fetal calf serum (199 + 2) (GIBCO, Grand Island). Viability of the cells is greater than 90% by trypan blue dye exclusion.

51 Cr Release Cytotoxicity Test. Sera to be tested are titrated in duplicate by doubling dilution in 10ul aliquots to a final dilution of 1/32, utilizing wells of microtiter test plates. 10 ul of target cells are added to each aliquot of serum dilution, mixed well, and incubated 30 min at room temperature. 0.2 ml 199 + 2 is added and the plates centrifuged in carriers (Cooke Engineering Co., Alexandria, VA.). The supernatant with unbound serum components and released ^{51}Cr is aspirated, and the cells are resuspended in a complement source; 25 ul non-immune rabbit serum pre-absorbed with target cells, diluted 1/5 in 199 + 2. After 30 min at 37° C, 125 ul of 0.25% trypsin and 0.025% DNase in EBSS is added to each well and incubation is continued an additional 15 min to facilitate release of ^{51}Cr from lysed cells. The plates are centrifuged at 70 g, sedimenting the remaining unlysed cells, and 95 ul of the supernatant is transferred from each well to a 11 x 75 mm test tube. The released ^{51}Cr is counted (Bio Gamma 11, Beckman Instruments, Wakefield, Mass.) for 1 min. Each serum is also tested at a 1/4 dilution in the absence of exogenous complement for complement independent cytotoxicity. In addition, each plate of sera includes wells controlling for the release of ^{51}Cr by complement without serum and for background release by test cells in medium alone. With every 12 sera, a positive control serum is included to give the level of maximal antibody mediated ^{51}Cr release. For each dilution of serum the cytotoxic index is calculated as follows:

$$C.I. = 100 \times \frac{^{51}Cr \text{ released by serum dilution} - ^{51}Cr \text{ released by complement alone}}{\text{maximal } ^{51}Cr \text{ release} - ^{51}Cr \text{ release by complement alone}}$$

Two independent determinations at each dilution are averaged. The titer of the serum is calculated as the dilution giving a cytotoxic index of 50. These calculations are performed semi-automatically on a Hewlett-Packard model 9830A calculator and the data for each serum indexed and stored.

Tissue Absorptions. Specific absorptions of cytotoxic antibody activity by tissues is performed as previously described[28]. Briefly, C57BL/6J mouse tissues are homogenized gently; the cells and large fragments are washed repeatedly to remove soluble material and are packed at 700 g to measure their volume in microliters. Resuspension allows accurate aliquoting of tissue fragments. These are again packed in microfuge tubes (Beckman Instrument Co.) the supernatant removed, and are resuspended in an equal volume of antiserum at a critically chosen dilution close to the serum titer value. Following incubation with tissue for 30 min at 4° C, the serum is recovered nearly quantitatively by centrifugation and is diluted for testing residual cytotoxic activity. Very little diminution of activity by non-specific absorption or dilution occurs and serum incubated with antigen negative tissues retains titers comparable to serum aliquots incubated without tissue.

RESULTS

When tested in this assay system, sera from some apparently normal humans show titers as high as 1/200. The assay is specific for complement dependent antibodies against cell surface antigens and measures them quantitatively. A titration curve of one human serum, shown in Figure 1, demonstrates the limits of accuracy of this measure. The curve is the mean of 15 separate determinations, the lines show the range of values at each dilution and represent the sum of variability in different target cell preparations and in the many pipetting steps in the assay, and is less than the variability calculated from the accuracy of the instruments used for the measuring steps. The titer of an individual serum is accurate only within ± one dilution, but high titer sera can be reliably distinguished from low titer sera.

65

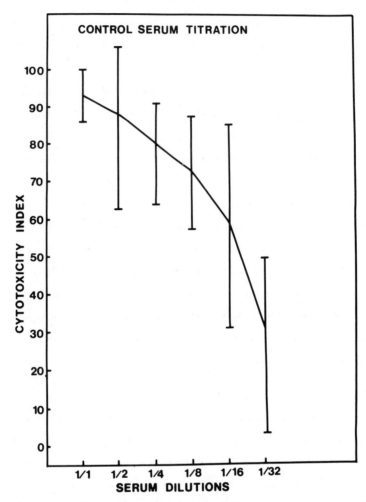

Fig. 1. This is the mean of 15 separate titrations of the same normal human serum. The error bars represent the range of values at each dilution. This variability is actually better than the variability calculated from the accuracy of the instruments used in the pipetting steps.

When normal human sera from individuals of different ages are tested, some individuals of each age group have high titers, while others of the same age have low titers, or no measurable activity. However, the incidence of higher than average titer is age related. Figure 2 presents some preliminary results from the

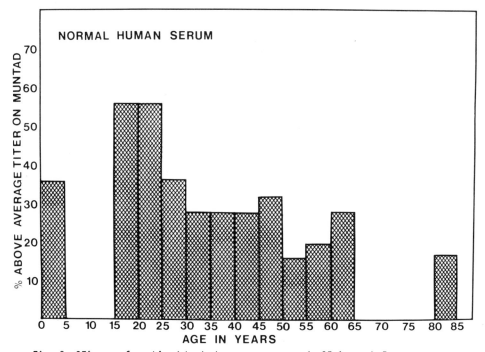

Fig. 2 271 sera from blood bank donors were tested, 25 in each 5 year span
except 0-5(18), 15-20(16) and 80-85(12). Insufficient numbers of sera were
tested in the 5-15 and 65-80 year spans to report. The average titer of the
whole group was 1/12. The data are presented as the proportion of individuals with titers above average. Despite the large variability between individuals in the same age span, the obvious differences between 20-25 year
olds and 50-55 year olds yield a P < .005.

testing of many normal sera. The percentage of individuals with titers

above the average for the whole group is highest in sera from people aged

20 to 25, lowest in people aged 50-55. These two age groups are different

with a P value of < .005 despite the variability of titers in each age

group. Because there are some age groups in which insufficient numbers of

individuals have been tested, data has not been presented for these ages,

and the data has not been subjected to complete statistical analysis.

What antigens are these antibodies directed against? Absorption of some

of the high titer sera from different aged individuals showed complete ab-

sorption of activity by brain and thymus. Figure 3 shows one selected

absorption of a single serum.

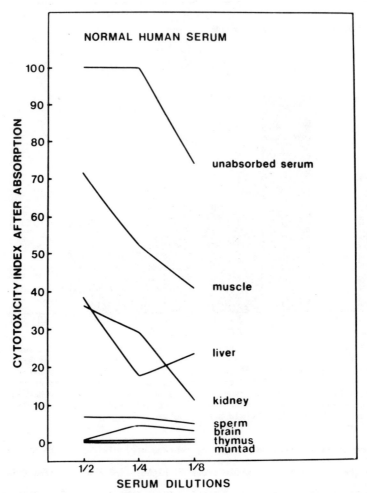

Fig. 3. The residual cytotoxicity for MUNTAD target cells remaining in aliquots of a single human serum after absorption with different C57BL/6J mouse tissue homogenates. Sperm, brain and thymus absorb maximally, along with MUNTAD itself. Liver, kidney and muscle absorb some, but not all activity, possibly due to the presence of heterophile anti-mouse antibodies in the human serum.

Partial absorption by liver, and muscle shows a component of cytotoxic activity directed at non-specific antigens shared by most tissues. Kidney, in the different absorptions, segregated sometimes with positively absorbing brain, and sometimes with presumably non-specifically absorbing liver and muscle. Sperm absorbed whenever

tried. These absorptions have been carried out on a small number of sera, so
that the overall pattern is not yet disclosed.

DISCUSSION

The intent of these studies is to form a picture of the incidence of levels of
anti-brain autoantibody in normal people, against which to measure the incidence
in dementia and other disorders of brain function. The first unexpected result is
that, in contrast to reports of elevated levels of autoantibody in aged people[36],
the highest incidence of cytotoxic anti-brain autoantibody as measured in this
assay was found in younger people. One possible explanation is that the levels
of autoantibody reflect the levels of immunoglobulin in general, which in the
normal human population peak in the same age range, around age 20[37]. The distribution of incidence of cytotoxic titers shown in this preliminary data bears some
resemblance to the age relationship of the levels of IgM immunoglobulin in normal
humans[37]. IgM is known to be many times more effective than IgG in cytotoxicity.
Therefore, this assay may be measuring a component of the normal immune capability
which is proportionate to total IgM synthesis. These data are incomplete in the
range from 65-80 years, and thus are not necessarily in conflict with previous
reports of rising levels of autoantibody in this age range. In fact, during this
older age span both IgM and IgG levels rise from a low between ages 50 and 60[37].
The anti-brain autoantibodies may also be found to follow this pattern.

Preliminary data on the specificity of the autoantibodies is in agreement with
reports of antibody absorbed by brain and thymus in conjunction with neurologic
disorders[13,14,15,21]. Antibodies directed at thymocytes have the potential of
altering the function of the immune system, and theoretically might either amplify or
decrease autoantibody production. In mice, the alloantigen Thy 1 is shared
between brain and thymus cell surfaces[38], and a similar antigen is described in
humans[39]. Further serological testing would be required to demonstrate that a
single antigen of this type, shared by thymus and brain is the target in this case,
and not different antigens absorbing on the two tissues.

69

In mice the most common pattern of absorption of anti-brain autoantibodies seems to be different. Absorption by brain and kidney has been reported [2], or by brain, kidney, and sperm [4], but specifically not thymus. However, in NZB mice, thymocytotoxic antibodies appear which are also absorbed by brain[40,41]. Spermatozoa, which here is seen to absorb, has not usually been tested in conjunction with other tissues. The tissue specificity of autoantibodies may be even less sharply defined; often activity is somewhat absorbed by many tissues[42,43]. The occasional absorption by kidney seen in this study but not present in Figure 2 may be of this sort.

Another contribution to the total measured cytotoxic activity could be heterophile antibody, antibody present in human sera which reacts with all mouse tissues. This could account for absorption by liver and muscle, tissues which share few antigens with brain cell surfaces. Heterophile antibodies are unavoidable in tests using target cells from another species[44], but the difficulty of obtaining any standardized source of human brain derived cells comparable to the MUNTAD cells is even greater.

We have no idea what the consequences of high levels of anti-brain autoantibodies may be in normal individuals. Individuals with high titers occur in every age group. The implication of the data is that some individuals with high titers as young people will grow older and have lower titers; however, we have no actual longitudinal data on high titer individuals. We do not know what diseases they may have had or may be more likely to get. Finally, we have no information that high levels of this antibody correlate with any functional deficit in these normal people.

REFERENCES

1. Allerand, C.D. and Yahr, M.D. (1964) Science, 144, 1141-1142.

2. Martin, S.E. and Martin, W.J. (1975) Proc.Nat. Acad. Sci. USA, 72, 1036-1040.

3. Nandy, K. (1973) in Neurobiological Aspects of Maturation and Aging, Ford, D. H. ed., Elsevier, Amsterdam, pp. 437-454.

4. Chaffee, J. K. and Schachner, M. unpublished observations.

5. Cutler, R.W.P., Deuel, R.K. and Barlow, C.F. (1967) Arch. Neurol. (Chic.), 17, 261-270.

6. Hicks, J. T., Albrecht, P. and Rapoport, S.I. (1976) Exp. Neurol., 53, 768-779.

7. Bornstein, M.B. and Crain, S.M. (1971) J. Neuropathol. Exp. Neurol., 30, 129.

8. Bornstein, M.B. (1973) in Progress in Neuropathology, Zimmerman, H.M., ed., Grune and Stratton, New York, vol. 2, pp. 69-90.

9. Karpiak, S.E., Serokosz, M. and Rapport, M.M. (1976) Brain Res., 102, 313-321.

10. Mihailovic, L., Divac, I., Mitrovic, E., Milosevic D. and Jankovic, B.D. (1969) Exp. Neurol., 24, 325-336.

11. Heath, R.G. (1970) in Biochemistry, Schizophrenia and Affective Illnesses, Himwich, H.W., ed., Williams and Wilkins, Baltimore, pp. 171-197.

12. Baron, M., Stern, M., Anavi, R., and Witz, I.P. (1977) Biol. Psych. 12, 199-219.

13. Husby, G., Li, L., Davis, L.E., Wedege, E., Kokmen, E. and Williams, R.C. Jr. (1977) J. Clin. Invest.,59, 922-932.

14. Bluestein, H.G. and Zvaifler, N.J. (1976) J. Clin. Invest., 57, 509-516.

15. Bresnihan, B., Oliver, M., Grigor, R. and Hughes, G.R.V. (1977) Clin. Exp. Immunol., 30, 333-337.

16. Kaufman, D.B. and Miller, H.C. (1977) Clin. Immunol. Immunopath., 7, 288-299.

17. Adams, R.D. and Kubic, C.S. (1952) Amer. J. Med., 12, 510-546.

18. Tourtellotte, W. (1970) J. Neurol. Sci., 10, 279-304.

19. Caspary, E.A. (1977) Br. Med. Bull., 33, 50-53.

20. Lisak, R.P., Zweiman, B. and Norman, M. (1975) Arch. Neurol. (Chic.), 32, 163-167.

21. Van den Noort, S. and Stjerholm, R.L. (1971) Neurology, 21, 783-793.

22. Schachner, M. (1973) Brain Res., 56, 382-386.

23. Schachner, M. and Hammerling, U. (1974) Brain Res., 73, 362-371.

24. Schachner, M. and Sidman, R.L. (1973) Brain Res., 60, 191-198.

25. Schachner, M. (1974) Proc. Nat. Acad. Sci. USA, 71, 1795-1799.

26. Schachner, M. and Carnow, T.B. (1975) Brain Res., 88, 394-402.

27. Schachner, M. and Wortham, K.A. (1975) Brain Res., 99, 201-208.

28. Schachner, M., Wortham, K.A., Carter, L.D. and Chaffee, J.K. (1975) Develop. Biol., 44, 313-325.

29. Zimmermann, A. and Schachner, M. (1976) Brain Res., 115, 297-310.

30. Chaffee, J.K. and Schachner, M. (1978) Develop. Biol., 62, 173-184

31. Chaffee, J.K. and Schachner, M. (1978) Develop. Biol., 62, 185-192.

32. Campbell, G. LeM., Schachner, M. and Sharrow, S.O. (1977) Brain Res., 127, 69-86.

33. Schachner, M., Ruberg, M.Z. and Carnow, T.B. (1976) Brain Res. Bull., 1, 367-378.

34. Yuan, D., Vitetta, E.S. and Schachner, M. (1977) J. Immunol., 118, 551-557.

35. Chaffee, J.K., Schachner, M. and Sidman, R.L., in preparation.

36. Strickland, R.G. and Hooper, B.M. (1972) Pathology, 4, 259-263.

37. Buckley, C.E., III, Buckley, E.G. and Dorsey, F.C. (1974) Fed. Proc., 33, 2036-2039.

38. Reif, A.E. and Allen, J.M.V. (1964) J. Exp. Med. 120, 413-433.

39. Arndt, R., Stark, R. and Thiele, H.G. (1977) Immunology, 33, 101-107.

40. Parker, L.M., Chused, T.M. and Steinberg, A.D. (1974) J. Immunol., 112, 285-292.

41. Shirai, T. and Mellors, R.C. (1971) Proc. Natl. Acad. Sci. USA, 68, 1412-1415.

42. Schlesinger, M. (1965) Nature (London), 207, 429-430.

43. Kidd, J.G. and Friedewald, W.F. (1942) J. Exp. Med. 76, 543-556.

44. Makinodan, T. (1972) in Tolerance, Autoimmunity and Aging, Sigel, M.M. and Good, R.A. eds., C.A. Thomas, Springfield, pp. 3-17.

IMMUNOLOGICAL PERTURBATION OF NEUROLOGICAL FUNCTIONS

MAURICE M. RAPPORT and STEPHEN E. KARPIAK
Division of Neuroscience, New York State Psychiatric Institute and Department
of Biochemistry, Columbia University College of Physicians and Surgeons.
722 West 168th Street, New York, N.Y. 10032

The painstaking microchemical analyses by Bass[1] of specimens of isocortex from
patients with senile dementia and elderly non-demented persons indicate that in
these brains the loss of neuronal cells is small compared with loss of synaptic
contacts, and that in dementia the loss of synaptic contacts (and of myelinated
axons) is much greater than in age-matched controls. Measurements of DNA, numbers
of cells, and gangliosides support the notion that "the dying back of neuronal
processes ... appears to be a critical factor in senile dementia"[1]. One may therefore regard any consideration of pathological processes that are detrimental to
synaptic connections as highly relevant for the problem of senile dementia and related disorders. The studies we have been engaged in for the past 8 years are concerned with immunological mechanisms that may be involved in synaptic pathology[2].
Our studies have shown that the introduction into the brain of antisera containing
antibodies directed against synaptic antigens can alter brain functions, and these
alterations reveal a degree of specificity. Although similar observations have
been reported a number of times, their depth and breadth have not yet been successful either in establishing the validity of this method of inducing synaptic changes
or of examining the mechanisms involved[3,4,5,6,7,8].

It is perhaps worth noting that changes induced by passive transfer of antibodies
should be considered separately from the question of whether auto-antibodies are
responsible for the pathological process in senile dementia. To detect autoimmunity
will require a different kind of measurement, one that can, perhaps, be more readily
undertaken once we have built a proper foundation with passive transfer studies.

Rather than present a review of the literature, we describe in this paper a
series of studies in our laboratory that serve as a foundation for our hypothesis
that the mechanism underlying immunological alteration of brain functions involves
interference in synaptic function. We wish to emphasize that this has been the
primary goal of our work, namely, to establish this mechanism by determining which
molecular constituents of synaptic membranes are intimately involved in neuronal
transmission.

Since our studies have developed through several stages in which the questions
have changed, the logic will be easier to understand by following the sequential
development. Our initial premises were two: first, that if the dissection of
brain functions or the establishment of regional specificity for such functions is

possible by using antibodies as an interventive agent, as suggested by the experiments of Mihailovic and Jankovic[3] and Jankovic et al.[4], then these antibodies
should work by altering synaptic activity; and second, that the most logical antigen to use for raising the required antibodies should be the synaptic membrane
fraction (SMF). Although this fraction is a complex mixture of antigens (and
therefore cannot be used in a systematic way to standardize antibodies against it)
the antisera it generates do permit initial approaches to the problem, especially
those concerned with technical details. Since antibodies do not cross the blood
brain barrier in adult animals, they must be injected directly into the brain, and
this procedure is inherently so unphysiologic that it is singularly unattractive
to physiologists and psychologists alike, and provokes their skepticism.

ANTI-SMF, EPILEPTIFORM ACTIVITY IN THE RABBIT

Initial questions, then, are concerned with techniques -- volume of antiserum,
its route and rate of administration, tissue damage, impairment of the blood brain
barrier, non-specific reactions and the like. In our first studies[9] we injected
rabbit antiserum into a rabbit brain, and since previous reports had not used such
a homologous system, we felt we were at least "improving the breed". In these
studies 50 μl of antiserum was injected on each of 2 successive days into rabbits
through a cannula in the lateral ventricle. Recurrent epileptiform spiking in the

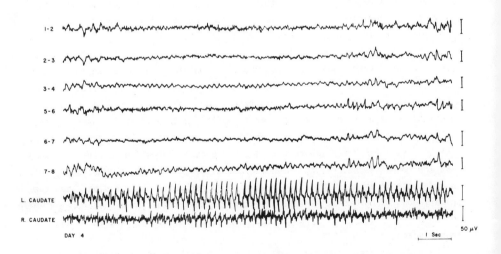

Fig. 1. EEG of rabbit injected intraventricularly with anti-SMF showing continuous spiking activity bilaterally in caudate nucleus. Cortical EEG was normal
during this period.

EEG (Fig. 1) was induced by antiserum to a rat synaptic membrane fraction (anti-SMF) whereas no effect was seen with antiserum to rat erythrocyte membranes. The abnormality occurred both cortically and subcortically and lasted up to 8 days. Both antisera had substantial antibody titers against their respective antigens as determined by complement fixation[10], the most convenient method for establishing a quantitative measure of antibody activity when the antigen is particulate. No convulsions were seen, and it was of considerable interest that when the seizure activity subsided, the abnormal EEG discharge could be reactivated with subthreshold intramuscular injections of pentylenetetrazol. These sustained effects in a chronic preparation, which were not the result either of mechanical damage or of non-specific toxic substances in the antiserum (in our judgment antiserum against a different type of antigen is a superior control to normal rabbit serum), encouraged us to extend these studies to rats where both EEG and behavioral effects could be studied conveniently[11].

ANTI-SMF; EPILEPTIFORM ACTIVITY; BASAL GANGLIA BEHAVIORS

Since the primary EEG abnormalities had been recorded from the caudate nuclei, it was reasonable to test caudate-mediated tasks, so-called because lesions of the caudate alter performance. In designing this experiment we also wished to assure ourselves that any observed alteration in behavioral response could not be attributed to irritative effects that might inhibit performance non-specifically. For this purpose we selected two behavioral paradigms that could be tested in the same animal: one, spontaneous alternation, a non-learned behavior which is caudate-mediated, and the other, a simple delayed response (a learned visual discrimination task) that is reported not to be caudate-mediated[12]. The anti-SMF serum (25 μl) was injected intraventricularly on each of 2 successive days. Behavioral training began on day 2, (prior to the second injection) and was repeated on days 3, 4 and 5. The control antiserum for these studies was antiserum to rat erythrocytes. EEG was also monitored. The learning curve for conditioned alternation (Fig. 2) showed that injection of anti-SMF serum had a marked effect, but injection of the anti-erythrocyte serum had no effect. Furthermore, rats receiving anti-SMF serum but not anti-erythrocyte serum showed a perseverative response to either the right or left side in the spontaneous alternation test. However the learning curve for delayed response, the control task in these same rats, was not altered (Fig. 3). As in the rabbits, antiserum to synaptic membranes induced recurrent epileptiform activity in the EEG whereas antiserum to rat erythrocytes was without effect. EEG changes began one day after the first injection and were characterized initially by intermittent spiking in the caudate nuclei, followed by continuous bursts of spikes lasting 2 to 5 sec. Surface activity at this time was that of an awake animal. This spiking disappeared three to four days after injection, but could be locally reactivated (after 3 weeks) by intramuscular injection of pentylenetetrazol

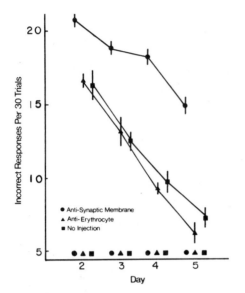

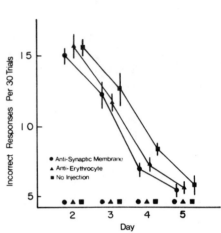

Fig. 2. Conditioned alternation learning curves showing inhibition after intraventricular injection of anti-SMF serum.

Fig. 3. Delayed response learning curves showing no inhibition after intraventricular injection of anti-SMF serum.

(40 mg/kg). This was not seen in control rats. A question that frequently arises in this connection concerns the relation of the behavioral interference to the abnormal EEG activity. This question cannot be answered decisively, but the failure to detect interference in such animals in performance of the delayed response task indicates that the EEG disturbance does not play an overriding role.

ANTI-SMF, ANTI-CEREBROSIDE; DRL BEHAVIOR; PRENATAL ADMINISTRATION

The next stage in the development of this work was directed to several new questions[13]: 1) could antisera be administered in such a way as to eliminate all mechanical brain damage and 2) could the effects be related to specific immunological systems, i.e. would antiserum against any constituent of brain membranes also produce alterations. The experimental design for this experiment (Fig. 4) was to administer the antiserum intravenously to the pregnant female in a very late stage of pregnancy (19 days), thus taking advantage of two biological phenomena: the absence of an intact blood brain barrier in the fetus and the fact that antibodies are one of the few protein molecules that do cross the placenta. In this experiment surrogate mothering was employed to avoid the possibility of antibodies being transferred postnatally in the milk. Delivery was normal, and male rats were

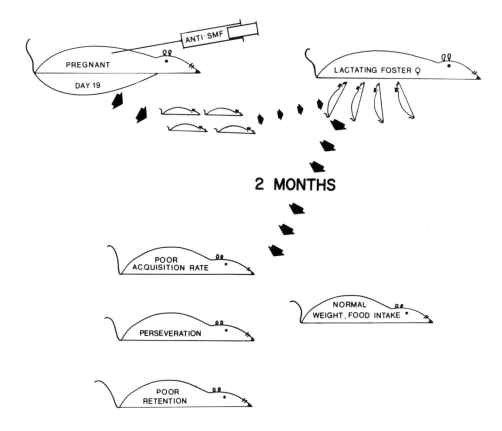

Fig. 4. Effect of anti-SMF serum administered prenatally; experimental design and results.

selected from the litters and fed by an untreated lactating female until they were weaned. The animals in experimental and control groups grew normally, showing the same food intake and weight gain. They were tested at two months of age on a vigilance task. This task, differential reinforcement at low rates (DRL), requires alertness and timing: the animal presses a lever for a food reward, but must wait a fixed time interval following the previous success. Animals from mothers injected with anti-SMF serum showed several behavioral deficits including perseveration, slow acquisition rates, and poor retention when compared with those from mothers injected with either saline or antiserum to galactocerebroside. In the initial training period every lever press produced a pellet. Normal rats showed a high percentages of responses between 2 and 4 seconds, whereas the group treated with anti-SMF serum showed no particular inclination to alter their perseverative behavior in order to obtain the food reward. When the assigned task was to wait for

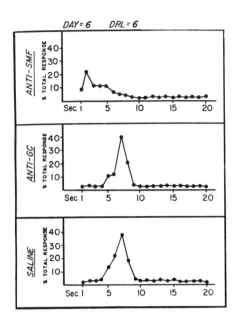

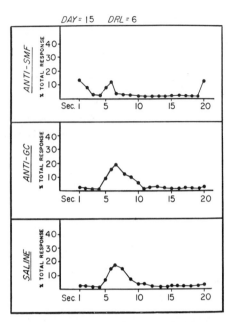

Fig. 5. DRL performance showing poor acquisition in rats receiving anti-SMF serum prenatally.

Fig. 6. DRL performance showing poor retention in rats receiving anti-SMF serum prenatally. (see text)

6 seconds after receiving a food pellet before pressing the lever again, (if pressed too soon, the automated apparatus recycled without delivery of the pellet), normal animals responded by the sixth day with a fairly good percentage of correct responses, whereas the anti-SMF animals did not seem to learn. They either pressed the lever too soon or did not show any interest (Fig. 5). With sufficient training (12 days) the treated animals were brought to the same response as the normal rats[13], but when then tested after a 3 day interval without training, the treated rats showed poorer retention than controls (Fig. 6). The conclusions to be derived from this experiment were somewhat different from those of the previous one. Since the antibodies were acting at a time of rapid brain development, we cannot distinguish between an action of these antibodies in preventing the formation of synaptic contacts and an action directed against contacts already formed. The deficit produced is a subtle one, but such impairment suggests that environmental factors evoking an antibody response in the mother may exert serious and irreversible changes in the brain of a developing fetus. The mother's brain is, of course, protected by a well-developed barrier that is impermeable to antibodies. This would represent a special case of an autoimmune mechanism directed against the developing brain.

ANTI-SMF; ANTI-S-100; ANTI-MYELIN; MAZE PERFORMANCE

In our next study[14] we extended the base in three ways: we altered the technique of administration, we tested a different type of behavior, and more particularly, we tested, as controls, antisera against a new group of "antigenic receptors" in the CNS. Our purposes were 1) to determine the biological activities of antisera against two other brain constituents: rat CNS myelin, a relatively homogeneous membrane preparation, and S-100 protein, a pure protein which is specific for nerve tissue, 2) to utilize an intracortical route of injection of the antibody, a route which causes much less damage to tissue and to the blood brain barrier than that caused by the insertion of a cannula into the ventricle, 3) to observe the effects of antibodies on a behavioral task (maze performance) known to be affected by cortical lesions and 4) to determine if this type of localized injection would affect EEG and behavior in a manner comparable to that used previously (which permitted much greater diffusion of antibody molecules). Antiserum to myelin was selected for comparison with antiserum to SMF because both types of antibodies were directed against specific membrane structures. Antiserum to S-100 protein was selected for three reasons: 1) this protein was one of the relatively few brain proteins for which specific antisera were then available 2) recent evidence[15] had indicated that S-100 protein was bound to membranes and 3) it had been reported that anti-S-100 protein affected behavior[6].

Adult male rats were trained on a Lashley III maze to a food reward. Immediately following training they were injected intracortically (through a carefully placed cannula) with 25 µl (at a rate of 3 µl/min) of one of the following three types of antisera: anti-SMF, anti-myelin, anti-S-100. On day 2 the rats were tested on the maze and then given a second injection of 25 µl of antiserum. Testing continued on days 3 to 5 with no further injections. EEG was monitored daily.

Only the rats injected with anti-SMF showed changes in the EEG. Epileptiform spiking began after 24 hours and was characterized initially as sporadic spiking localized to the area of injection; on subsequent days the spiking became more sustained and of higher amplitude, spreading ipsilaterally and contralaterally (Fig. 7). This abnormal activity receded by the 7th day. Four weeks after return to normal, the spiking could be reactivated at the site of antibody injection by pentylenetetrazol (20 mg/kg, intramuscular). With respect to maze running, on day 1 all rats performed the task at the same rate. On subsequent days, testing for latency showed a significant difference across groups (Fig. 8). Whereas there were no differences between the uninjected and the anti-myelin serum injected groups, those injected with antisera to either SMF or S-100 protein were both learning the maze more slowly than the other two groups. These differences were also seen by analysis of errors: a significantly larger number of errors were made by the anti-SMF and anti-S-100 injected groups compared with the uninjected or anti-myelin injected animals. Motor activity in all animals was judged to be

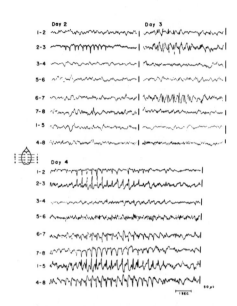

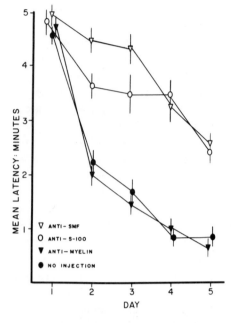

Fig. 7. Cortical EEG tracings after intracortical injection of anti-SMF serum showing focal spiking at injection site (day 2) followed by ipsilateral and contralateral spreading (days 3 and 4).

Fig. 8. Maze performance curves showing inhibition by both anti-SMF serum and anti-S-100 protein serum injected intracortically. Anti-myelin serum showed no effect.

normal. No clinical signs were associated with the epileptiform discharges, and no specific morphological changes were seen in brain on histological examination. These results showed clearly that the more localized subcortical route of injection produced readily detectable functional alterations, that antibodies against S-100 protein as well as antibodies against SMF would slow the learning process, and, what was most interesting, that EEG and behavioral effects could be dissociated, since anti-S-100 serum did not induce EEG changes but did interfere with learning. This observation indicates the potential for specificity that is inherent in the technique of immunological perturbation.

ANTI-SMF; ANTI-S-100; ANTI-14-3-2; ANTI-MYELIN; ANTI-CEREBROSIDE; PASSIVE AVOIDANCE

Since we had now found that CNS functions could be altered by antisera against two antigens (synaptic membrane fraction and S-100 protein) but not by antisera to three other antigens (erythrocyte membrane, myelin, galactocerebroside) we felt it was important to have available a convenient test for rapidly screening antisera against a number of different antigens that have become or are becoming available as progress continues in the isolation of nervous system constituents. For this

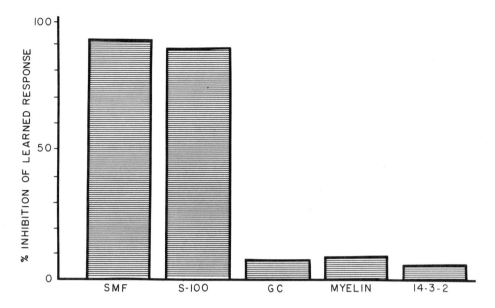

Fig. 9. Passive avoidance behavior. Almost complete inhibition by intraventricular injection of anti-SMF serum and anti-S-100 protein serum. Antisera to galactocerebroside (GC), rat CNS myelin, and bovine 14-3-2 protein had no effect.

purpose we adopted the passive avoidance paradigm, a behavior that can be taught to the animals in a single trial and which has proved useful in studies of the different phases of learning. We tested antisera to 5 different nervous system antigens, four that were mentioned previously plus bovine 14-3-2 protein, a neuronal protein isolated by Dr. B.W. Moore (and to whom we are indebted for supplying the high-titered antiserum). Antisera were injected intraventricularly immediately following training. The two types of antisera that proved to be effective inhibitors in this test were those previously found effective in other tests (anti-SMF and anti-S-100 protein) whereas the other three types of antisera (anti-14-3-2 protein, anti-myelin, anti-galactocerebroside) were without effect[2] (Fig. 9).

This series of studies was now sufficiently extensive to convince us of the merits of the immunoneurological attack on problems of brain function: the specificity was real, and the probability for a locus of action of the antibodies on the process of synaptic transmission was high. There was clearly now a need to persuade a larger scientific community that this was correct, not only to obtain the intellectual support required by a new area whose reliability had been questioned, but because survival of interdisciplinary efforts such as this depends on the development of a "critical mass" of scientific effort, a mass that can rarely be mounted by a single group.

In order to ensure reproducibility of the experiments, it was essential a) to find an antiserum reagent that could be obtained conveniently and b) to establish criteria that would serve to define such reproducibility. This cannot yet be done with antiserum to the synaptic membrane fraction for two reasons: 1) the antigen contains too many constituents and 2) immunological response to such a complex mixture of antigens is too variable (the response differs not only from one rabbit to the next, but in the same rabbit as a function of time). Even S-100 protein is not a satisfactory antigen for this purpose because, in our experience, the antibody response to this specific nervous tissue protein does not meet the criteria of frequency and intensity to allow a convenient accumulation of a large number of high-titered antisera. However, one of the molecules that is known to be present in synaptic membranes in relatively high concentration is G_{M1} ganglioside. We have recently shown, by labeling techniques using membrane-impermeable reagents, that G_{M1} ganglioside is present and accessible for reaction on the intact membrane of synaptosomes[16,17] and can therefore readily react with antibodies that may have access only to the synaptic cleft and other intercellular spaces. Antibodies against G_{M1} ganglioside can be readily prepared[18,19] and although the quantities of ganglioside required to obtain these antibodies are large, the immunizing antigen can be conveniently isolated in gram quantities. For this purpose the total

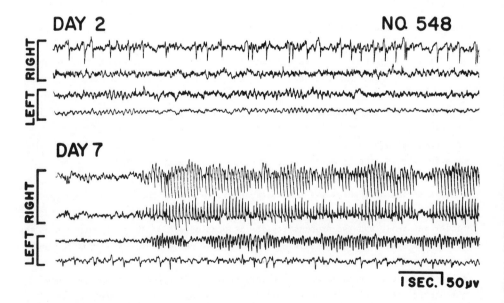

Fig. 10. Recurrent seizure activity induced by single intracortical injection (10 μl) of antiserum to G_{M1} ganglioside. Cortical EEG tracings.

ganglioside mixture from bovine brain can be used[20], and this antigen will induce antibody formation in almost all rabbits[21]. We therefore decided to examine the activity of antiganglioside sera in altering brain functions.

In the first of these studies[22] it was shown that a single injection of 10 μl of anti-ganglioside serum into the sensorimotor cortex of rats would induce epileptiform seizures lasting several weeks. Three different anti-ganglioside sera were tested and all were found to be effective: seizure activity was induced in 26 of the 28 animals injected. For these studies an ideal control was now available, namely, absorbed antiserum: the very same antisera that had produced the effects but from which the anti-G_{M1} ganglioside antibodies had been removed by absorption with small quantities of pure G_{M1} ganglioside. These absorbed antisera were without effect in all 16 of the rats into which they were injected. With native (untreated) antisera, seizures did not begin until about 24 hours after intracortical injection, and then were usually seen on the ipsilateral side, spreading on subsequent days both ipsilaterally and contralaterally, and increasing in frequency and amplitude (Fig. 10). Tissue damage at the site of injection was minimal, no differences being detectable between injections that caused seizures and those that did not.

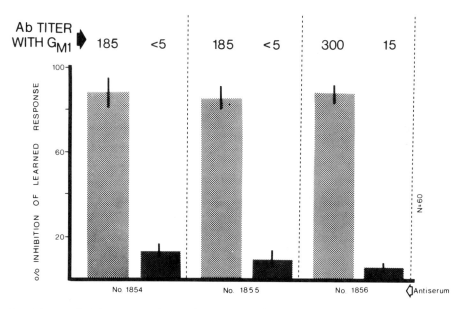

Fig. 11. Inhibition of passive avoidance behavior by intraventricular injection of anti-ganglioside serum immediately after training. Antiserum absorbed with pure G_{M1} ganglioside had no effect. Also shown are the antibody titers (of the three different antisera tested) with pure G_{M1} ganglioside determined by complement-fixation before and after absorption with G_{M1} ganglioside.

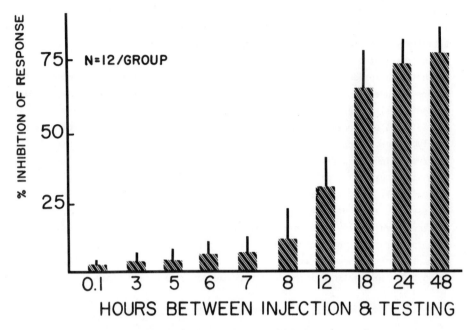

Fig. 12. Antiganglioside serum inhibits the consolidation phase of memory. Animals (mice) injected immediately after training on a passive avoidance paradigm did not show memory loss until 8 to 12 hours.

ANTI-G_{M1} GANGLIOSIDE; PASSIVE AVOIDANCE

In our next study these anti-ganglioside sera were shown to inhibit passive avoidance learning by intraventricular injection immediately after training.[23] Again, the absorbed antisera used as controls were without effect (Fig. 11). In these studies of passive avoidance memory, animals are usually tested for their ability to remember their training after 7 days. When, however, we tested them at much shorter intervals after injection, it was possible to determine whether the effect of the antiserum was on the acquisition or on the consolidation phases of learning. In this experiment (Fig. 12), we found that the effect of the anti-ganglioside serum in inhibiting the memory function was not seen until about 8 hours after injection[24]. Since it is known that, in this single trial learning, acquisition is almost immediate, the antiserum must have produced its inhibition of learning by interfering with the consolidation phase. There is no reason to suspect that the antibodies interfere with protein synthesis, and therefore the immunological method and the use of protein synthesis inhibitors (such as acetoxycyclohexi-mide[25] and anisomycin[26]) are independent methods of blocking consolidation of memory.

We have now reviewed all of our studies that have been published. They show that alteration of brain functions both in adult and developing rats can be induced by antibodies directed against three different antigens but not by antibodies against four other antigens. The three "antigenic receptors" that produce positive effects, namely, SMF, G_{M1} ganglioside, and S-100 protein have all been localized in synaptic membranes, albeit with great differences in the reliability of the evidence for such localization. The four "antigenic receptors" that do not produce positive effects, namely, galactocerebroside, 14-3-2 protein, myelin, and erythrocyte membrane are presumably not present in synaptic membranes. The total presumptive evidence is therefore reasonably strong that these antibodies are producing their effects by acting on synaptic membranes and causing interference with synaptic transmission. Similar studies in the literature also permit this interpretation[27,28,29,30,31,32]. The most useful reagent for securing more rigorous evidence for this hypothesis appears to be the antiserum to G_{M1} ganglioside. Pure antibody to G_{M1} ganglioside can now be prepared by affinity chromatography on acrylamide gels polymerized in the presence of pure G_{M1}[33]. Although G_{M1} ganglioside is only a fraction of the total ganglioside mixture, the other components can be converted to G_{M1} by either enzymic hydrolysis with commercially available neuraminidase or by mild acid hydrolysis. Pure G_{M1} ganglioside can then be readily obtained by recrystallization. G_{M1} ganglioside free of other gangliosides is also available commercially, but it is still too costly for most purposes. The specificity of the antibody has also been carefully studied. Antisera prepared against the total ganglioside mixture react with both G_{M1} and G_{D1b} gangliosides but not with G_{D1a} or G_{T1} gangliosides[34]. Absorption of the sera with pure G_{M1} ganglioside removes the reactivity to both G_{M1} and G_{D1b} gangliosides[21]. We are therefore dealing with antibodies that cross-react with two molecular species. In view of the known presence of G_{M1} ganglioside in glial cells, in myelin, and presumably in dendrites as well as in synaptic membranes, it is not yet clear that localization studies per se will provide the necessary evidence to prove that biological changes stem from alteration of synaptic connections. However, the availability of pure reagents may permit such evidence to be obtained through measurements of the turnover of various neurotransmitters, and we are now proceeding in this direction. In addition to this aspect of mechanism, we must also address the question of persistence of antibodies and the processes that can be initiated by binding of the antibody molecule as a "ligand" to a membrane antigen as a "receptor". Does this involve lateral movement of antigens? internalization of the immune complex? "receptor" turnover? accessory factors such as complement? If answers to these questions can be found, they will surely contribute to our confidence in a synaptic site of action for the antibodies.

What degree of dissection is attainable with immunoneurological methods? This is still a difficult area in which to make predictions. Synaptic membranes contain many polypeptides[35], all of which are potentially antigenic, and it seems likely that differences in function among synapses will be reflected in differences in membrane composition. To detect such differences may require the development of very discriminating behavioral tests.

Even though G_{M1} ganglioside is widely distributed, antibodies against G_{M1} ganglioside have not shown activity in a number of _in vivo_ tests such as pain threshold, pattern discrimination, and fixed reinforcement schedules, or affected _in vitro_ synaptic activity of adult cerebellar cultures[36] or neurite growth of chick embryonic dorsal root ganglion cells[37]. Some of this specificity may be attributed to the inability of the methods used thus far to detect consequences of antibody binding to the antigenic site. One would certainly not expect the binding of antibodies to G_{M1} ganglioside in the synaptic membrane, in dendrites, in glial cells and in myelin to have the same consequences. So the chemical specificity of antibodies for structural elements in the nervous system must be combined with a concept of specificity of functional alteration in relation to anatomical localization in order to develop a useful framework of reference.

Our studies show that the interventive approach to brain function using antibodies has a broad base and can be sufficiently sensitive to overcome many of the usual obstacles (for weak antisera non-specific effects may still be a problem). The immunological foundations are rapidly becoming stronger although this important aspect has received much too little attention. If the aging process leads to an increased circulation of brain-reactive bodies[38], and if, in a disorder like senile dementia, the blood brain barrier loses its efficacy, then some of the observed loss of cognitive and motor functions may well be made more severe by immunological attack on synaptic connections.

Although there may be a close relation between such immunological studies and disease processes, the power of immunological methods is even greater. These methods may provide the bridge between morphology and the underlying biochemical process. The creation of such a bridge may be an even more ambitious goal than selective blocking of functional pathways. It is, however, encouraging to invoke Toynbee's dictum namely, that "It is a paradoxical but profoundly true and important principle of life that the most likely way to reach a goal is to be aiming not at that goal itself but at some more ambitious goal behind it".

ACKNOWLEDGMENTS

The studies were supported in part by a grant from the USPHS (NS-13762).

Figures 2 and 3 were reprinted with permission from Neuropsychologia, Volume 12, S. E. Karpiak, M. M. Rapport, and F. P. Bowen, 1974, Pergamon Press, Ltd.

REFERENCES

1. Bass, N.H. (1978) Paper presented at 11th Annual Winter Conference on Brain Research, Keystone, Colorado.

2. Rapport, M.M. and Karpiak, S.E. (1976) Res. Comm. in Psychol., Psychiat., and Behav., 1, 115-134.

3. Mihailovic, L. and Jankovic, B.D. (1961) Nature, 192, 665-666.

4. Jankovic, B.D., Rakic, L., Veskov, R. and Horvat, J. (1968) Nature, 218, 270-271.

5. DeRobertis, E., Lapetina, E., Saavedra, J.P., and Soto, E.F. (1966) Life Sci., 5, 1979-1989.

6. Hyden, H. and Lange, P. (1970) Exp. Cell Res., 62, 125-132.

7. Heath, R.G. and Krupp, I.M. (1967) Am. J. Psychiat., 123, 1499-1504.

8. MacPherson, C.F.C. and Chinerman, J. (1970) Exp. Neurol., 31, 45-52.

9. Karpiak, S.E., Bowen, F.P. and Rapport, M.M. (1973) Brain Res., 59, 303-310.

10. Rapport, M.M. and Graf, L. (1957) Annals. N.Y. Acad. Sci., 69, 608-632.

11. Karpiak, S.E., Rapport, M.M. and Bowen, F.P. (1974) Neuropsychologia, 12, 303-322.

12. Chorover, S. and Gross, C. (1963) Science, 30, 826-827.

13. Karpiak, S.E. and Rapport, M.M. (1975) Brain Res., 92, 405-413.

14. Karpiak, S.E., Serokosz, M. and Rapport, M.M. (1976) Brain Res., 102, 313-321.

15. Rusca, G., Calissano, P. and Alema, S. (1972) Brain Res., 49, 223-227.

16. Rapport, M.M., Hungund, B.L. and Mahadik, S.P. (1975) Neurosci. Abst., 1, 616.

17. Rapport, M.M., and Mahadik, S.P. (1977) in Mechanisms, Regulations and Special Functions of Protein Synthesis in the Brain, Roberts, S., Lajtha, A. and Gispen, W.H. eds., Elsevier, Amsterdam, pp. 221-230.

18. Rapport, M.M. and Graf, L. (1969) Progr. Allergy, 13, 273-331.

19. Naiki, M., Marcus, D.M. and Ledeen, R. (1974) J. Immunol., 113, 84-93.

20. Pascal, T.A., Saifer, A., and Gitlin, J. (1966) Proc. Soc. Exptl. Biol. Med. 121, 739-742.

21. Rapport, M.M., Graf, L., Huang, Y. and Yu, R.K. (1978) Fed. Proc., 37, in press.

22. Karpiak, S.E., Graf, L. and Rapport, M.M. (1976) Science, 121, 735-737.

23. Karpiak, S.E., Graf, L. and Rapport, M.M. (1978) Brain Res., in press.

24. Karpiak, S.E., Sowin, T. and Rapport, M.M. (1977) Neurosci. Abstr. 3, 236.

25. Agranoff, B.W. (1972) in Basic Neurochemistry, Albers, R.W., Siegel, G.J., Katzman, R. and Agranoff, B.W. eds., Little, Brown and Co., N.Y. pp. 645-665.

26. Flood, J.F., Bennett, E.L., Orne, A.E., Rosenzweig, M.R. and Jarvik, M.E. (1977) Science, 199, 324-326.

27. Bowen, F.P., Kosarova, J., Casella, D., Nicklas, W.J., and Berl, S. (1976) Brain Res., 102, 363-367.

28. Kobiler, D., Fuchs, S. and Samuel, D. (1976) Brain Res., 115, 129-138.

29. Shashoua, V.E. (1977) Proc. Nat. Acad. Sci., 74, 1743-1747.

30. Williams, C.J. and Schupf, N. (1977) Science, 197, 328-330.

31. Blessing, W.W., Costa, M., Geffen. L.B., Rush, R.A. and Fink, G. (1977) Nature, 267, 363-369.

32. Fillenz, M., Gagnon, C., Stoeckel, K. and Thoenen, H. (1976) Brain Res., 114, 293-303.

33. Marcus, D.M. (1976) in Glycolipid Methodology, Witting, L.A. ed., Amer. Oil Chem. Soc., Champaign, Ill., pp. 243-245.

34. Rapport, M.M., Graf, L. and Ledeen, R. (1968) Fed. Proc. 27, 463.

35. Mahadik, S.P., Korenovsky, A. and Rapport, M.M. (1976) Anal. Biochem., 76, 615-633.

36. Crain, S., personal communication.

37. Roisen, F., personal communication.

38. Nandy, K. (1973) in Neurological Aspects of Maturation and Aging, Ford, D.H. ed., Elsevier, Amsterdam, pp. 437-454.

HISTOTOPOGRAPHY OF CELLULAR CHANGES IN ALZHEIMER'S DISEASE

MELVYN J. BALL, M.D., F.R.C.P.(C),

Departments of Pathology and Clinical Neurological Sciences,

University of Western Ontario, London, N6A 5C1, Canada.

ABSTRACT

The topographic distribution of neurofibrillary tangles of Alzheimer, granulovacuolar degeneration of Simchowicz, and rod-like bodies of Hirano was analysed in
the hippocampal cortex of patients with Alzheimer's dementia and mentally normal,
aged controls. A semiautomated scanning stage microscope (Wild) linked potentiometrically to an XY pen recorder (Rikadenki) permitted the plotting of cytoarchitectonic "scattergrams" from the sequentially screened hippocampal formations. The
density of all three histological lesions per cubic mm. of cortex was quantified by
measuring the area of each of six "zones", using a digitizer and programmable
calculator (Hewlett-Packard).

In elderly normal brains as well as those of Alzheimer's disease, the statistically most representative ranking order of predilection (in decreasing severity) for
neurofibrillary tangles was: entorhinal cortex>subiculum>H_1>endplate>presubiculum>
H_2. For granulovacuolar degeneration the best rank order was: subiculum>H_1>H_2>end-
plate>entorhinal cortex>presubiculum. For Hirano bodies the best rank order was:
H_1>subiculum>H_2>entorhinal cortex>endplate>presubiculum. The similarities between all
three orders of predilection and the "selective vulnerability" of certain hippocampal
foci to hypoxic, ischemic and epileptic effects raise the possibility that a focally
accentuated cytotoxic mechanism might be operating in all such regional predisposi-
tions.

INTRODUCTION

The degree of neurofibrillary tangle formation, of granulovacuolar degeneration of
Simchowicz and of Hirano body formation has been quantified in several studies[1-13].
However, the pertinent literature contains very few observations on the exact topo-
graphic distribution of such changes within areas of involvement.

Hirano and Zimmerman[14], reporting on the localization of neurofibrillary tangles,
examined the hippocampus, hypothalamus, midbrain, pontine tegmentum and medulla. In
silver stains of mesial temporal tissue from 28 mentally normal elderly and 97 neurologically ill patients, they observed that pyramidal neurones in two regions -- the
glomerular formation of the hippocampal gyrus, and the H_1 field of Rose (Sommer
sector) in Ammon's horn -- were more affected by tangles than all other foci. No
quantitative data accompanied this impression, however. Earlier, Goodman[15] had made
a similar comment on 23 cases of Alzheimer's disease, stating that tangle formation

was worst in the glomeruli substantiae reticulatae Arnoldi and next most severe in the cornu Ammonis.

From the hippocampi of 200 unselected autopsies in a state mental hospital, Woodard[1] calculated the percentage of neurones showing Alzheimer tangles in an area he called the ventrolateral quadrant, which included some of Rose's H_1 field and some of the prosubiculum. In a single coronal section through the mid-hippocampus, he noted tangles were "usually more prevalent there" than in the rest of the hippocampal and parahippocampal cortex; and that granulovacuolar degeneration was never focal except for this prevalence in the ventrolateral quadrant.

In 219 consecutively autopsied patients of a general hospital, Tomlinson and Kitchener[7] quantified granulovacuolar change in one section of each hippocampus. The distribution was felt to be the same as in the brains of 30 non-demented old people and 25 proven dements with Alzheimer's disease: areas H_1 and H_2 were most afflicted, whereas the other fields (H_3, H_4 and H_5) were involved only if the percentage of all the neurones in H_1 and H_2 also affected reached or exceeded 10%. "Small numbers" of subicular neurones were "occasionally" degenerated with granulovacuoles.

From 48 demented peoples' brains, Jamada and Mehraein[16] measured tangle distribution in two sections of the limbic cortex. In 22 cases of "presenile" dementia, the rank order of severity was H_1>presubiculum>subiculum>H_3 and H_2. In 28 cases of "senile dementia" the order was H_1>presubiculum, subiculum and H_3>H_2. In 8 cases of Alzheimer's disease, Hooper and Vogel[10] quantified tangle formation as 0 to +4, and granulovacuolar degeneration from 0 to +3, in just 5 microscopic fields per hippocampus. Tangles were "generally severe" in hippocampus proper; and in entorhinal, parasubicular and presubicular cortex, the subiculum was "better preserved" between the "confluently involved" prosubiculum and the altered presubiculum. Granulovacuoles were "most commonly found" in Rose's H_1 field. This predilection of tangles and granulovacuoles for the Sommer sector (H_1) and adjacent medial subiculum, with much less involvement of H_2, the endplate, or the lateral subiculum had already been noted by Corsellis[4].

McLardy[6], observing the brains of 85 Alzheimer dements, claimed that in the subiculum the "vast majority" of cells showed no neurofibrillary tangles "of significance", whereas in the lateral entorhinal cortex they were "at least as widespread and advanced" as in H_1. The medial entorhinal, H_2, and the endplate zones were "strikingly spared" in most cases.

The topography of Hirano bodies has been mentioned in three recent papers. Hirano[17], recognizing these rod-like inclusions initially in cases of amyotrophic lateral sclerosis - Parkinsonism dementia complex from Guam, reported that also in Alzheimer's (presenile) disease, senile dementia, Pick's disease and even normal brains of elderly people they were confined solely to Sommer sector and the immediately adjacent areas. In 152 pathological and 50 normal brains, randomly chosen, Ogata et al[8] felt similarly that these rod-like structures were confined to the

pyramidal layer of Sommer's sector and the stratum lacunosum subjacent to it.
Gibson and Tomlinson[12], examining the brains of 34 dements with Alzheimer's disease
(presenile and senile), 24 non-demented people over age 60 years, and 27 intellectually normal younger subjects, commented that Hirano bodies occur "particularly" in
Sommer's sector of the hippocampus.

During quantitative analyses in our laboratory of neurofibrillary tangles[11] and
granulovacuoles[13] in serially sectioned hippocampi of mentally normal patients'
brains and of some cases of Alzheimer's disease, a tendency for regional predilection was apparent for all three types of histological abnormality. The following
approach was taken to quantify this striking topographic phenomenon.

METHODS

The brains of four patients, ages 63 to 83 years (mean 72.8), judged mentally
sound and neurologically normal from clinical data, served as controls (Table 1).
Pertinent clinical and neuropathological details were reported earlier[11,13]. From a
psychiatric institute and a veterans' hospital the brains of eight patients dying at
ages 56 to 91 years (mean 74.6) with dementia of Alzheimer disease type were also
examined (Table 1). These latter manifested abundant senile plaques and neurofibrillary tangles in their cortex[18], decreased brain weight, generalized cortical
atrophy, and no arteriolosclerosis or significant infarction from appreciable cerebrovascular disease.

TABLE 1

CLINICAL DATA

	Case	Sex	Age (years)
Cont.	1	M	63
	2	M	69
	3	M	76
	4	F	83
Alzs.	5	F	56
	6	F	67
	7	F	71
	8	M	77
	9	F	77
	10	M	78
	11	M	80
	12	F	91

Each entire formalin-fixed hippocampus (from 2 cm. behind the temporal lobe's
rostral tip to the level of the splenium) was excised, cut sequentially in the
coronal plane, and all paraffin blocks serially sectioned at 6μ.

The middle section from each tissue block[11] was stained with hematoxylin-eosin-
Luxol fast blue; the very next serial section was stained by Congo-red-gallocyanin
for visualizing neurofibrillary tangles with polarized light[19]. The region to be

screened encompassed the hippocampal formation (Ammon's horn), the prosubiculum, the subiculum and presubiculum of the hippocampal gyrus, and the parahippocampal gyrus as far laterally as the collateral sulcus.

This entire area (outlined with ink on the coverslip) was scanned sequentially using the semi-automated Wild M501 microscope, at 400X magnification, with a square (Weibel) ocular graticule. Neurones with granulovacuoles, and rod-like Hirano bodies, were easily seen in H and E/LFB sections; adding a red interference filter gave neurofibrillary tangles in the Congo red sections a congophilic birefringence and a yellow-green dichroism against the blue-orange background. An X-Y pen recorder (Rikadenki BW-200) linked potentiometrically to the gears of the microscope stage permitted the production of one dot of ink on recording paper corresponding to the location of each visual field containing one or more neurones bearing a tangle (Figure 1), or granulovacuole(s) (Figure 2), or containing one or more Hirano bodies (Figure 3). Such fields were considered "positive" whether or not the tangle-bearing or granulovacuole-bearing cells also manifested a nucleus or a nucleolus in the section. A total of 221,443 microscopic fields was examined (each 0.051 mm^2 in a section 5.85μ in true thickness).

The outer edge of the hippocampal cortex and the configuration of the dentate fascia (d) were also inked on these "scattergrams" by tracking them with the microscope. These anatomical markings made it easy to compare each "scattergram" (Figures 1, 2 and 3, left-hand rows) with the histological sections from which they had been made (Figures 1, 2 and 3, right-hand rows). Six coronal sections of each left hippocampus were thus surveyed -- one from more anteriorly (upper rows), one closer to the middle (middle rows), and one from more posteriorly in the hippocampus (lower rows) for tangle formation (Figure 1); the next three serial sections respectively for granulovacuoles (Figure 2); and these latter three sections once more for Hirano bodies (Figure 3). Coronal sections from six samples of right hippocampi were analysed in the same manner; but since there were no differences in those additional 11,477 microscopic fields, the results are presented for left hippocampi only. Boundaries around these six "zones" were drawn onto the "scattergrams", and the cortical area within each border was measured (in sq. mm.) with a digitizer linked to a (Hewlett-Packard) calculator. As the "scattergram" magnification from the actual glass slides was known (X64), as well as the paraffin sections' true thickness, it was possible to calculate the number of positive fields per cu. mm. of tissue --- an "Adjusted Field Index" --- for each "zone". The Adjusted Field Indices of the three sections of each case were then averaged to get a Mean Adjusted Field Index for each "zone" (Tables 2, 3 and 4).

The total area of hippocampal grey matter scanned was divided into six "zones" -- the endplate (Rose's fields H_3, H_4 and H_5); H_2; the lateral part of H_1 (Sommer sector), corresponding to CA_1 of Lorente de Nó's cornu Ammonis; the medial part of H_1 (prosubiculum) and contiguous subiculum; the presubiculum; and the entorhinal region, including parasubiculum and the parahippocampal gyrus (Figure 4).

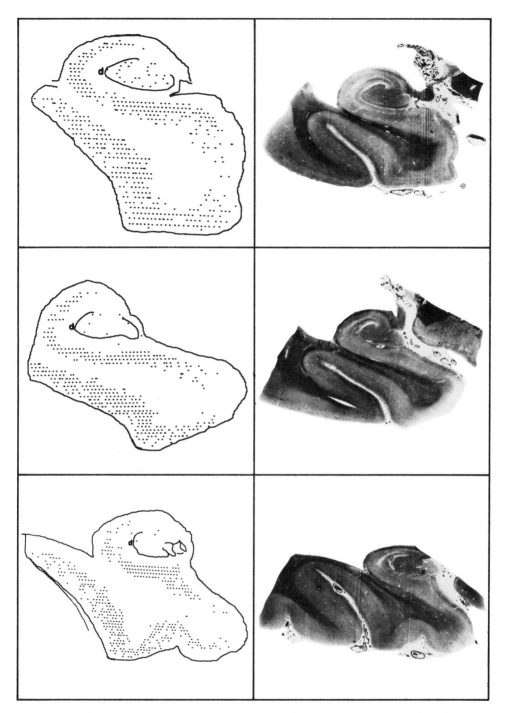

Fig. 1. "Scattergrams" of the topographic distribution of neurofibrillary tangles of Alzheimer in the hippocampal formation (left), each with photomicrograph of the histological section from which it was derived (right). Every dot represents one 'positive' microscopic field (at 400 X) containing at least one tangle-bearing neurone. Fascia dentata, d.

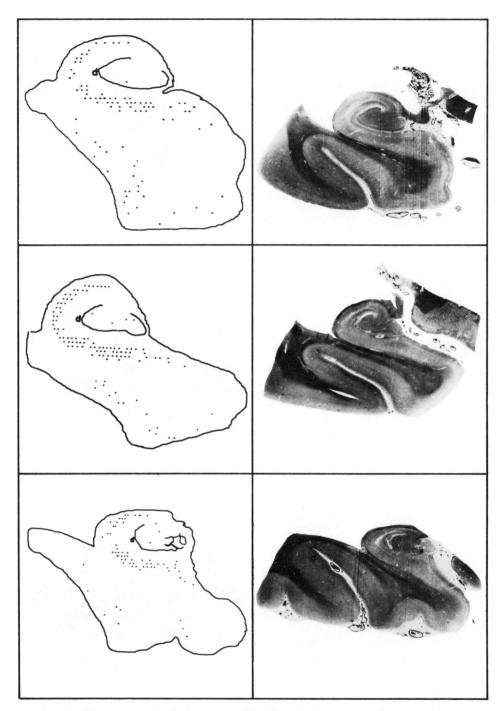

Fig. 2.   "Scattergrams" of the topographic distribution of granulovacuolar degeneration of Simchowicz in the hippocampal formation (left), each with photomicrograph of
the histological section from which it was derived (right).   Every dot represents one
'positive' microscopic field (at 400 X) containing at least one neurone with granulovacuolar change.   Fascia dentata, d.

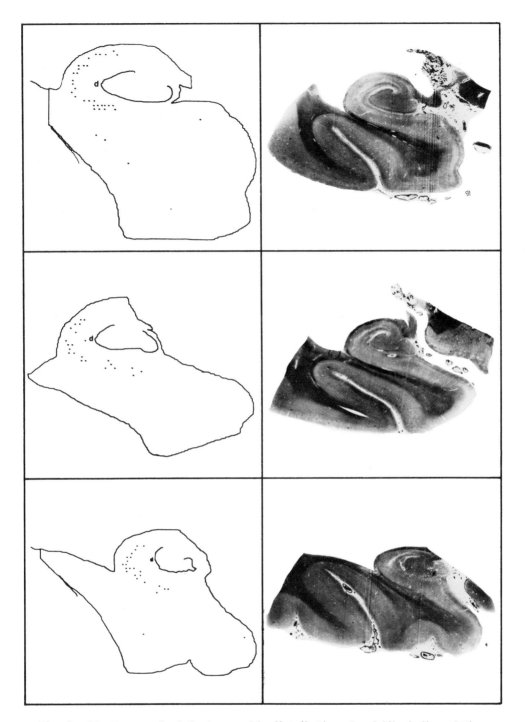

Fig. 3. "Scattergrams" of the topographic distribution of rod-like bodies of Hirano in the hippocampal formation (left), each with photomicrograph of the histological section from which it was derived (right). Every dot represents one 'positive' microscopic field (at 400 X) containing at least one Hirano body. Fascia dentata, d.

TABLE 2

MEAN ADJUSTED FIELD INDEX, NEUROFIBRILLARY TANGLES

CASE	ZONE					
	Endplate	H_2	H_1	Subic.	Presubic.	Entorhin.
1	26.88 (2)	4.11 (6)	14.99 (5)	20.53 (4)	21.15 (3)	199.23 (1)
2	8.08 (5)	0 (6)	12.69 (4)	14.08 (3)	61.60 (2)	70.40 (1)
3	15.71 (4)	11.12 (5)	57.60 (1)	28.35 (3)	9.68 (6)	28.56 (2)
4	8.88 (6)	10.27 (5)	36.77 (2)	33.71 (3)	27.25 (4)	58.05 (1)
5	73.68 (6)	83.52 (5)	259.95 (3)	635.57 (1)	163.23 (4)	305.84 (2)
6	192.59 (4)	58.59 (6)	277.47 (3)	393.39 (2)	99.00 (5)	458.19 (1)
7	353.92 (2)	115.41 (4)	63.23 (6)	98.29 (5)	331.25 (3)	434.37 (1)
8	639.79 (3)	472.91 (5)	873.65 (2)	1001.57 (1)	290.45 (6)	630.24 (4)
9	410.16 (4)	192.77 (6)	926.16 (3)	1420.48 (2)	346.99 (5)	1493.76 (1)
10	59.52 (6)	63.17 (5)	100.00 (4)	292.29 (1)	143.04 (3)	163.95 (2)
11	249.71 (5)	472.21 (3)	820.67 (2)	878.72 (1)	108.48 (6)	430.41 (4)
12	265.96 (5)	620.91 (3)	1177.01 (1)	939.31 (2)	189.73 (6)	442.08 (4)

(Numbers in parentheses indicate rank order within each case.)

TABLE 3

MEAN ADJUSTED FIELD INDEX, GRANULOVACUOLAR DEGENERATION

CASE	ZONE					
	Endplate	H_2	H_1	Subic.	Presubic.	Entorhin.
1	19.68 (3)	7.01 (5)	24.99 (2)	8.88 (4)	0 (6)	26.59 (1)
2	14.03 (3)	8.88 (4)	20.43 (2)	22.69 (1)	0 (6)	5.20 (5)
3	0 (6)	30.48 (2)	25.97 (3)	38.21 (1)	2.77 (5)	14.45 (4)
4	39.49 (4)	7.63 (6)	78.80 (1)	51.41 (3)	14.61 (5)	58.59 (2)
5	143.81 (4)	333.25 (3)	627.81 (2)	637.81 (1)	53.87 (6)	93.31 (5)
6	103.31 (4)	175.76 (3)	352.40 (2)	364.48 (1)	0 (6)	96.37 (5)
7	77.15 (3)	58.61 (4)	105.97 (1)	81.41 (2)	24.56 (6)	57.49 (5)
8	314.93 (3)	177.76 (4)	625.25 (1)	608.93 (2)	9.57 (6)	40.13 (5)
9	78.11 (5)	255.36 (3)	576.51 (1)	462.32 (2)	17.15 (6)	103.28 (4)
10	3.87 (5)	4.37 (4)	0 (6)	56.77 (1)	7.84 (3)	18.13 (2)
11	102.61 (4)	326.67 (1)	176.53 (2)	130.13 (3)	42.96 (5)	35.95 (6)
12	103.08 (4)	147.52 (3)	378.65 (1)	340.96 (2)	6.83 (6)	12.08 (5)

(Numbers in parentheses indicate rank order within each case.)

TABLE 4 MEAN ADJUSTED FIELD INDEX, HIRANO BODIES

CASE	Endplate	H_2	H_1	Subic.	Presubic.	Entorhin.
				ZONE		
1	0 (5)	11.95 (2)	15.38 (1)	10.17 (3)	0 (5)	0 (5)
2	0 (4)	0 (4)	13.31 (1)	0 (4)	0 (4)	0 (4)
3	0 (5)	18.23 (2)	19.81 (1)	13.78 (3)	0 (5)	0 (5)
4	0 (5)	6.98 (3)	40.08 (1)	36.20 (2)	0 (5)	0 (5)
5	0 (5.5)	255.11 (3)	714.41 (1)	263.88 (2)	12.50 (4)	0 (5.5)
6	12.03 (3)	0 (5.5)	195.58 (1)	56.03 (2)	0 (5.5)	6.57 (4)
7	0 (5)	3.79 (3)	45.21 (1)	27.93 (2)	0 (5)	0 (5)
8	0 (4.5)	0 (4.5)	72.10 (2)	119.53 (1)	0 (4.5)	0 (4.5)
9	0 (6)	26.91 (3)	401.46 (1)	65.61 (2)	6.89 (5)	7.54 (4)
10	10.67 (3)	0 (5)	11.42 (2)	70.50 (1)	0 (5)	0 (5)
11	0 (5)	0 (5)	18.84 (2)	28.53 (1)	0 (5)	6.28 (3)
12	0 (5)	20.43 (3)	191.44 (1)	177.98 (2)	0 (5)	0 (5)

(Numbers in parentheses indicate rank order within each case.)

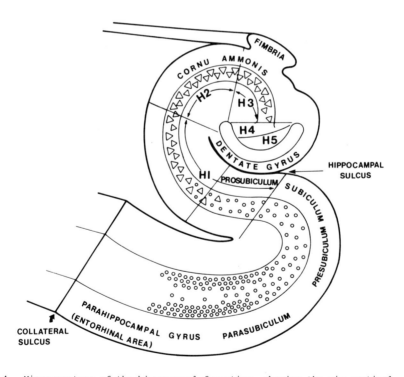

Fig. 4. Micro-anatomy of the hippocampal formation, showing the six cortical
"zones" surveyed: endplate (Rose's H_3, H_4 and H_5 fields); H_2; lateral part of H_1
(Sommer sector); medial H_1 and subiculum; presubiculum; entorhinal area.

The relative density of positive <u>fields</u> is a reasonable reflection of the relative density of actual histological lesions, since the <u>mean</u> number of tangle-bearing neurones per field varied very little, ranging in the ten cases re-examined for this purpose only from 1.15 to 2.81 (Table 5); the mean number of granulovacuolar neurones per field in the eight cases reviewed from only 1.10 to 1.69 (Table 6); and the mean number of Hirano bodies in any one field from only 1.03 to 1.54 in the three cases reviewed (Table 7). Hence, a <u>rank order number</u> could be assigned to each Mean Adjusted Field Index (see subscripts in parentheses, Tables 2, 3 and 4), with "1" indicating the largest and "6" the smallest Field Index of each case.

TABLE 5

VARIATION OF TANGLE DENSITY IN POSITIVE FIELDS

CASE	Number of Positive Fields	Number of Tangled Neurones	Mean Number of Tangled Neurones per Field (+ S.D.)
3	27	31	1.15 (+0.36)
4	119	170	1.43 (+0.88)
5	311	657	2.11 (+1.83)
6	597	1180	1.98 (+1.47)
7	175	276	1.58 (+0.99)
8	634	1315	2.07 (+1.57)
9	974	2740	2.81 (+2.16)
10	165	320	1.94 (+1.26)
11	144	279	1.94 (+1.45)
12	315	716	2.27 (+1.53)

TABLE 6

VARIATION OF GRANULOVACUOLAR DENSITY IN POSITIVE FIELDS

CASE	Number of Positive Fields	Number of Neurones with Granulovacuoles	Mean Number of Neurones with Granulovacuoles per Field (+1 S.D.)
5	73	120	1.64 (+0.95)
6	48	60	1.25 (+0.48)
7	10	11	1.10 (+0.32)
8	95	131	1.38 (+0.64)
9	32	54	1.69 (+0.93)
10	10	11	1.10 (+0.32)
11	13	15	1.15 (+0.38)
12	41	57	1.39 (+0.80)

TABLE 7

VARIATION OF HIRANO BODY DENSITY IN POSITIVE FIELDS

CASE	Number of Positive Fields	Number of Hirano Bodies	Mean Number of Hirano Bodies per Field (+1 S.D.)
5	204	315	1.54 (+0.84)
10	93	117	1.26 (+0.49)
12	29	30	1.03 (+0.19)

RESULTS

The actual ranking orders of the Mean Adjusted Field Indices for neurofibrillary tangles (Table 2, numbers in parentheses) were compared by means of Spearman's rank correlation test against each possible order of permutation within each of the six "zones". That particular rank order with the best statistically significant correlation was "entorhinal>subiculum>H_1>endplate>presubiculum>H_2", in diminishing magnitude of density of tangle-positive microscopic fields. For this permutation the mean of all six r_S coefficients of correlation was 0.910; and in all six of those situations $p<0.01$. (This best order could also have been anticipated from the rank order of magnitude of the six means of all twelve rank numbers in each "zone".) Thus in each "zone" the likelihood that all twelve actual ranking numbers in the vertical column would have so closely approached the best rank number of each "zone" merely by chance is less than 1 in 100.

For granulovacuoles, the rank order of Mean Field Indices (from Table 3, numbers in parentheses) having the best statistically significant correlation was a little different -- "subiculum>H_1>H_2>endplate>entorhinal>presubiculum". For this permutation the mean of the six r_S correlation coefficients was even higher, at 0.929; and once more in all six "zones" $p<0.01$.

For Hirano bodies, the rank order of Mean Field Indices (from Table 4, numbers in parentheses) with the best statistically significant correlation was somewhat different yet again -- "H_1>subiculum>H_2>entorhinal>endplate>presubiculum". This permutation gave a mean for the six r_s correlation coefficients of 0.959; again in all six "zones" $p<0.01$.

Previous workers[14,15] had found tangle formation to be worst in the glomerular formations of Arnold. As many of these clustered neurones are situated in the parahippocampal gyrus, their impression would be in accord with our observations that the entorhinal cortex most often exhibits the heaviest density of tangle-positive fields, although the same region is much less involved by granulovacuoles. Woodard[1] had also noted granulovacuolar degeneration to be considerably less prevalent in the parahippocampal cortex.

Our rank orders indicate that both the H_1 zone of Rose and the adjacent subiculum are virtually always severely afflicted by tangles, as Goodman[15], Hooper and Vogel[10], and Hirano and Zimmerman[14] had commented; by granulovacuoles, as Corsellis[4], Tomlinson and Kitchener[7] had remarked; and by Hirano bodies, as Hirano et al[17], Ogata and co-workers[8], and Gibson and Tomlinson[12] claimed.

By contrast both the H_2 "zone" and the endplate (Rose's H_3, H_4 and H_5) are less severely affected by these same three changes. Earlier investigators had also suggested this decreased predilection for tangles and granulovacuoles[4,6,7,10,14], and by implication a similar low predilection for Hirano bodies in these regions as well[8,12,17].

McLardy's comment[6] that the "medial entorhinal cortex" was strikingly spared of neurofibrillary tangles may also be in agreement with our ranking numbers for the presubiculum (probably the same area), which has remarkably little involvement by tangles, granulovacuoles or Hirano bodies in our material.

Although the best rank orders obtain for all three histological parameters both in control brains and those from demented patients of similar age with Alzheimer's disease, the magnitude of such involvement, as the "scattergrams" indicated, is very different. In Table 8 is listed the mean of the Mean Adjusted Field Indices (from Tables 2,3 and 4) for the four controls, and for the eight Alzheimer cases, in each of the six geographic "zones". The values as would be expected are larger in the brains of Alzheimer's disease than in age-matched controls. However, the increment attributable to the Alzheimer process varies from a 6-fold increase (entorhinal) to a more than 40-fold increase (H_2) for tangles; from a 2-fold (entorhinal) to a 14-fold increase (H_2) for granulovacuoles; and from a 4-fold (H_2) to a 9-fold increment (H_1) for Hirano bodies (Table 8).

TABLE 8

MEAN VALUE OF THE MEAN ADJUSTED FIELD INDICES

	Endplate	H_2	H_1	Subic.	Presubic.	Entorhin.
		NEUROFIBRILLARY TANGLES				
Controls	14.89	6.38	27.34	24.17	29.92	89.06
Alzheimer's	280.66	259.94	562.27	707.45	209.02	544.87
Increment:	x18.8	x40.7	x20.6	x29.3	x7.0	x6.0
		GRANULOVACUOLAR DEGENERATION				
Controls	18.30	13.50	37.55	30.30	4.35	26.21
Alzheimer's	115.86	184.91	356.51	335.35	20.35	57.09
Increment:	x6.3	x13.7	x9.5	x11.1	x4.7	x2.2
		HIRANO BODIES				
Controls	0	9.29	22.15	15.04	0	0
Alzheimer's	2.84	38.28	206.31	101.25	2.42	2.55
Increment:	N/A	x4.1	x9.3	x6.7	N/A	N/A

For both of the first two parameters mentioned, the entorhinal indices increase by the smallest increment, those of the presubiculum by the next largest, the end-plate by the next, H_1 the next, subiculum by the next (second greatest) and H_2 by the biggest increment (Table 8). All six hippocampal "zones" thus apparently maintain a similar relative susceptibility to the degree of augmented involvement by these two different lesions. However, the increments in affliction by Hirano bodies are smallest in H_2, larger in subiculum, and the largest in H_1 (Table 8).

DISCUSSION

As yet there is no solid explanation for the striking histotopographic predilections in location of these three degenerative phenomena in the hippocampi of aged or demented people's brains. There is clearly a preferential affliction of Rose's H_1 field both in the Sommer sector of its lateral part and in its medial end with contiguous subiculum; a notable sparing of the presubiculum; and a relatively mild involvement of H_2 and of the endplate.

The clinical neuropathologist is immediately reminded of an analogous focal phenomenon, the so-called "selective vulnerability" of different parts of hippocampal cortex to hypoxic or epileptic insults[20,21]. In those events, H_2, the 'resistant zone', is less vulnerable, while H_1 and the end-folium are the most vulnerable. The entorhinal region is frequently involved when H_1 is affected. The dentate gyrus is least vulnerable of all.

Our best ranking orders in aged and demented cases do suggest likewise that H_2 is less vulnerable to all three histological changes; that H_1 (and the adjacent subiculum) are highly at risk; that the entorhinal neurones are frequently involved, by neurofibrillary tangles at any rate; and that the fascia dentata is least vulnerable, since no tangles, granulovacuoles or Hirano bodies have ever been noted there in our material to date.

The data comparing the quantitative changes in density of positive microscopic fields (Table 8) have not, of course, been corrected for potential differences in neuronal packing densities within the six different "zones". The same reservation applies to our rank order tests. On the other hand, a "zone" with fewer neurones per unit volume than its neighbours might actually not contain the expectedly fewer tangles, granulovacuoles or Hirano bodies per unit volume. In another study[22] we in fact found that tangles and granulovacuoles (in the posterior hippocampus) are proportionately more common in Alzheimer brains compared to controls than the relative differences in neurone population densities would have predicted from the same sections.

Given these limitations, there may be some import to the finding that while the superimposition of the Alzheimer process on physiological ageing augments the density both of tangles and of granulovacuoles most markedly in the H_2 "zone", dementia appears to be accompanied by the largest increment of Hirano body density in H_1

instead. Furthermore, the maximal change there may be only a 9-fold increase, while the maximal increment for granulovacuoles may be 14 times, and for tangles 40 times. These differences in the locations at greatest risk and in the magnitude of this increased risk might explain such findings as that of Ogata and co-workers[8], who reported no difference in the number of rod-like structures of Hirano between 50 normal brains and 31 cases of "senile brain" disease (or any other pathological condition). Even when the Hirano body counts in elderly dements have significantly exceeded normal controls, as Gibson and Tomlinson[12] noted in their comparison of 16 dements and 6 normals age 60 years and over, the suggestion has been made that Hirano bodies are less likely than tangles to be important in the development of dementia because of their virtual restriction to the hippocampus. Also, whereas tangles and granulovacuoles are clearly intraneuronal (perikaryal) abnormalities, Hirano bodies may be extra-neuronal and there is even considerable uncertainty about which cells produce them[12]. If they were produced by glial cells[12,23], our noting their greatest propensity for H_1 in dementia would agree with Morel and Wildi's observation[24] that of 233 "ischemic glial scars" in 128 brains both from older controls and psychiatric patients (including dements), the H_1 zone with subiculum was the most heavily involved (102 lesions), with the H_2 area less so (95), and still less the endplate (18) or presubiculum (6).

Two main theories have been advanced to explain the cytoarchitectonic selectivity of hypoxic cortical lesions[20]: the anatomic 'vascular' hypothesis originally popularized by Spielmeyer[25], and the physicochemical notion of 'pathoclisis' put forward by the Vogts[26]. Neither hypothesis completely accounts for the phenomenon. Rather than branching dichotomously like most other parts of the cerebral arteriolar tree, the terminal hippocampal arterioles are believed to divide into a series of arcades arranged in a rake-like pattern[27]. It has been suggested that hypotensive episodes exert a much larger hydrodynamic effect on the vascular bed of such rake-like configurations than in dichotomously dividing vessels where the falling intravascular pressure is equally distributed[27]. Angioarchitectonic studies of the hippocampal microvasculature should determine if such anastomotic arcades are more prevalent in the vascular supply to the regions of greatest predilection for the histological changes already discussed. In any case, it is by no means established whether regional cortical hypoperfusion or hypoxia predisposes to tangles, granulovacuoles or Hirano bodies.

A second possibility is that the phenomenon of chemical specificity of "chains" of neurones functionally linked by a common neurotransmitter substrate underlies these regional hippocampal variations. If the memory circuitry of the limbic system proves dependent on cholinergic synapses[28], and if a cortical deficiency of choline acetyltransferase in Alzheimer's disease[29,30,31,32] indicates a particular jeopardy of one neurochemical system, the sparing of some hippocampal "zones" from these lesions may mean the neurotransmitter for that afferent path is resistant, while another transmitter utilized by a different set of afferents (perhaps choline-dependent) is especially at risk[33].

Whatever the explanation, some focally accentuated mechanism appears to involve some hippocampal regions both in ageing and in the dementing process far more selectively than their close neighbours.

ACKNOWLEDGEMENTS

This investigation was supported by the Canadian Geriatrics Research Society; and also by the University Hospital Research Trust Fund. The assistance of Drs. B. Flumerfelt, L. Beattie, M. Smout, B. Adilman, W.F.E. Brown, J. Allcock, H.J.M. Barnett and R. Goyer is gratefully acknowledged.

The author thanks Charles Vis and Mary A. Bell for technical assistance; Mr. B. Greyson for constructing the microscope-pen recorder interface; and Mr. M. Donnelly, Mr. G. Moogk, Mrs. V. Bruckschwaiger and Mr. G. Pettigrew for graphics.

REFERENCES

1. Woodard, J.S. (1962) Clinicopathological significance of granulovacuolar degene-ration in Alzheimer's disease. J. Neuropath. Exp. Neurol., 21, 85-91.

2. Tomlinson, B.E., Blessed, G. and Roth, M. (1968) Observations on the brains of non-demented old people. J. Neurol. Sci., 7 , 331-356.

3. Tomlinson, B.E., Blessed, G. and Roth, M. (1970) Observations on the brains of demented old people. J. Neurol. Sci., 11, 205-242.

4. Corsellis, J.A.N. (1970) The limbic areas in Alzheimer's disease and in other conditions associated with dementia. In: Alzheimer's disease: A Ciba Foundation Symposium, G.E.W. Wolstenholme and M. O'Connor, eds., J. and A. Churchill, London, pp. 37-50.

5. Dayan, A.D. (1970) Quantitative histological studies on the aged human brain. II. Senile plaques and neurofibrillary tangles in senile dementia. Acta Neuropath. (Berl.), 16, 95-102.

6. McLardy, T. (1970) Memory function in hippocampal gyri but not in hippocampi. Intern. J. Neuroscience, 1, 113-118.

7. Tomlinson, B.E. and Kitchener, D. (1972) Granulovacuolar degeneration of hippo-campal pyramidal cells. J. Path., 106, 165-185.

8. Ogata, J., Budzilovich, G.N., and Cravioto, H. (1972) A Study of Rod-like Structures (Hirano Bodies) in 240 Normal and Pathological Brains. Acta Neuropath. (Berl.), 21, 61-67.

9. Tomonaga, M., Yamanouchi, H., Mannen, T. and Kameyama, M. (1975) On the Hirano bodies observed in the brains of the aged. Japanese J. Geriatrics, 12, 13-17.

10. Hooper, M.W. and Vogel, F.S. (1976) The limbic system in Alzheimer's disease. Amer. J. Pathol., 85, 1-19.

11. Ball, M.J. (1976) Neurofibrillary tangles and the pathogenesis of dementia: a quantitative study. Neuropath. Appl. Neurobiol., 2, 395-410.

12. Gibson, P.E. and Tomlinson, B.E. (1977) Numbers of Hirano bodies in the hippo-campus of normal and demented people with Alzheimer's disease. J. Neurol. Sci., 33, 199-206.

13. Ball, M.J. and Lo, P. (1977) Granulovacuolar degeneration in the ageing brain and in dementia. J. Neuropath. Exp. Neurol., 36, 474-487.

14. Hirano, A. and Zimmerman, H.M. (1962) Alzheimer's neurofibrillary changes; a topographic study. Arch. Neurol., 7, 227-242.

15. Goodman, L. (1953) Alzheimer's disease: a clinicopathological analysis of 23 cases with a theory on pathogenesis. J. Nerv. Ment. Dis., 118, 97-130.

16. Jamada, M. and Mehraein, P. (1968) Verteilungsmuster der senilen Veränderungen im Gehirn. Arch. Psychiat. Nervenkr., 211, 308-324.

17. Hirano, A., Dembitzer, H.M., Kurland, L.T. and Zimmerman, H.M. (1968) The Fine Structure of Some Intraganglionic Alterations. J. Neuropath. Exp. Neurol., 27, 167-182.

18. Corsellis, J.A.N. (1976) Ageing and the dementias. In: Greenfield's Neuro-pathology, W. Blackwood and J.A.N. Corsellis, eds., E. Arnold, London, 3rd edition, p. 813.

19. Stokes, M.I. and Trickey, R.J. (1973) Screening for neurofibrillary tangles and argyrophilic plaques with Congo red staining and polarized light. J. Clin. Path., 26, 241.

20. Brierley, J.B. (1976) Cerebral hypoxia. In: Greenfield's Neuropathology, W. Blackwood and J.A.N. Corsellis, eds., E. Arnold, London, 3rd edition, pp. 43-85.

21. Corsellis, J.A.N. and Meldrum, B.S. (1976) Epilepsy. In: ibid, pp. 771-795.

22. Ball, M.J. (1977) Neuronal loss, neurofibrillary tangles and granulovacuolar degeneration in the hippocampus with ageing and dementia -- a quantitative study. Acta Neuropath. (Berl.), 37, 111-118.

23. Field, E.J., Mathews, J.D. and Raine, C.S. (1969) Electron microscopic observations on the cerebellar cortex in Kuru. J. Neurol. Sci., 8, 209-224.

24. Morel, F. and Wildi, E. (1955) Contributions à la connaissance des différentes altérations cérébrales du grand âge. Arch. Suisses Neurol. Psychiat., 76, 174-223.

25. Spielmeyer, W. (1925) Zur Pathogenese örtlich elektiven Gehirnveränderungen. Zeitschrift für die gesamte Neurologie und Psychiatrie, 99, 756-776.

26. Vogt, C. and Vogt, O. (1937) Sitz und Wesen der Krankheiten im Lichte der topostischen Hirnforschung und der Variierens der Tiere. Journal für Psychologie und Neurologie (Leipzig), 47, 237-457.

27. Scharrer, E. (1940) Vascularization and vulnerability of the cornu Ammonis in the opposum. Arch. Neurol. Psychiat., 44, 483-506.

28. Drachman, D.A. (1977) Memory and cognitive function in man: Does the cholinergic system have a specific role? Neurology, 27, 783-790.

29. Bowen, D.M., Smith, C.B., White, P. and Davison, A.N. (1976) Neurotransmitter-related enzymes and indices of hypoxia in senile dementia and other abiotrophies. Brain, 94, 459-496.

30. Davies, P. and Maloney, A.J.F. (1976) Selective loss of central cholinergic neurones in Alzheimer's disease. Lancet, 2, 1403.

31. Perry, E.K., Perry, R.H., Blessed, G. and Tomlinson, B.E. (1977) Necropsy evidence of central cholinergic deficits in senile dementia. Lancet, 1, 189.

32. Perry, E.K., Gibson, P.H., Blessed, G., Perry, R.H. and Tomlinson, B.E. (1977) Neurotransmitter Enzyme Abnormalities in Senile Dementia. J. Neurol. Sci., 34, 247-265.

33. Perry, E.K., Perry, R.H., Gibson, P.H., Blessed, G. and Tomlinson, B.E. (1977) A cholinergic connection between normal ageing and senile dementia in the human hippocampus. Neurosci. Letters, 6, 85-89.

SENILE DEMENTIA: A FOCAL DISEASE IN THE TEMPORAL LOBE

THOMAS L. KEMPER

Boston City Hospital, Boston, Massachusetts

INTRODUCTION

In the brains of elderly presumed normal individuals, in senile dementia, and in

Alzheimer's presenile dementia a variety of changes have been noted. Of these,

neurofibrillary tangles, neuronal cell loss, granulovacuolar degeneration, and senile

(neuritic) plaques have received the widest attention. Although these changes are

often present in small number in patients without clinical evidence of dementia, they

are more marked in patients with senile dementia and Alzheimer's disease[1,2]. Of

particular interest for the present study and of presumed importance for the patho-

genesis of the dementia, is the regional distribution of these various changes. In

the forebrain they appear to occur in greater concentrations in the hippocampal form-

ation (used here for the hippocampus and subicular fields), parahippocampal gyrus,

and amygdala than in the cerebral cortex . At the level of the reticular formation

of the forebrain and brain stem they are primarily confined to monoaminergic nuclei.

This pattern of distribution can be most readily seen in regional studies of the

occurrence of neurofibrillary tangles. In a systematic survey of their distribution

in the brains of elderly individuals, patients with Alzheimer's disease, and those

with senile dementia, Hirano and Zimmerman[3] noted a preponderance of this change in

these areas. The regional specificity of the various monoaminergic brain stem and

basal forebrain areas in senile dementia was confirmed by Ishii[4] and the relatively

greater involvement of the hippocampal formation, parahippocampal gyrus, and amygdala

than of the cerebral cortex was corroborated by the semiquantitative study of

Hooper and Vogel[5]. The greater vulnerability of the hippocampal formation than the

cerebral cortex in senile dementia was also noted in the quantitative studies of

Dayan[6,7]; according to Ball[8] their density in the hippocampal formation in patients

with senile dementia is six-to-forty times greater than in age-matched controls.

A similar relatively greater vulnerability to neuronal loss also appears to occur

in these same regions. Shefer[9] determined the absolute number of neurons in six

neocortical areas and in the hippocampal formation in "healthy old age," senile

dementia, and Alzheimer's disease. He found that the most marked cell loss in all
three groups was in the hippocampal formation and that in both dementias the neuronal
cell loss was greater in this area than in aged controls. This latter finding has
been recently confirmed by Ball[10]. In our own material the amygdala shows marked
neuronal cell loss only in cases of senile dementia, with the most marked loss in
the monoamine-containing medial, medial central, and cortical nuclei[11]. In the
brain stem age-related neuronal loss has been shown only in the monoaminergic locus
coeruleus, while the other nuclei for which information is available, the inferior
olive, facial nucleus, ventral cochlear nucleus, and abducens and trochlear nuclei
all failed to show age-related cell loss[12].

Granulovacuolar degeneration is confined primarily to hippocampal formation.
There it is found in small numbers in control aged brains, while in patients with
senile dementia it occurs in significantly greater concentrations[13]. According to
Ball[10] both the density of this change and the neurofibrillary tangle are both
positively correlated with the extent of neuronal cell loss in the hippocampus in
senile dementia.

Senile plaques, which occur predominantly in the cortex and amygdala,[2]
apparently do not show the same regional specificity shown by the other changes noted
above[7].

The present study was undertaken to explore in greater detail the distribution
of the neurofibrillary tangle in two of these vulnerable zones, the hippocampus and
parahippocampal gyrus. It was hoped that such an analysis, taken together with the
known connectivity of this region, might provide some further insight into the
pathology of senile dementia.

MATERIALS AND METHODS

The material for this study came from routine autopsies done at the Boston City
Hospital. Fourteen cases were randomly selected with the only criteria used being
the presence of neurofibrillary tangles, freedom from other pathological changes in
the regions studied, and the availability of paried silver (Bodian) and Nissl-stained
sections of the hippocampal formation and parahippocampal gyrus. For each brain
identically processed histological sections from the frontal cortical area FD of

von Economo and Koskinas were also surveyed. The hippocampal areas and the subiculum (subiculum and prosubiculum) were identified according to Lorente de No[14] and the entorhinal areas 28 and Pr2 and the perirhinal area 35 of Brodmann according to Van Hoesen and Pandya[15]. In some sections, areas 28 and Pr2 were not present due to the caudal location from which the block was taken, but all contained all other cyto-architectonic areas. In order to avoid bias all sections were studied without ref-erence to the clinical records.

For each case a template negative image enlargement was made at a fixed magnifi-cation using the Nissl-stained section as a negative in a conventional darkroom enlarger and directly exposing high-contrast enlarging paper. With the aid of a stereomicroscope the limits of each cytoarchitectonic area were identified on the Nissl-stained section and then indicated on the templates and silver-stained sections. Then at a magnification of 100x, with the aid of an ocular reticle, the number of neurofibrillary tangles was counted in a 1 mm wide column throughout the total thick-ness of the central part of each cytoarchitectonic area. The average depth of the column was then determined and the results expressed as the number of tangles per mm^2 of the histological section.

RESULTS

The results are shown in the table together with the age of patients. Cases 1-5 are patients for whom there was no evidence of dementia in the clinical records and are presumed, but not definitely known, to be mentally normal. Cases 6-14 all had clear clinical documentation of senile dementia. In the table these are arbitrarily ranked according to the density of neurofibrillary tangles in the neocortex. The mean age in both groups was similar, respectively 86 and 88 years. It can be seen that in the first group that there were no neurofibrillary tangles in the sample area in the neocortex. Within the study area their highest concentration occurred in areas Pr2 and area 35, followed in decreasing concentrations by the subiculum, CA1, and area 28. None were found in CA2-4 or in the presubiculum. In the patients with senile dementia there was a marked increase in density of neurofibrillary tangles in all areas showing this change in the presumed non-demented individuals. In addition they appeared in small numbers in the temporal neocortex and presubiculum. The most marked increase occurred in CA1 and the subiculum and these two cytoarchitectonic areas had by far the highest density of tangles of any areas studied.

TABLE 1

Table to show the distribution of neurofibrillary tangles according to anatomical location in the hippocampus and parahippocampal gyrus and in the frontal lobe. The data is expressed as the number of neurofibrillary tangles per mm^2 of the histological section.

Case No.	Age	Hippocampal formation			Presubic.	28	Pr2	35	Neocortex	
		CA2-4	CA1	Subiculum					Temporal	Frontal
Presumed non-demented patients										
1	70+	0	0	0.6	0	0	1.7	12.1	0	0
2	83	0	1.0	7.3	0	1.2	3.8	5.5	0	0
3	91	0	0.8	0	0	-	-	4.7	0	0
4	83	0	0	0	0	0.4	1.4	1.3	0	0
5	86	0	2.9	2.7	0	-	-	0	0	0
Average	86	0	0.9	2.1	0	0.5	2.3	4.7	0	0
Senile dementia										
6	90	0	10.0	12.2	0	2.7	4.0	2.1	0	0
7	75	0	2.9	14.3	0.4	8.2	12.3	9.2	1.0	0
8	79	0	1.8	12.7	0	2.2	4.4	1.9	1.2	0
9	89	0	16.7	8.9	0.6	-	-	5.2	1.3	0
10	102	0	3.9	6.4	0	1.0	6.8	4.3	2.1	0
11	84	0	5.0	10.0	2.3	-	-	10.6	2.8	0
12	90	0	46.7	33.3	0	13.8	20.8	11.7	3.2	0
13	92	0	19.0	15.0	1.8	-	-	17.9	4.1	0
14	95	0	116.2	71.3	0	-	-	5.8	7.1	0
Average	88	0	24.7	20.5	1.1	5.6	9.7	7.6	2.5	0

The next highest concentration was in areas Pr2 and 35 followed by 28, the temporal cortex, and the presubiculum. As in the first group, neurofibrillary tangles were not found in CA2-4 of the hippocampus or frontal neocortex. In order to better visualize the selective distribution of the neurofibrillary tangles in these patients with senile dementia, a camera lucida drawing was made of silver-stained section of case 12 (Figure 1). In it the location of each tangle is indicated by a small black dot.

DISCUSSION

This study was designed to determine the relative density of neurofibrillary tangles as an index of severity of involvement of neurons in different cytoarchitectonic areas of the temporal lobe in aged and senile individuals. Although the individual sample areas were small, the results of this study are in agreement with others[6, 7, 8] in that there is a marked increase in the density of neurofibrillary tangles in the hippocampus in senile patients as compared to aged controls, and that the former group is further characterized by the occurrence of neurofibrillary tangles in the neocortex[16].

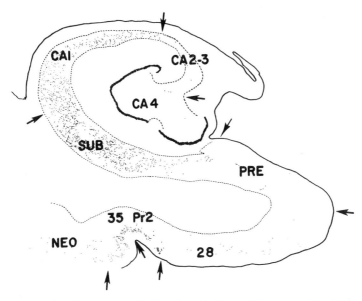

Figure 1. Camera lucida drawing of the distribution of the neurofibrillary tangles in case 12. The location of each neurofibrillary tangle is shown by a small black dot. Neo = Neocortex, PRE = Presubiculum, and SUB = Subiculum. The limits of the cytoarchitectonic areas are indicated by arrows.

Before proceeding with the discussion of the data, it will be useful at this time to review the connectivity of the hippocampus and parahippocampal gyrus[15,17,18,19,20]. This is summarized in Figure 2. All data shown in these diagrams are from the primate experiments and the templates made to correspond to the camera lucida drawing in Figure 1. The location of the cytoarchitectonic areas is shown in Figure 2A. In 2B is shown the neocortical input to this area. It is from limbic cortex and temporal associated cortices. The cingulate cortex projects to the presubiculum via the cingulum bundle. The frontal area FF and the temporal areas TE, TG, TF, and TH project to areas 35 and Pr2 and to a lesser extent to area 28. These various neocortical areas in turn receive projections from association cortices from all

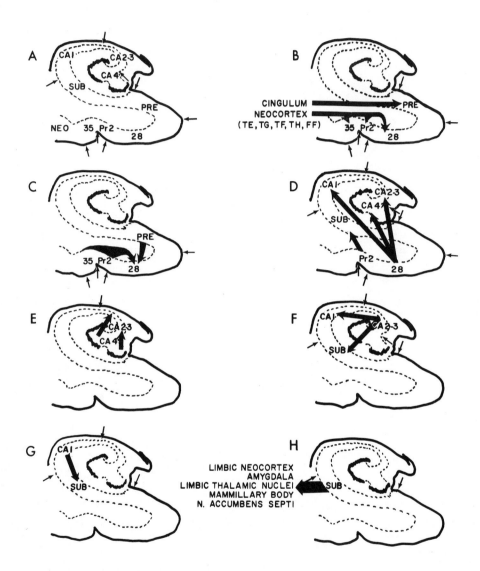

Figure 2. Diagram to show the circuitry of the hippocampus and parahippocampal gyrus. See text for explanation. Abbreviations in figure 1.

lobes of the forebrain[15, 17]. The presubiculum, Pr2,and 35 all project to area 28 (Figure 2C), which in turn projects to the fascia dentata and CA1-4 of Ammon's horn. Pr2 projects to the subiculum (Figure 2D). Figures 2E and 2G show the intrinsic circuits of the hippocampal formation. It can be seen that these are sequential, all eventually projecting to the subiculum with the heaviest projection to this area from CA1. Thus the neocortical input to this region, after complex sequential processing eventually converges on a single area, the subiculum. The subiculum in turn provides virtually the entire efferent (projection) pathway from this entire area, projecting to the limbic neocortical area FL of the frontal lobe, the cingulate cortex, the limbic nuclei of the thalamus (anterior tubercule and nucleus lateralis dorsalis), the amygdala, mammillary body, and nucleus accumbens septi. The only apparent exception is the projection to the septum which comes from a wide area of the hippocampal formation.

In the present study the patients without clinical evidence of dementia showed most marked involvement of the frontal and temporal neocortical input zone, Pr2 and area 35, with preservation of the input zone for the cingulum bundle, the presubiculum. The output zone of this region, the subiculum, and CA1 which has a dense projection to it, showed a smaller number of tangles. All other areas were essentially unaffected. In the patients with senile dementia the highest density of neurofibrillary tangles was in the subiculum and CA1. The average density of tangles in these locations was respectively, 9.8 x to 8.2 x greater than that found in the adjacent temporal lobe neocortex. The average density of tangles in these patients in Pr2 and areas 35 and 28 were intermediate between that found in the neocortex and that found in CA1 and the subiculum. As was also noted in the presumed non-demented elderly patients, both CA2-4 and the frontal cortex appear to be resistant to the formation of tangles in these individuals. In the presubiculum they occurred in only small numbers. Thus in both groups of patients the same four cytoarchitectonic areas, CA1, the subiculum, Pr2, and area 35 appear to be most susceptible to the development of neurofibrillary tangles. The differences were in the relative emphasis on the neocortical input zone in presumed non-demented individuals, and the increase in numbers of tangles and their marked preponderance in the output (projection) zone of

111

of this area in the senile patient.

Although the significance of the location of the neurofibrillary tangle in these locations is unknown, they appear to be in strategic location to interface with the orderly flow of information in this area. Much of it is derived from limbic cortical areas which in turn receive wide projections from neocortical association areas. Its major cotrical efferent projections are back to limbic cortices and its subcortical projections to areas implicated Papez[21] as the anatomical substrate of emotion. This circuit described by Papez consists of the sequential projection of the mammillary body to the anterior nucleus of the thalamus, to cingulate cortex, to hippocampus, and from here closing the loop by its projection to the mammillary body.

The relationship of a lesion in this location to the memory deficit appears to be well documented[22, 23] and it seems likely that the changes noted in these brains are in some way related to this prominent and early feature of senile dementia. Only with careful attention to the pathological changes in these and other areas of brain in well documented individuals with and without senile dementia will it be possible to begin to understand the relationship between structural changes in the brain and the clinical manifestations of this dementing process.

Although neurofibrillary tangle appears to have a strikingly selective predilection for certain cytoarchitectonic areas in the hippocampus and parahippocampal gyrus and apparently elsewhere in the brain, it is not clear in what way these areas of predilection are related. In the reticulate core of the forebrain and brain stem the predilection is for the monoaminergic system. It is possible that the selective changes noted in the various areas of the cerebral cortex and in the amygdala are in some way related to these subcortical monoaminergic cell groups. In this regard it is of interest to note that in eleven of the fourteen brains used for the present study sections from the upper pons and mesencephalus were available. In all cases one or several of the monoaminergic nuclei showed neurofibrillary tangles.

ACKNOWLEDGEMENT

The author would like to thank Gary W. Von Hoesen for his help in the preparation of figure 2.

REFERENCES

1. Tomlinson, B.E. (1977) in Dementia, Wells, C. ed., F.A. Davis Co., Philadelphia, pp. 113-153.

2. Corsellis, J.A.N. (1976) in Greenfield's Neuropathology, Blackwood, W. and Corsellis, J.A.N. eds., Year Book Medical Publishers, Chicago, pp. 796-848.

3. Hirano, A. and Zimmerman, H.M. (1962) Arch. Neurol., 7, 227-242.

4. Ishii, T. (1966) Acta Neuropath., 6, 181-187.

5. Hooper, W.M. and Vogel, F.S. (1976) Amer. J. Path., 85, 1-13.

6. Dayan, A.D. (1970) Acta Neuropath., 16, 95-102.

7. Dayan, A.D. (1970) Acta Neuropath., 1970, 85-94.

8. Ball, M.J. (1976) Neuropath. Appl. Neurobiol., 2, 395-410.

9. Shefer, V.F. (1972) Zh. Nevropat. Psikhiat. Korsakov., 72, 1024-1029.

10. Ball, M.J. (1977) Acta Neuropath., 37, 111-118.

11. Herzog, A.G. and Kemper, T.L. Unpublished observation.

12. Brody, H. and Vijayashankar, N. (1977) in The Aging Brain and Senile Dementia, Nandy, K. and Sherwin, I. eds., Plenum Press, New York, pp. 15-21.

13. Ball, M.J. and Lo, P. (1977) J. Neuropath. Exsp. Neurol., 36, 474-487.

14. Lorente de No, R (1934) J. Psychiat. Neurol., 46, 113-177.

15. Van Hoesen, G.W. and Pandya, D.N. (1975) Br. Res., 95, 1-24.

16. Tomlinson, B.E. et al. (1970) J. Neurol. Sc., 11, 205-242.

17. Van Hoesen, G.W. et al. (1972) Science, 175, 1471-1473.

18. Van Hoesen, G.W. et al. (1975) Br. Res., 95, 25-38.

19. Van Hoesen, G.W. and Pandya, D.N. (1975) Br. Res., 95, 39-59.

20. Rosene, D.L. and Van Hoesen, G.W. (1977) Science, 198, 315-317.

21. Papez, J.W. (1937) Arch. Neurol. Psychiat., 38, 725-743.

22. Van Buren, J.M. and Borke, R.C. (1972) Brain, 95, 599-632.

23. Penfield, W. and Mathieson, G. (1974) Arch. Neurol., 31, 145-154.

CONSIDERATIONS OF TRANSMISSIBLE SUBACUTE AND CHRONIC INFECTIONS, WITH A SUMMARY
OF THE CLINICAL, PATHOLOGICAL AND VIROLOGICAL CHARACTERISTICS OF KURU,
CREUTZFELDT-JAKOB DISEASE AND SCRAPIE

CLARENCE J. GIBBS JR., D. CARLETON GAJDUSEK and COLIN L. MASTERS
National Institute of Neurological and Communicative Disorders and Stroke, National
Institutes of Health, Bethesda, Maryland 20014

I.   INTRODUCTION

Transmissible subacute progressive degenerative diseases of the nervous system
represent an important category of disease, particularly as many of these diseases
were once thought to be "degenerative" in nature. One of the most challenging
aspects in studying these diseases is the elusive nature of the "unconventional"
viruses of kuru, Creutzfeldt-Jakob disease, and scrapie. Observations on their
unusual physicochemical properties and apparent lack of immunogenicity has led to
the possibility that they may represent a new class of microbiologic agent. In
this chapter, we summarize the basic features of subacute and chronic viral diseases
in general, and present in tabular form our current knowledge on the viruses of
kuru, Creutzfeldt-Jakob disease, and scrapie. Recent detailed reviews of these
subjects are available[24-26].

II.   PERSISTENT VIRAL INFECTIONS: GENERAL CONSIDERATIONS[18]
    A.   Terminology
        1.   Viral infection does not necessarily imply disease.
            a.   Apparent or clinical infection is accompanied by disease.
            b.   Inapparent or subclinical infection is silent.
        2.   Latent viral infection is chronic inapparent infection in which there
is a state of equilibrium established between virus and host.
            a.   In some latent infections virus may be easily demonstrable at all
times.
            b.   In an occult infection no infectious virus can be demonstrated,
and the presence of masked virus is only inferred from indirect tests or
circumstantial evidence.
    B.   Patterns of Disease Associated with Persistent Infections of Man or Animals
        1.   Acute clinical illness followed by persistent latent infection with
demonstrable virus
            a.   Prenatal rubella
            b.   Perinatal cytomegalovirus
            c.   ?Infectious and serum hepatitis
            d.   Equine infectious anemia

115

2. Acute clinical illness followed by persistent latent occult infection with one or more recurrences of acute disease during which infectious virus is again demonstrable

      a. Varicella-zoster

      b. Herpes simplex

      c. Herpes B. (H. Simiae of macaque monkeys)

3. Chronic disease in which virus is demonstrable at first, but later becomes masked

      a. Rabbit papilloma

4. Prolonged occult latent infection followed by acute disease during which infectious virus is demonstrable

      a. Swine influenza

      b. Rabies

5. Protracted progressive infection followed by subacute or chronic disease, with infectious virus demonstrable throughout both phases

      a. Kuru

      b. Creutzfeldt-Jakob disease

      c. Scrapie

      d. Transmissible mink encephalopathy

      e. Lymphocytic choriomeningitis of mice

      f. Mouse mammary tumor

      g. Wild mouse ecotropic C-type RNA virus

6. Acute apparent infection with subsequent prolonged occult inapparent infection followed by subacute or chronic disease in which virus remains masked

      a. Subacute sclerosing panencephalitis (Dawson's encephalitis)

7. Protracted or life-long latent infection without apparent disease at any time (virus known to be present only because it has accidentally infected less tolerant hosts which show disease; or, immunosuppressive therapy unmasks the virus)

      a. Rabies in rabbit endothelium tissue culture

      b. Paracrinkle virus in King Edward potatoes

      c. Progressive multifocal leukoencephalopathy

C. Postulated Causes of Virus Masking

1. Virus bound to antibody

2. Virus present in amounts too small to be detected by technique used

3. Virus present only in incomplete and noninfectious form

4. Virus noninfectious during vegetative phase

5. Virus has become "moderate" (adapted to the host cells in which it can no longer initiate recognizable evidence of disease)

6. Virus has been incorporated into the genetic material of the host (provirus)

III. GENERAL CRITERIA OF "SLOW INFECTIONS"[14]

    A. A very long initial period of latency, lasting from several months to several years

    B. A protracted course of illness following the appearance of clinical signs with progression to death

    C. Primary anatomical lesions limited to a single organ system

    D. Limited range of susceptible hosts

IV. SUBACUTE OR CHRONIC ANIMAL DISEASES KNOWN TO BE OF VIRAL ETIOLOGY

    A. Diseases of the Nervous System

        1. Scrapie (sheep, goats, rodents, non-human primates, ?man?)

        2. Mink encephalopathy (mink, ferrets, non-human primates, hamsters)

        3. Visna (sheep)--the same as Maedi and Montana sheep disease

        4. Lymphocytic choriomeningitis (mice)

        5. Virus-induced hind limb paralysis (mice)

        6. Chronic arbovirus encephalitis

            a. Russian spring-summer encephalitis (monkeys, rodents)

            b. Kyasanur Forest disease (mice)

            c. Louping ill (sheep)

    B. Diseases of Other Systems

        1. Maedi hemorrhagic pneumonia; the same as Visna and Montana sheep disease

        2. Aleutian mink disease (mink, ferrets)

        3. Infectious pulmonary adenomatosis (sheep)

        4. Lymphocytic choriomeningitis renal disease (mice)

        5. Neoplastic diseases of rodents, fowl, etc.

            a. DNA oncogenic viruses

                polyoma, papilloma, SV-40

                Shope fibroma

                human adenoviruses

                Lucke frog kidney carcinoma

                Marek's disease of chickens

            b. RNA oncogenic viruses

                mouse leukemia

                avian leukosis

                Rous sarcoma

                mouse mammary tumor

                wild mouse ecotropic virus

                wild mouse amphotropic virus

V. SUBACUTE OR CHRONIC HUMAN DISEASES KNOWN OR SUSPECTED TO BE OF VIRAL ETIOLOGY

    A. Diseases of the Nervous System

        1. Infectious Virus Demonstrated

            a. Kuru

            b. Creutzfeldt-Jakob disease (subacute spongiform encephalopathy or subacute presenile polioencephalopathy)

            c. Progressive multifocal leukoencephalopathy

            d. Familial Alzheimer's disease?

            e. Subacute sclerosing panencephalitis (Dawson's encephalitis)

            f. Chronic arbovirus encephalitis (Kozhevnikov's epilepsy or chronic Russian spring-summer encephalitis with epilepsia partialis continua)

            g. ?Vilyuisk encephalitis

        2. Viral Etiology sometimes Postulated on Histopathological and/or Epidemiological Grounds (without direct demonstration of virus)

            a. Encephalitis lethargica (von Economo's encephalitis)

            b. Presenile dementias (Alzheimer's and Pick's diseases)

            c. Progressive cerebral poliodystrophy (Alper's disease)

            d. Amyotrophic lateral sclerosis and the amyotrophic lateral sclerosis-parkinsonism-dementia complex of Guam

            e. Multiple sclerosis

            f. Leucodystrophies (Schilder's and Krabbe's diseases)

            g. Progressive Supranuclear Palsy (Steele-Richardson syndrome)

            h. Huntington's chorea

    B. Diseases of Other Systems

        1. Virus Demonstrated

            a. Warts

            b. ?Burkitt's lymphoma (Epstein-Barr virus of the herpes group)

        2. Viral Etiology sometimes Postulated because of Histopathology, Epidemiology or Similarity to Known Viral Disease of Animals without other evidence

            a. Leukemias and lymphomas

            b. Other neoplastic diseases

            c. Chronic hepatitis

            d. Chronic connective tissue, cardiac, pulmonary, renal diseases

VI. KURU IN MAN

    A. Major Clinical Manifestations

        1. Clinical course

            a. Insidious onset without fever or systemic illness

            b. Emotional changes

            c. Progressive ataxia and incoordination

d. Fine shivering tremor of extremities, trunk and head, increasing with exertion or fatigue

e. Immobile facies with slow relaxation of emotional expressions, diminished blinking

f. Progressive dysarthria

g. Flexed posture with rigidity (sometimes "cogwheel") later in disease

h. Convergent strabismus

i. Repetitive choreiform and athetoid movements

j. Incontinence

k. Decubitus ulcers

l. Impaired deglutition, starvation and bronchopneumonia

m. Death (3 to 6 months after onset if patients remain in the villages, up to a year in hospital)

2. Negative Findings

a. No fever

b. No convulsions

c. No sensory changes

d. Normal (variable) deep tendon reflexes and plantar responses

e. Normal EEGs

f. Normal blood, urine, CSF studies

g. No demonstrable humoral or cellular antibody to kuru virus

B. Pathology

1. Major neuropathological changes

a. Severe neuronal loss and degeneration

b. Glial proliferation (astrocytes, microglial)

c. Other common findings

Torpedoes of Purkinje cell axons, and antler-like swellings of dendrites

Homogeneous PAS-positive amyloid plaques, doubly birefringent

Moderate spongiform change of cerebral gray matter

Changes are most severe in the cerebellum which may show gross atrophy. There is especially striking reduction in neurons of the granular layer (also marked in the basal ganglia and pontine nuclei).

2. No consistent pathological findings in other systems

VII. TRANSMISSIBLE CREUTZFELDT-JAKOB DISEASE IN MAN

A. Major Clinical Manifestations

1. Clinical course

a. Insidious onset, usually without fever or systemic illness

  b. Behavioral disturbance (confusion, emotional liability, depression, withdrawal)

  c. Progressive dementia

  d. Pyramidal tract signs

  e. Myoclonus and occasionally fasciculations

  f. Characteristic EEG (high voltage periodic synchronous spikes; spike and wave or triphasic complexes on a slow background)

  g. Cerebellar dysfunction

  h. Extrapyramidal signs (ridigity, dystonia, tremor)

  i. Visual abnormalities (including blindness, dyschromatopsia, blurring)

  j. Early higher cortical dysfunction (dysphasia, apraxia, agnosia)

  k. Upper and occasionally lower motor neuron signs

  l. Seizures

  m. Stuporous state followed by coma

  n. Decubitus ulcers

  o. Impaired deglutition, starvation and bronchopneumonia

  p. Liver dysfunction (non-specific)

  q. Familial occurrence

  r. Death (on average, 7 months after onset, but may persist in vegetative state for more than 2 years)

  s. Pneumoencephalopathy and CT scan may show ventricular enlargement, cerebral cortical atrophy, or cerebellar atrophy

 2. Negative Findings

  a. No fever

  b. Normal blood and sugar

  c. CSF usually normal but may occasionally have elevated protein and γ-globulin

  d. No demonstrable humoral or cellular antibody to the CJD virus

B. Pathology

 1. Major neuropathological changes

  a. Spongiform change (variation in intensity and distribution)

  b. Neuronal loss (severity related to duration of illness)

  c. Astrocytic hypertrophy and proliferation (severity related to duration of illness)

  d. Variable degree of gross brain atrophy

  e. Reduction of cortical ribbion of gray matter

  f. Variable PAS-positive plaques

 2. No consistent pathological features in other systems

TABLE 1

COMPARISON OF KURU, CJD AND SCRAPIE

		KURU	CJD	SCRAPIE
A.	Clinical Manifestations in Natural Disease			
	1. Course of Illness			
	a. Long asymptomatic incubation	?5 yrs	+	?2-4 yrs
	b. Insidious onset	+	+	+
	c. Progressive ataxia	+	+	+
	d. Tremors	+	+	+
	e. Behavioral changes	+	+	+
	f. Relentless progression	+	+	+
	g. Dementia	±	+	±
	h. Myoclonus	±	+	±
	i. Characteristic EEG changes	-	+	+
	j. Fasciculations	-	+	+
	k. Somnolence	-	+	±
	l. Death	3-12 mo	1mo->2yrs	2-6 mo
	2. Negative Findings			
	a. Afebrile course	+	+	+
	b. No convulsions	+	±	+
	c. Normal blood, CSF findings	+	+	+
B.	Histopathological Findings			
	1. Distribution			
	a. Primarily gray matter disease	+	+	+
	b. Cerebellum much more severely affected than cerebrum	+	-	+
	c. No significant pathology outside the nervous sytem	+	+	+
	2. Cellular Changes			
	a. Neuronal loss and degeneration	+	+	+
	b. Astrocytic hypertrophy, proliferation	+	+	+
	c. Vacuolated neurons	+	+	+
	d. Spongiform change in gray matter	+ moderate	+ minimal to severe	+ minimal
	e. PAS-positive plaques in some cases	+	+	+
	3. Negative Findings			
	a. No inflammation	+	+	+
	b. No primary demyelination	+	+	+

TABLE 1 (continued)

COMPARISON OF KURU, CJD AND SCRAPIE

	KURU	CJD	SCRAPIE
C. Epidemiology			
1. Endemic enzootic in confined populations	+	- exception[19]	+
2. Disease may appear years after individual leaves the original population	+	?	+
3. Genetic predisposition of the natural host apparently required	?	?	+
4. Familial patterns	+	+	+

TABLE 2

A. SYNONYMS FOR CJD

Disseminated encephalomyelopathy

Spastic pseudosclerosis

Creutzfeldt-Jakob disease

Cortico-pallido-spinal degeneration

Cortico-striata-spinal degeneration

Jakob's syndrome

Presenile dementia with cortical blindness

Heidenhain's syndrome

Subacute vascular encephalopathy with mental disorder, focal disturbances, and
    myoclonus epilepsy

Subacute spongiform encephalopathy

Subacute progressive encephalopathy

Subacute presenile spongiosus atrophy

Nevin-Jones disease

Brownell-Oppenheimer syndrome

B. SYNONYMS FOR SCRAPIE

Tremblante (France)

Polioencephalomyelitis

Convulsive disease

Crazy disease

Nervous disease

Disease of the nerves

Vertigo

TABLE 2 (continued)

B.   SYNONYMS FOR SCRAPIE

Lumbar prurigo

Lumbar neuralgia

Jumping disease

Enzootic peripheric neuritis

Traberkrankheit (Germany)

Guubberkrankheit (Germany)

Wetzkrankheit (Germany)

Surlokozjanka (Hungary)

Rida (Iceland)

TABLE 3

ILLUSTRATIVE DATA ON THE RANGES OF THE INCUBATION AND THE DURATION OF CLINICAL
DISEASE (IN MONTHS) OF VARIOUS SPECIES OF NONHUMAN PRIMATES SUSCEPTIBLE TO THE
SUBACUTE SPONGIFORM VIRUS ENCEPHALOPATHIES

HOST	KURU		CJD		SCRAPIE	
	INCUBATION PERIOD	DURATION PERIOD	INCUBATION PERIOD	DURATION PERIOD	INCUBATION PERIOD	DURATION PERIOD
APES:						
Chimpanzee	10-82	<1-15	11-71	<1-6	(137)	
Gibbon	+(10)	<1	NT		NT	
NEW WORLD MONKEYS:						
Capuchin	10-92	<1-2	29-34	5-11	(28)	
Capuchin	11-71	<1-23	11-47.5	<1-27	32-35.5	3-5
Marmoset	1-76	<1-3.5	18-54	<1-2	NT	
Spider	10-85.5	<1-13	4-50	<1-7.5	38	10.5
Squirrel	8-53.5	<1-5	5-35.5	<1-8.5	8-63	<1-4
Woolly	33	4	21	4.5	NT	
OLD WORLD MONKEYS:						
African green	18	<1	25-57	<1-12	(126)	
Baboon	(124)		47.5	<1	NT	
Bonnet	19-27	<1-2.5	31.5-37	1-2	NT	
Bushbaby	(114)		16	2	NT	
Cynomolgus macaque	16	<1	52.5-60	5-7	27-72	2-22
Patas	(120)		47-60.5	5.5-8	NT	
Pig-tailed macaque	70	7	+(2)	<1	NT	
Rhesus	15-103	<1-2	43-73	<1-12	30-37	11.5-17
Sooty mangabey	+(2)	<1	+(2)-41.5	<1-2.5	NT	

TABLE 3 (continued)

	KURU		CJD		SCRAPIE	
	INCUBATION PERIOD	DURATION PERIOD	INCUBATION PERIOD	DURATION PERIOD	INCUBATION PERIOD	DURATION PERIOD
Stump-tailed macaque (130)			60	6-12	NT	
Vervet	NT		45	<1	NT	

+(n) = the number of months following inoculation before death due to an intercurrent infection in which the animals' brain had histological evidence of spongiform encephalopathy. (n) = the number of months animals have been under observation following inoculation. (n)- = the number of months following inoculation that animal(s) were under observation before dying of intercurrent infections and whose tissues showed no histopathological evidence of spongiform encephalopathy. Numbers shown represent a range in the number of months before onset of clinical diseases and the number of months duration before death or elective killing. NT = not tested.

TABLE 4

NONPRIMATE HOST RANGE OF SUBACUTE SPONGIFORM VIRUS ENCEPHALOPATHIES AND INCUBATION PERIODS IN MONTHS BEFORE ONSET OF CLINICAL DISEASE

HOST	KURU INCUBATION PERIOD	CJD INCUBATION PERIOD	SCRAPIE INCUBATION PERIOD
Cat	(59)	18.5-24	(34)
Ferret	18-70.5	24	(51)+
Gerbil	(24)+	(24)+	4-5
Goat	(104)+	(43)+	8-17
Guinea pig	(27)	14-17	(27)
Hamster	(28)	18	4-12
Mink	45	(36)+	12-19
Mouse	$22-1/2^a$	20^b	4-17
Opossum	(22)+	(12)+	NT
Raccoon	NT	NT	NT
Rat	(51)	4	7-10
Sheep	(63)+	(63)+	5-12
Skunk	NT	NT	NT
Vole	NT	NT	2-4

[a] Spongiform encephalopathy developed in one mouse (Balb C strain) 22-1/2 months following intracerebral inoculation of human brain from kuru patient IGIERAKABA; however, spongiform encephalopathy has not been observed in several hundred additional mice of several strains inoculated with suspensions of brain from an additional 8 patients and 6 animals affected with kuru.

TABLE 4 (continued)

[b] Spongiform encephalopathy developed in one mouse (C3H strain) 20 months following inoculation of human brain from CJD patient M. Ma.; however, spongiform encephalopathy has not been observed in several hundred additional mice of several strains inoculated with suspensions of brain from an additional 4 patients and 2 animals affected with CJD. Transmission of CJD to mice has been independently reported by other investigators[57].

NT = Not tested.

TABLE 5

TRANSMISSION OF KURU AND CJD BY VARIOUS ROUTES OF INOCULATION SHOWING RANGE OF ASYMPTOMATIC INCUBATION PERIODS IN MONTHS ASSOCIATED WITH EACH ROUTE

ROUTE	KURU	CJD
i.c. (intracerebral)	+(2)-103[a]	+(2)-73
i.v. (intravenous)	11	+(5)-44
i.p. (intraperitoneal)	27	(94)
s.c. (subcutaneous)	32	(18)
i.m. (intramuscular)	24	11
p.o. (by mouth)	(110)	(17)
i.d. (intradermal)	(36)	(37)
i.n. (intranasal)	(6)-	(NT)
i.o. (intraocular)	(5)-	(5)-
i.s. (intraspinal)	(NT)	(85)
i.n., i.o.	(66)	(NT)
i.d., vac. (vaccination)	(66)	(NT)
s.c., i.d.	(NT)	24
i.v., i.p., i.m.	(NT)	16
i.p., s.c., i.m.	18	(32)-
i.v., i.p., s.c., i.m.	13-82	(NT)
transfusion	(NT)	(39)
corneal transplant	(NT)	(40)

[a] A plus sign followed by a number in parentheses, +(n), indicates positive histopathologic lesions in brain of animals dying of intercurrent infection; (n) = number of months following inoculation that animal(s) have remained asymptomatic; (n)- = number of months animal(s) were on test before dying with nonspecific illnesses and whose CNS tissues were histopathologically negative for kuru and/or CJD.

TABLE 6

DETECTION OF VIRUS IN INDIVIDUAL ORGANS OR FLUIDS OF PATIENTS AND NONHUMAN PRIMATES WITH KURU OR CJD

	KURU (origin of specimens)		CJD (origin of specimens)	
	HUMANS	ANIMALS	HUMANS	ANIMALS
Adrenal			NA[a]	
CSF	−	−	+	
Cord	+		NA	
Cornea			−	−
Diaphragm			NA	
Eyeball			NA	
Feces			NA	
Heart			NA	
Kidney	+	−	+	−
Liver	−	−	+	
Lung			+	
Lymph node	+	−	+	−
Lymphocytes			NA	
Milk	−			
Muscle	−		NA	
Peripheral nerve			NA	
Placenta amnion	−			
Saliva			NA	
Semen			NA	
Spleen	+	−	NA	
Testes			NA	
Thyroid			NA	
Urine	−		NA	
Blood (transfusion unit)[b]			NA	−
Corneal transplant				−
Liver-spleen-kidney-node	−	+	+	
Muscle-lung-heart			−	
Serum/blood	−		−	

[a] Indicates recently initiated experiments in which the incubation periods have not been of long enough duration to warrant a negative result.

[b] 500 ml of whole blood containing anticoagulant transfused from patient to chimpanzee.

TABLE 7

ATYPICAL PROPERTIES OF UNCONVENTIONAL VIRUSES

PHYSICAL AND CHEMICAL PROPERTIES

Resistant to:

    Formaldehyde

    β-Propiolactone

    EDTA

    Proteases (trypsin, pepsin)

    Nucleases (ribonucleases A and III, deoxyribonuclease I)

    Heat (80°C); incompletely inactivated at 100°C

    Ultraviolet radiation: 2540 Å

    Ionizing radiation (γ rays): equivalent target 150,000 d

    Ultrasonic energy

Atypical ultraviolet action spectrum: 2370 Å = 6x2540 Å inactivation

Invisible as recognizable viron by electron microscopy (only plasma membranes, no
    cord and coat)

No nonhost proteins demonstrated

BIOLOGIC PROPERTIES

Long incubation period (months to years; decades)

No inflammatory response

Chronic progressive pathology (slow infections)

No remissions or recoveries: always fatal

"Degenerative" histopathology: amyloid plaques, gliosis

No visible virion-like structures by electron microscopy

No inclusion bodies

No interferon production or interference with interferon production by other viruses

No interferon sensitivity

No virus interference (with more than 30 different conventional viruses)

No infectious nucleic acid demonstrable

No antigenicity

No alteration in pathogenesis (incubation period, duration, course) by immuno-
    suppression or immunopotentiation:

    ACTH, cortisone

    Cyclophosphamide

    X-ray

    Antilymphocytic serum

    Thymectomy or splenectomy

    Nude athymic mice

    Adjuvants

TABLE 7 (continued)

BIOLOGIC PROPERTIES (continued)

Immune B-cell and T-cell functions intact *in vivo* and *in vitro*

No cytopathic effect in infected cells *in vitro*

Varying individual susceptibility to high infection dose in some host species (as scrapie in sheep)

---

c The Nobel Foundation 1977.

TABLE 8

CLASSIC VIRUS PROPERTIES OF UNCONVENTIONAL VIRUSES

Filterable to 25 nm average pore diameter (APD) (scrapie, TME), 100 nm APD (kuru, CJD)

Titrate "cleanly" (all individuals succumb to high LD_{50} in most species)

Replicate to titers of 10^8/g to 10^{12}/g in brain

Eclipse phase

Pathogenesis: first replicate in spleen and elsewhere in the reticuloendothelial system, later in brain

Specificity of host range

"Adaptation" to new host (shortened incubation period)

Genetic control of susceptibility in some species (sheep and mice for scrapie)

Strains of varying virulence and pathogenicity

Clonal (limiting dilution) selection of strains from "wild stock"

Interference of slow-growing strain of scrapie with replication of fast-growing strain in mice

---

c The Nobel Foundation 1977.

REFERENCES

1. Abinanti, F.R. (1967) The possible role of microorganisms and viruses in the etiology of chronic degenerative diseases of man. Ann. Rev. Microbiol. 21: 467-493.

2. Alper, T., Haig, D.A., and Clarke, M.C. (1966) The exceptionally small size of the scrapie agent. Biochem. Biophys. Res. Commun. 22: 278-283.

3. Gajdusek, D.C. (1967) Slow virus infections of the nervous system. New Eng. J. Med. 276: 392-400.

4. Gajdusek, D.C., Gibbs, C.J. Jr., and Alpers, M. (1967) Transmission and passage of experimental "kuru" to chimpanzees. Science 155: 212-214.

5. Gibbs, C.J. Jr. (1967) Search for infectious etiology in chronic and subacute degenerative diseases of the central nervous system. Current Topics in Microbiol and Immunology 40: 44-58.

6. Gibbs, C.J. Jr., Alpers, M., and Gajdusek, D.C. (1967) Attempts to transmit subacute and chronic neurological diseases to animals. With a progress report on the experimental transmission of kuru to chimpanzees. Presented at the Workshop on "Contributions to the Pathogenesis and Etiology of Demyelinating Diseases", Locarno, Switzerland, May 31-June 3.

7. Gibbs, C.J. Jr. and Gajdusek, D.C. (1966) General considerations of slow virus infections. Symposia Series Immunobiological Standardization 1: 131-146.

8. Gibbs, C.J. Jr. and Gajdusek, D.C. (1967) The epidemiology of slow virus infections. Transactions of the Thirty-second North American Wildlife and Natural Resources Conference, pp 396-404.

9. Gibbs, C.J. Jr. and Gajdusek, D.C. (1967) Kuru--a prototype subacute infectious disease of the nervous system as a model for the study of amyotrophic lateral sclerosis. Presented at the Symposium of Amyotrophic Lateral Sclerosis and Related Disorders, The Institute of Medical Sciences, Presbyterian Medical Center, San Francisco, and the National Multiple Sclerosis Society, Inc., April 29-May 1, San Francisco. In: Contemporary Neurology Symposia.

10. Gibbs, C.J. Jr., Gajdusek, D.C., Asher, D.M., Alpers, M.P., Beck, E., Daniel, P., and Matthews, W.B. (1968) Creutzfeldt-Jakob disease (spongiform encephalopathy): transmission to the chimpanzee. Science 161: 388-389.

11. Gajdusek, D.C. and Zigas, V. (1957) Degenerative disease of the central nervous system in New Guinea. (The endemic occurrence of "kuru" in the native population). New Eng. J. Med. 267: 974-978.

12. Hadlow, W.J. (1959). Scrapie and kuru. Lancet 2: 289-290.

13. Hunter, G.D. and Millison, G.C. (1964) Studies on the heat stability and chromatographic behavior of the scrapie agent. J. Gen. Microbiol. 37: 251-258.

14. Sigurdsson, B. (1954) Observations on three slow infections of sheep. Brit. Vet. J. 110(7,8,9): 255-270, 307-322, 341-354.

15. Chronic Infectious Neuropathic Agents (CHINA) and other Slow Virus Infections. Edited by J.A. Brody, W. Henle and H. Koprowski. Springer-Verlag, New York. 1967.

16. Conference on Measles Virus and Subacute Sclerosing Panencephalitis. Edited by J.L. Sever and W. Zeman, Neurology 18(part 2), 1968.

17. Slow, Latent and Temperate Virus Infections. Edited by D.C. Gajdusek, C.J. Gibbs, Jr. and M. Alpers. Washington, D.C. Government Printing Office, 1965. (NINDB Monograph No. 2, PHS Publication No. 1378).

18. Symposium on Latency and Masking in Viral and Rickettsial Infections. Edited by D.L. Walter, R.P. Hanson and A.S. Evans. Burgess, Minneapolis, 1957.

19. Kahana, E., Alter, M., Braham, J., and Sofer, D. (1974) Creutzfeldt-Jakob disease: Focus among Libyan Jews in Israel. Science 183: 90-91.

20. Roos, R., Gajdusek, D.C., and Gibbs, C.J. Jr. (1973) The clinical characteristics of transmissible Creutzfeldt-Jakob disease. Brain 96:Part I, 1-20.

21. Ferber, R.A., Wiesenfeld, S.L., Roos, R.P., Bobowick, A.R., Gibbs, C.J. Jr., and Gajdusek, D.C. (1974) Familial Creutzfeldt-Jakob disease: transmission of the familial disease to primates. Internat'l Congress Series No. 319, Neurology pp 358-380.

22. Gajdusek, D.C. and Gibbs, C.J. Jr. (1975) Familial and sporadic chronic neurological degenerative disorders transmitted from man to primates. In: Primate Models of Neurological Disorders, B.S. Meldrum and C.D. Marsden, editors. Advances in Neurology 10: 291-317. Raven Press, New York.

23. Gibbs, C.J. Jr. and Gajdusek, D.C. (1975) Studies on the viruses of subacute spongiform encephalopathies using primates their only available indicator. In: Proceedings of the First Inter-American Conference on Conservation and Utilization of American Non-Human Primates in Biomedical Research, Lima, Peru, June 2-4.

24. Traub, R.D., Gajdusek, D.C., and Gibbs, C.J. Jr. (1977) Transmissible virus dementias. The relation of transmissible spongiform encephalopathy to Creutzfeldt-Jakob disease. In: Aging, Dementia and Cerebral Function, M. Kinsbourne and L. Smith, editors. Charles C. Thomas Publishing, Springfield, Illinois. Spectrum Publishing Company, Flushing, New York.

25. Gajdusek, D.C. (1977) Unconventional viruses and the origin and disappearance of kuru. In: Les Prix Nobel en 1976, pp. 167-216. P.A. Norstedt and Soner, Stockholm. Also: Science 197:4307(September 2), 943-960.

26. Gibbs, C.J. Jr. and Gajdusek, D.C. (1978) Atypical viruses as the cause of sporadic, epidemic, and familial chronic diseases in man: slow viruses and human diseases. In: Perspectives in Virology, Volume 10, edited by Morris Pollard. Raven Press, New York. In press.

27. Manuelidis, E.E., Gorgacz, E.J., and Manuelidis, L. (1978) Transmission of Creutzfeldt-Jakob disease with scrapie-like syndromes to mice. Nature 271: 778-779.

28. Tateishi, J., Koga, M., Ohta, M., Yamashita, Y., Shibisaki, H., and Kuroiwa, Y. An animal experiment of spongiform encephalopathy associated with kuru plaques and degeneration of the white matter: the first report. Presented at the ALS Meeting in Tokyo, Japan, February 2-3, 1978.

CEREBRAL HEMODYNAMICS AND METABOLISM IN DEMENTIA: FEATURES DISTINGUISHING NORMAL
PRESSURE HYDROCEPHALUS FROM ATROPHY

MARCUS E. RAICHLE, M.D., ROBERT L. GRUBB, JR., MOKHTAR H. GADO, M.B., B.CH.,
F.F.R., JOHN O. EICHLING, PH.D., CHARLES P. HUGHES, M.D.
Mallinckrodt Institute of Radiology, Washington University School of Medicine,
510 South Kingshighway, St. Louis, Missouri 63110 (USA)

ABSTRACT

Cerebral atrophy and normal pressure hydrocephalus cause significant decreases
in cerebral blood flow and $CMRO_2$ and a mild, not significant increase in cerebral
blood volume. Similar changes in cerebral hemodynamics and metabolism were seen in
both groups of patients. These studies were not found to be useful in distinguishing
patients with cerebral atrophy from those with normal pressure hydrocephalus.
Changes in cerebral blood flow after acute decreases in the intracranial pressure
also were not useful in distinguishing these two groups of patients and, thus, are
not likely to be helpful in identifying patients that would have a favorable
outcome of CSF-shunting.

INTRODUCTION

Since the description of the syndrome of normal pressure hydrocephalus in
1965[1,2], there has been enthusiastic use of cerebrospinal fluid (CSF) shunting
procedures in dementia patients with normal CSF pressure. Unfortunately, clinical
signs and several diagnostic procedures, such as pneumoencephalography, isotopic
cisternography, and CSF infusion studies, are not always reliable in differentiating
normal pressure hydrocephalus from dementias of other etiologies[3,4]. Furthermore,
the diagnostic procedures commonly used to establish the diagnosis of idiopathic
normal pressure hydrocephalus often fail to predict which patients will improve
after shunting of the CSF[5].

It has been proposed that the symptoms and signs of normal pressure hydrocephalus
are produced by reduced cerebral blood flow secondary to distention of the
ventricles[6]. Cerebral blood flow was found to be reduced in normal pressure
hydrocephalus, and CSF shunting procedures were reported to restore cerebral blood
flow values to normal levels. Clinical improvement and reduced ventricular size
were described when cerebral blood flow increased following the placement of a
CSF shunt[7-9]. In patients with normal pressure hydrocephalus after the CSF pressure
was lowered by lumbar puncture, increased cerebral blood flow and cerebral blood
volume were reported to be good indicators of successful outcome of CSF shunting
and useful aids in differentiating normal pressure hydrocephalus from other
dementias[10].

We therefore measured cerebral blood flow, cerebral oxygen utilization ($CMRO_2$) and cerebral blood volume in patients with dementia to see if these studies would be of value in differentiating normal pressure hydrocephalus from dementia caused by cerebral atrophy. In several patients, we obtained a second measurement of cerebral blood flow, $CMRO_2$, and cerebral blood volume after acutely lowering the intracranial pressure to determine if this procedure could be of use in predicting the clinical outcome of CSF shunting.

METHODS

Forty-nine studies of regional cerebral blood flow (rCBF), regional cerebral oxygen utilization ($rCMRO_2$), and regional cerebral blood volume (rCBV) were performed in 30 unselected, but not formally randomized, patients undergoing diagnostic cerebral angiography for evaluation of dementia. Informed consent for measurements of cerebral blood flow, $CMRO_2$, and cerebral blood volume was obtained from the responsible relative of the patients studied. The procedures and consent form used were approved by the Washington University School of Medicine Human Studies Committee. The clinical history, neurologic signs, pneumoencephalography, and isotopic cisternography were used to divide the patients into two groups: normal pressure hydrocephalus and cerebral atrophy. Clinical symptoms and signs used to distinguish normal pressure hydrocephalus patients from those with cerebral atrophy were progressive dementia, gait disorders, and urinary incontinence. Pneumoencephalographic signs of normal pressure hydrocephalus were hydrocephalus with little or no air seen in the sulci over the cerebral convexities, rounding of the lateral angles of the lateral ventricles, a callosal angle of less than 120°, disproportionate enlargement of the trigones of the lateral ventricles, and enlargement of the third and fourth ventricles. Isotopic cisternogram signs of normal pressure hydrocephalus employed were retention of isotope in the lateral ventricles at 72 hours or longer and a block of isotope flow at the mid-convexity or parasagittal regions of the cerebral hemispheres. All patients meeting all these criteria were classified as having normal pressure hydrocephalus and the remainder were considered to have cerebral atrophy. Severity was scored on a formal dementia rating scale[11], administered by one of the investigators (C.P.H.).

By these criteria, 11 patients were classified as having normal pressure hydrocephalus. Ten of these patients were believed to have idiopathic normal pressure hydrocephalus and in one patient the normal pressure hydrocephalus was secondary to a subarachnoid hemorrhage. Ten of these 11 patients underwent a CSF-shunting procedure.

Nineteen patients were included in the cerebral atrophy group. A diagnosis of Alzheimer's disease was made in 13 patients; two patients had Jakob-Creutzfeldt disease, one patient had Huntington chorea, one patient had presenile dementia associated with Whipple disease, one patient had marked cerebral atrophy following a severe diffuse head injury, and one patient had severe presenile dementia associated with a left frontotemporal arachnoid cyst. Seven patients with cerebral atrophy had histologic confirmation of the diagnosis by a brain biopsy. None of the patients with a diagnosis of cerebral atrophy had a CSF-shunting procedure.

The methods employed for the measurement of regional CBF, $CMRO_2$ and CBV are described elsewhere[12-19]. The measurements of regional CBF, volume, and metabolism were averaged for each patient to obtain mean hemispheric values for cerebral blood flow, cerebral blood volume, and $CMRO_2$. This was done for two reasons: (1) The number of regions studied in each hemisphere varied from three in our earliest studies to 13 in our latest studies, thus precluding systematic regional comparison. (2) The resultant changes in flow, volume, and metabolism often occurred diffusely throughout the cerebral hemisphere.

In seven patients in the normal pressure hydrocephalus group and 12 patients in the cerebral atrophy group, the intracranial pressure was lowered by removing 30 to 40 ml of CSF via a lateral C1-C2 spinal tap following baseline studies of rCBF, $rCMRO_2$ and rCBV. However, in three patients this did not significantly improve cerebral perfusion pressure, and these patients were not included in Figure 2. Repeat studies of cerebral hemodynamics and metabolism were then immediately performed. Since the carbon dioxide reactivity of cerebral blood flow was not measured in these patients, cerebral blood flow was corrected for changes in $PaCO_2$ by an increase or decrease in cerebral blood flow of 1 ml per 100 gm per minute for each increase or decrease, respectively, in $PaCO_2$ of 1 mm Hg[20].

T tests were used to test the significance of observed changes in CBF, CBV, and $CMRO_2$ in each group from normal values, and to test the significance of changes seen after the intracranial pressure was lowered by CSF removal.

RESULTS

Cerebral atrophy and normal pressure hydrocephalus produced significant decreases in cerebral blood flow and $CMRO_2$ (p<0.001) (Figure 1). Small, but not significant, increases in cerebral blood volume were seen in both groups of patients (Figure 1). There were not significant differences in the mean values of cerebral blood flow, $CMRO_2$, and cerebral blood volume between patients with cerebral atrophy and normal pressure hydrocephalus. Most patients with both cerebral atrophy and normal pressure hydrocephalus had diffuse changes in cerebral blood flow, $CMRO_2$, and cerebral blood volume. In the patients with focal changes (10% or greater change in rCBF, $rCMRO_2$, and rCBV, as compared with mean hemispheric values of cerebral blood flow, $CMRO_2$,

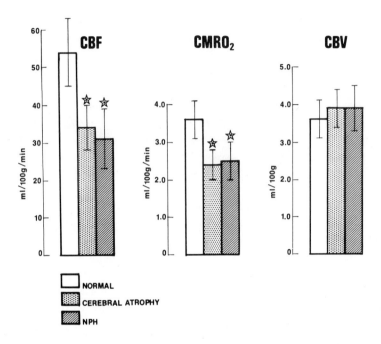

Fig. 1. Mean values of cerebral blood flow, $CMRO_2$, and cerebral blood volume in patients with cerebral atrophy and normal pressure hydrocephalus. Standard deviation of mean values shown by vertical bars. Mean values significantly different from normal values are indicated by stars.

and cerebral blood volume) in cerebral hemodynamics and metabolism, no consistent pattern in the location of focal changes was noted. There was no definite correlation between degree of dementia, as shown by the dementia rating scale score[11], and the amount of depression of cerebral blood flow and $CMRO_2$.

Following the removal of 30 to 40 ml of CSF, there was a small but significant ($p<0.05$) increase in cerebral blood flow in patients with normal pressure hydrocephalus (Figure 2). A similar small, but significant ($p<0.01$) increase in cerebral blood flow also was seen in patients with cerebral atrophy. In both groups of patients there was also improvement in $CMRO_2$ after 30 to 40 ml of CSF was removed (Figure 2). This increase in $CMRO_2$ was significant ($p<0.05$) in the cerebral atrophy group of patients, but $CMRO_2$ was not monitored in enough normal pressure hydrocephalus patients following CSF removal to make a statement about the significance of changes in $CMRO_2$. We must conclude that no distinction could be made between patients with normal pressure hydrocephalus and patients with cerebral atrophy by changes seen in CBF after the intracranial pressure was lowered (Figure 2).

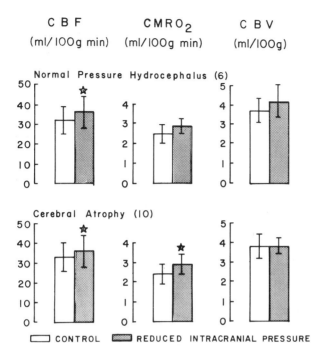

Fig. 2. Mean values of cerebral blood flow (CBF), cerebral metabolic rate for oxygen (CMRO₂), and cerebral blood volume (CBV) before and after acutely lowering cerebrospinal fluid pressure by withdrawal of fluid. Standard deviation of mean values are shown by vertical bars. Mean values significantly different from control values are indicated by stars.

DISCUSSION

Cerebral blood flow was reduced 37% in patients with cerebral atrophy and 42% in patients with normal pressure hydrocephalus. CMRO₂ was reduced 33% in the cerebral atrophy patients and 31% in the normal pressure hydrocephalus patients. Similar degrees of reduction of cerebral blood flow have been reported in patients with cerebral atrophy[3,10,20-25] and normal pressure hydrocephalus[3,7,10,22]. CMRO₂ also has been found to be significantly reduced in demented patients[2,8,26]. It is assumed that cerebral blood flow is reduced as a consequence of the decreased metabolism seen in these patients. This synergism between cerebral blood flow and metabolism is thought to be mediated by metabolically generated hydrogen ions acting on cerebral resistance vessels[27,28]. As metabolism falls, less hydrogen ion is generated. Vasoconstriction occurs, leading to increased cerebrovascular resistance and a fall in cerebral blood flow.

While many patients with dementia due to either cerebral atrophy or normal pressure hydrocephalus have diffuse reductions of cerebral blood flow, many have focal reductions of cerebral blood flow[10,20-22,24,25]. No consistent pattern of focal cerebral blood flow reductions has been reported. Some series of patients had highly variable areas of cerebral blood flow reduction[24], while others had focal cerebral blood flow reductions, predominantly frontal and temporal[21,24,25]. Some severely affected patients with presenile dementia were found to have low blood flow mainly in the occipito-temporal-parietal regions[21]. Most of our patients, with either cerebral atrophy or normal pressure hydrocephalus, had diffuse reductions of cerebral blood flow and $CMRO_2$. However, early in this series we monitored only three to six areas of the cerebral hemisphere. For this reason, it is not possible for us to make a definitive statement about regional cerebral hemodynamics and metabolism in demented patients.

The mild, but not significant, increase in cerebral blood volume seen in both groups was unexpected. It would be anticipated that the decline in cerebral blood flow of 37% in patients with cerebral atrophy and 42% in patients with normal pressure hydrocephalus would be accompanied by a decline in cerebral blood volume of 15% in the cerebral atrophy patients and 18% in the normal pressure hydrocephalus patients[17]. Mathew and co-authors[10] also noted a small (9%) increase in patients with cerebral atrophy, but found a modest (8%) decrease in cerebral blood volume in patients with normal pressure hydrocephalus.

There are three hypothetical explanations for this apparent paradoxical increase in cerebral blood volume observed. First, as tissue atrophies, blood vessels may remain, thus increasing the *relative* vascular density of the tissue. In this regard, the observations of Hassler[29] and Fang[30] on changes of the microvasculature in senile brains are of considerable interest. They have reported an increase in the coiling and looping effects of perforating arteries, arterioles, and venules, sometimes leading to increased length of these vessels. Also small knoblike formations and sinusoidal enlargements along the course of draining venules have been observed in senile brains. Second, it seems reasonable to suggest, although it remains to be proved, that as brain atrophies, the venous capacitance vessels may dilate in response to the alteration in pressure-volume relationships in the closed cranial cavity (i.e., ex vacuo dilation of venous capacitance vessels). Third, the increased cerebral blood volume could be due to a normal autoregulatory response of brain resistance vessels caused by a reduction in perfusion pressure[29-31]. Normally, brain resistance vessels constrict in response to an increase in cerebral perfusion pressure (increased blood pressure or decreased intracranial pressure) and dilate in response to a decrease in cerebral perfusion pressure in order to maintain cerebral blood flow constant. If one assumes that a reduction in cerebral perfusion pressure is involved in the pathophysiology of at least some cases of dementia (e.g., normal pressure hydrocephalus), then an increase, relative to expectation, in cerebral blood volume would not be too surprising. This hypothesis would be supported by, for example, a higher resting cerebral blood volume in demented patients with normal pressure hydrocephalus than in those with atrophy. Furthermore, if this is the explanation, an acute reduction in intracranial pressure by spinal fluid drainage, which in effect increases cerebral perfusion pressure, should be accompanied by a reduction in cerebral blood volume. Unfortunately, our data do not indicate which of these three explanations might be correct, as all three types of response of cerebral blood volume and cerebral blood flow to an acute fall in intracranial pressure were noted in individual patients, and no particular pattern of response emerged in either group of patients in this study (Figure 2).

Mathew and co-workers[10] stated that changes in cerebral blood flow and cerebral blood volume after lowering CSF pressure were useful in differentiating normal pressure hydrocephalus from cerebral atrophy. In their series, patients with normal pressure hydrocephalus had significant increases in cerebral blood flow and cerebral blood volume after the CSF pressure was lowered. These changes were not seen in their patients with cerebral atrophy. This test was also considered a reliable indicator of successful CSF shunting results. The normal pressure hydrocephalus patients with the best clinical outcome after a shunt had the largest cerebral blood flow increases when the CSF pressure was lowered preoperatively. Our results do not support the findings of these authors. We found changes in cerebral blood flow after lowering the intracranial pressure to be of no help in differentiating patients with normal pressure hydrocephalus from patients with cerebral atrophy (Figure 2). Cerebral blood flow increased significantly in both groups of patients.

ACKNOWLEDGEMENTS

This work was supported by U.S. PHS Grants No. HL13851 and NSO 6833 (NINCDS); and by Teacher-Investigator Award No. NS11059 (NINCDS - Dr. Raichle).

REFERENCES

1. Hakim, S. and Adams, R.D. (1965) J. Neurol. Sci., 2, 307-327.
2. Adams, R.D., Fisher, C.M., Hakim, S. et al. (1965) NEJM 273, 117-126.
3. Coblentz, J.M., Mattis, S., Zingesser, L. et al. (1973) Arch. Neurol., 29, 299-308.
4. Messert, B., Wannamaker, B. (1974) Neurol. (Minneap), 24, 224-231.
5. Stein, S.C. and Langfitt, T.W. (1974) J. Neurosurg., 41, 463-470.
6. Greitz, T.V.B. (1969) Lancet, 1, 863-865.
7. Greitz, T.V.B., Grepe A.O.L., Kalmer, M.S.F. et al. (1969) J. Neurosurg., 31, 644-651.
8. Salmon, J.H. and Timperman, A.L. (1971) Neurol. (Minneap), 21, 33-42.

9. Salmon, J.H. and Timperman, A.L. (1971) J. Neurol. Neurosurg. Psychiat., 34, 687-692.

10. Mathew, N.T., Meyer, J.S., Hartmann, A. et al. (1975) Arch. Neurol., 32, 657-664.

11. Blessed, G., Tomlinson, B.E. and Roth, M. (1968) Br. J. Psychiat., 114, 797-811.

12. Eichling, J.O., Raichle, M.E., Grubb, R.L. Jr. et al. (1974) Circ. Res., 35, 358-364.

13. Ter-Pogossian, M.M., Eichling, J.O., Davis, D.O. et al. (1969) Radiol., 93, 31-40.

14. Carter, C.C., Eichling, J.O., Davis, D.O. et al. (1972) Neurol. (Minneap), 22, 755-762.

15. Raichle, M.E., Grubb, R.L. Jr., Eichling, J.O. et al. (1976) J. Appl. Physiol., 40, 638-640.

16. Ter-Pogossian, M.M., Eichling, J.O., Davis, D.O. et al. (1970) J. Clin. Invest., 49, 381-391.

17. Eichling, J.O., Raichle, M.E., Grubb, R.L. Jr. et al. (1975) Circ. Res., 37, 707-714.

18. Grubb, R.L. Jr., Raichle, M.E., Eichling, J.O. et al. (1974) Stroke, 5, 630-639.

19. Grubb, R.L. Jr., Phelps, M.E. and Ter-Pogossian, M.M. (1973) Arch. Neurol., 28, 38-44.

20. Gustafson, L., Risberg, J. (1974) Acta Psychiat. Scand., 50, 516-538.

21. Hagberg, B., Ingvar, D.H. (1976) Br. J. Psychiat., 128, 209-222.

22. Ingvar, D.H., Risberg, J. and Schwartz, M.S. (1975) Neurol. (Minneap), 25, 964-974.

23. Munck, O., Barenholdt, O. and Busch, H. (1968) Scand. J. Lab. Clin. Invest. Suppl 102, 12, A.

24. Obrist, W.D., Chivian, E., Cronquist, S. et al. (1970) Neurol. (Minneap), 20, 315-322.

25. Simard, D., Olesen, J. and Paulson, O.B. (1971) Brain, 94, 273-288.

26. Lassen, N.A., Feinberg, L. and Lane, M.H. (1960) J. Clin. Invest., 39, 491-500.

27. Lassen, N.A. (1968) Scand. J. Lab. Clin. Invest., 2, 247-251.

28. Raichle, M.E., Grubb, R.L. Jr., Gado, M. et al. (1976) Arch. Neurol., 33, 523-526.

29. Hassler, O. (1965) Acta Neuropathol (Berl), 5, 40-53.

30. Fang, H.C.H. (1976) in Neurobiology of Aging, Terry, R.D., Gershon, S. eds., Raven Press, New York, pp. 155-166.

31. Rapela, C.E. and Green, H.D. (1964) Circ. Res., 15 (Suppl), 205-212.

32. Grubb, R.L. Jr., Phelps, M.E., Raichle, M.E. et al. (1973) Stroke, 4, 390-400.

33. Grubb, R.L. Jr., Raichle, M.E., Phelps, M.E. et al. (1975) J. Neurosurg., 43, 385-398.

AGE DIFFERENCES IN CORTICAL EVOKED POTENTIALS: A COMPARISON OF NORMAL OLDER
ADULTS AND INDIVIDUALS WITH CNS DISORDERS

LARRY W. THOMPSON, HENRY J. MICHALEWSKI
Andrus Gerontology Center, University of Southern California, University Park,
Los Angeles, California 90007
RONALD E. SAUL
Department of Neurology, Rancho Los Amigos Hospital, 7601 Imperial Highway,
Downey, California 90242

ABSTRACT

Reliable age differences in event related potentials (ERP) are known to occur
during the adult years. Differences seen in elderly demented patients appear
as exaggerations of normal age differences. The pattern of differences is
influenced by the information value of the stimuli used to obtain the ERP. Two
studies with normal subjects are presented to illustrate this pattern. One
study involves the effects of stimulus repetition and stimulus change on the
ERP; the other examines the effects of uncertainty in making predictions of
stimulus events. The effects of simple auditory, visual, and auditory plus
visual stimulation on the ERP in young and old normals and elderly patients
with central nervous system disorders are also presented. The results emphasize
the need for controlling cognitive processing demands in ERP investigations.

Over 30 years ago Liberson[1] observed that changes evoked in the spontaneous
EEG as a result of sensory stimulation could provide a useful index of cerebral
dysfunction. Subsequent studies have shown decreased reactivity of the EEG to
sensory stimulation in subjects with brain damage,[2,3] in older community volunteers,[4] and in older "poor learners" when compared with older "good learners".[5]
Despite positive results such as these, there have been few investigations in
this area. The difficulties in quantifying the EEG, plus a lack of clinical
scientists who have the requisite skills in computer sciences and mathematics,
have contributed to the limited progress. Advances in computer technology
during the past 15 years, however, have greatly facilitated the study of
specific responses--event related potentials (ERP) which are embedded within
the spontaneous EEG. Computer averaging techniques enable one to extract
electrophysiological responses to repetitive stimuli from background "noise"
in the EEG. Typically, these are complex waveforms containing several positive
and negative components which are known to vary systematically with a number of
biological and behavioral measures, both between- and within-subjects.

139

A near incomprehensible proliferation of studies attest to the sensitivity of the ERP to changes in psychological state, and researchers have been encouraged that this technology might be useful in the diagnosis and prognosis of central nervous system dysfunction. Following the lead of earlier EEG research, a number of studies have demonstrated differences in various ERP components across a variety of patients with neurological disorders when compared with normal controls [6,7,8,9,10,11,12,13,14,15,16]. Some investigators have reported that ERPS are more sensitive than traditional EEG measures in detecting organic pathology,[17,18] and others have reported low correlations between the EEG and ERP.[6,19] While such findings suggest that evoked responses potentially may be a significant tool in clinical work, there are numerous discrepancies and ambiguities in the literature, rendering their usefulness in clinical settings yet unclear. It is surprising, therefore, that clinical research in this area has not progressed at a more rapid pace. With the possible exception of multiple sclerosis and recently brainstem far-field potentials, comparatively few of the evoked potential studies have focused on clinical neurological conditions.

Although technical and methodological differences among studies surely contribute to the confusion in this area, as Oosterhuis et al.[18] have pointed out, age differences may also be an important factor to consider. There are substantial age changes in evoked responses across the life span, and since many central nervous system disorders are age-related, appropriate controls for age should be introduced when attempting to examine the relationship of the ERP to organic pathology. With this in mind, we would like to present data from our laboratory illustrating various ERP changes observed during the late adult age range, with a view to the development of simple techniques for the exploration of evoked responses in central nervous system disorders.

Recent reviews[20,21] have emphasized that there is a consistent picture of change in evoked responses across the adult age range, even though relatively few investigations have been completed. Briefly, elderly individuals show increased amplitude of early components ($\approx < 100$ msec) and substantial decreases in amplitude of later components when passive stimulation is used. This trend is apparent with visual, auditory, or somatosensory stimulation. Latencies of both early and late components are longer for old than for young with visual stimulation. While a similar trend for latencies is seen in the auditory and somatosensory modalities, the picture appears less clear. When active processing of information contained in the stimulus presentation is called for, however, distinctly different patterns are apparent. Age differences in the later components are decreased, and there is some suggestion that the extent of the differences is negatively correlated with the difficulty of the processing task.

The distinction between passive stimulation and active processing clearly emphasizes the need to control for level of cognitive processing in evoked potential studies in attempting to unravel the functional significance of changes in ERP across the adult age range. This same problem also holds for the evaluation of patient groups. For example, studies involving elderly patients suffering from chronic brain syndrome secondary to cerebral arteriosclerosis,[13] and patients with senile dementia of the Alzheimer type,[15] indicate that the most substantial differences between patients and age matched controls occur in the amplitude and latency of later components. In fact, these differences appear on the surface to be exaggerations of the age differences seen in the normal elderly. Since these later components are believed to be implicated in higher cognitive and integrative activity, the trends across age and patient groups render compelling the interpretation that the changes observed are reflective of the dementia process in patients, as well as possible milder cognitive impairment in the normal elderly. On the other hand, the fact that they are so readily modifiable by experimental manipulation of cognitive processing leaves room for another interpretation, particularly if similar patterns of change in these components could be demonstrated in patients with central nervous system disorders. While probably not the case on the basis of the data available, one could convincingly argue that the decreased amplitudes seen in the later components of the elderly and elderly demented patients, may occur simply because they are disinterested in the seemingly irrelevant stimuli, characteristically used to produce the ERPs. A point to be emphasized here pertains to the complexity and dynamic nature of the system being studied, which is, as it should be, exquisitely sensitive to the slightest manipulation of external as well as internal events. As much care, therefore, should be given to the phenomenology of the stimulus complex in evoked potential studies, as is currently given to the elaborate analysis of the scalp potentials. Continued evaluation of psychological factors which affect ERPs is critical in developing an understanding of the mechanisms underlying changes observed in older adults and neurological patients. The basis for this contention may be made clearer by examining age differences in ERPs in experimental paradigms involving active processing.

It is often thought that the reaction of the central nervous system to stimulus repetition and to stimulus change may reflect basic processes associated with higher cognitive activity involved in attention and learning. In view of the cognitive changes which occur with age, it seemed reasonable to question whether older persons would have a different pattern of habituation and dishabituation in the ERP than younger individuals. To investigate this question, we used a paradigm patterned after a study by Ritter et al.[22]

Ten old community volunteers ($\overline{X}$ age = 71 yrs) and 10 young ($\overline{X}$ age = 21 yrs) college students participated. Subjects listened to pure tones (900 Hz) of 50 msec duration presented every 5 sec in blocks of 30 tones for 15 blocks. Three tones in each block were increased in frequency to 3,300 Hz; these occurred randomly between the 3rd and 27th tone of each block. Previous research in our laboratory revealed that these two tones yielded highly similar ERPs from the vertex recording site. By averaging the EEG associated with each tone across the 15 blocks (omitting any novel tone presentation), it is possible to obtain information regarding the change in ERP due to stimulus repetition (habituation). By averaging the 45 higher tones occurring within the 15 blocks, it is possible to obtain information regarding the responsivity of the ERP to stimulus change.

This paradigm was run under two conditions. In one (Ignore Condition) the subject was requested to read excerpts from Newsweek which were duplicated on 5" x 8" cards. In the other (Attend Condition) the subject was requested to count the number of standard tones occurring in each block. In this condition the number of tones in each block varied with a range of 28 to 32 ($\overline{X}$ = 30).

Recordings were obtained from F_z, C_z, and O_z with linked earlobes as the reference, using Grass model 7P122B amplifiers modified to provide a 12 sec time constant. Data were stored on FM tape and analyzed off-line by means of a Varian digital computer following editing for eye movement and other artifacts. ERPs were graphically displayed, and components were identified visually. Amplitude and latency of each of six components were determined and used in subsequent data analysis.

Brent et al.[23] analyzed the data obtained from the vertex placement. Analysis of variance for repeated measures was completed to make comparisons for age (young-old), conditions (Ignore-Attend), and trials. For considering the effects of stimulus repetition, the trial factor was Trial Blocks 1, 2, 5, 10, and 15. For looking at the effects of stimulus change the trial factor included the EP associated with the novel tone (N), the tone immediately preceding the novel tone (N-1), and the one immediately following (N+1).

The results of the overall age comparisons for the standard tones collapsed across conditions and blocks were consistent with other findings in the literature. The old had a larger P_1 amplitude (F = 11.49; df = 1/16; p < .01), and a smaller P_2 (F = 13.25; df = 1/16; p < .01). Latencies were longer in the elderly for P_2 (F = 49.25; df = 1/16; p < .01), N_2 (F = 19.42; df = 1/16; p < .01), P_3 (F = 12.15; df = 1/16; p < .01), and N_3 (F = 4.60; df = 1/16; p < .05). Thus, the data suggest that in the elderly early components (0-120 msec) are enhanced when compared with the young, but there is no change in latency. Intermediate components (120-250 msec) show both reduced amplitudes and prolonged latencies. Later components (250+ msec) show no age differences in amplitude, but latencies are substantially longer in the elderly group.

Age differences associated with stimulus change are illustrated in Figure 1. The mean amplitudes and latencies of the six ERP components are graphically presented for the N-1, N, and N+1 trials in the Ignore condition. Both N_2 and P_3 showed a significant quadratic trend across the three trials (F = 4.76;

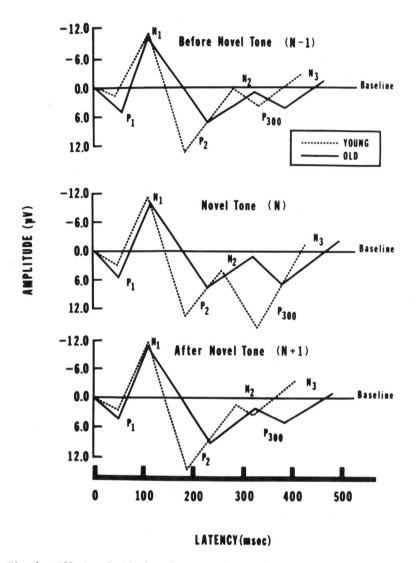

Fig. 1. Effects of stimulus change on the ERP in young and old community subjects. Graphic representation is comprised of mean amplitude and latency for each component in the ERP.

$df = 1/16$; $p < .05$, and $F = 30.88$; $df = 1/16$; $p < .01$, respectively), suggesting that an orienting or dishabituation occurred to the stimulus change. A significant Trials by Age interaction ($F = 10.76$; $df = 2/32$; $p < .05$) for P_3 indicates that the young showed a greater response to the novel tone than the old. No other components showed significant changes.

The only component that distinguished the Attend-Ignore conditions was P_3. A Condition by Trial quadratic trend ($F = 7.06$; $df = 1/16$; $p < .05$) was due to the larger P_3 to the novel tone in the Attend condition when compared to the Ignore condition. The age comparison revealed that while the young showed a P_3 to the novel tone in the Ignore condition, the old did not. In the Attend condition, the old clearly had a P_3 to the novel tone, but this was substantially smaller than the response for the young.

Figure 2 shows the effects of stimulus repetition on the ERP at the vertex recording site for a young and older subject. The decrement in the response of N_1 and P_2 is much more noticeable in the younger subject than in the older individual. While not clearly visible here, P_1 also was reduced across time. None of the other components demonstrated a significant change across blocks. Figure 3 provides the mean amplitude for the young and old groups of these two components plotted for Blocks 1, 2, 5, 10, and 15. The first two points represent the average across Trials 1-20 (20) and Trials 5-25 (25) of the first block. Analysis revealed significant linear trends for N_1 ($F = 14.43$; $df = 1/16$; $p < .01$) and P_2 ($F = 9.70$; $df = 1/16$; $p < .01$) which is due primarily to increased ERPs during the first two blocks. Age differences were also apparent with the young subjects showing a greater response amplitude initially and a more rapid decrement with repetition. Analysis of the F_z and O_z placements were reported in a separate paper,[24] but revealed trends similar to the vertex tracings.

As observed in Figure 2, stimulus repetition tends to make the ERP of old and young more similar. Along with decreased amplitudes, there is increased variability in the response suggesting that the cortical response may not be as systematically time-locked to the stimulus being presented. The general picture of these data makes it appear as if the older subjects were partially habituated at the outset. Similar findings have been reported in the habituation of the alpha blocking response by Obrist.[4]

In summary, it appears that the early and intermediate components are susceptible to change with stimulus repetition while the later components are less responsive. On the other hand, an abrupt change precipitates a greater response in the later components, particularly if the stimuli have some significance for the individual. In this regard P_3 seems to be most sensitive to stimulus change when processing of stimulus information is increased. Age differences are apparent to both stimulus repetition and stimulus change, and it is not clear that they are minimized by increased processing demands.

144

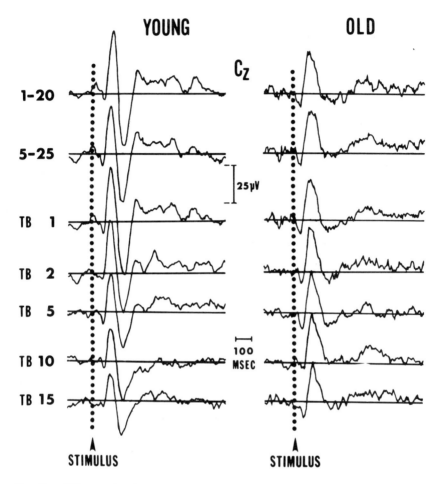

Fig. 2. Effects of stimulus repetition on the ERP in a young and old
community volunteer. TB refers to the average response to standard tones
in the respective trial blocks. The first two points refer to the average
of Tones 1 through 20 and 5 through 25 in the first TB.

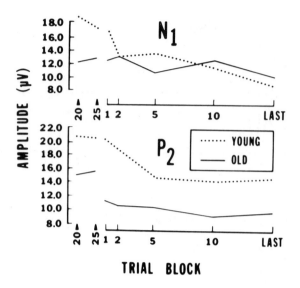

Fig. 3. Mean amplitude of components N_1 and P_2 plotted across trial blocks for both young and old community volunteers.

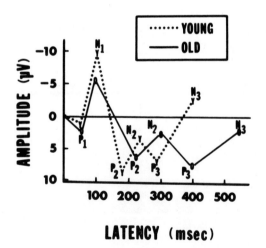

Fig. 4. Mean amplitude and latency for each component comparing young and old volunteers while predicting events in a certainty-uncertainty task.

The task, however, is a simple one (counting standard tones) and may not be of sufficient complexity to enhance ERP responses in the elderly. The old subjects did show evidence of a substantial change in the P_3 waveform to novel tones when required to count, whereas no change was discernible at times when the novel tone carried very little meaningful information.

This study agrees with the other findings in the literature that P_3 (often referred to as $P_{\overline{300}}$, $P_{3(00)}$, or the certainty wave) is associated with cognitive processing. In view of this, we felt that age differences in this waveform should be explored more fully. Smith et al.[25] used a paradigm developed by Sutton et al.[26] to study changes in this potential by manipulating the level of uncertainty of an event. The task consisted of paired signals presented through headphones at variable intervals. The first signal in each pair was 1, 2, or 3 clicks in rapid succession. Following a variable interval, either a low (900 Hz) or high (3,300 Hz) tone was presented. Four possible contingencies were presented to each subject: (1) one click always followed by a low tone; (2) two clicks always followed by a high tone; (3) three clicks followed by a low tone 50% of the time; (4) three clicks followed by a high tone 50% of the time. The subject's task was to predict which tone would be presented in each contingency. Thus, a subject could be certain which tone would follow when 1 or 2 clicks were presented, but uncertain when 3 clicks were presented. The four contingencies were randomly interspersed with the constraint that all would occur an equal number of times. The intertrial interval ranged from 6 to 9 sec, and the interstimulus interval was 3 to 5 sec.

Fifty presentations of each contingency were given to seven old community volunteers ($\overline{X}$ = 68.5) and seven young college students ($\overline{X}$ = 23.4). Both groups were comparable with respect to education and socio-economic status. Vertex ERPs were obtained for the four contingencies using the procedures described earlier.

Figure 4 provides a graphic presentation of the mean amplitudes and latencies for each component during the uncertain condition. In considering amplitude measures, only N_1 showed a significant age difference ($\underline{F}$ = 15.74; $\underline{df}$ = 1/10; $\underline{p}$ < .01). For the latency measures, there was no age difference at N_1, but both P_2 and P_3 were significantly longer in the elderly ($\underline{F}$ = 10.1; $\underline{df}$ = 1/10, $\underline{p}$ < .01 and $\underline{F}$ = 19.6; $\underline{df}$ = 1/10; $\underline{p}$ < .01, respectively). Changes from the certain to uncertain conditions were comparable for both age groups.

As previously noted, these data suggest that age differences in amplitude measures are minimized as task involvement increases. Marsh and Thompson[21] have reported similar trends for latency measures as well in auditory discrimination tasks. Thus, these findings are consistent with others in the literature, but insufficient data make any conclusions tenuous for the moment. Additional studies manipulating type and difficulty of cognitive processing are needed to provide a clearer understanding of how ERPs might be implicated in functional changes.

Such conclusions increase the complexities of devising ERP assessment measures which could be used throughout the life span, and, in particular, include clinical and patient populations. In clinical settings it is fully realized that it is not always possible to directly apply ERP techniques with the control and precision normally demanded, since patient groups differ markedly in their capacity to participate in experimentation. As a starting point, we have been collecting and analyzing ERPs in the normal aged and selected cerebrovascular patients and contrasting the results from these groups to normal young subjects. Initially, our experimental paradigm has been designed to gather bimodal ERPs consisting of responses to simple tones, flashes, and the combined simultaneous presentation of tones and flashes. With a small number of trials in the averaging process, the number of components (beyond 100 msec) which can be identified with certainty in each ERP waveform is limited, especially in patient populations. However, both auditory and visual responses usually exhibit characteristic polyphasic negative-positive waveforms which are prominent after 100 msec and which are separated in time or latency as they appear over the scalp. The ability to keep these simple responses separate or distinct might serve as an index of the brain's integrative capacity or a breakdown in that function. An experiment currently in progress in our laboratories attempts to examine these variables, and some preliminary results are described.

Findings for seven old subjects ranging in age from 70 to 77 years ($\overline{X}$ = 73.7 yrs), five cerebrovascular patients ranging in age from 48 to 69 years ($\overline{X}$ = 61.8 yrs), and five young subjects ranging in age from 17 to 28 years ($\overline{X}$ = 24.4 yrs) are considered. Older subjects were volunteers recruited at the Andrus Gerontology Center and were in excellent health with minimal auditory or visual loss. Young subjects were recruited from the University of Southern California campus.

Recordings of both old and young groups were carried out at the Andrus Gerontology Center, while cerebrovascular patients were recorded at Rancho Los Amigos Hospital after normal clinical EEG testing was performed. Electrode sites F_3, F_4, P_3, and P_4 referred to linked ears were used in the old and young groups, and these same sites referred to the ear contralateral to injury were used in the cerebrovascular cases. Stimulation at both laboratories consisted of 1,000 Hz tones (100 msec, 80 dB), flashes (photic stimulators, intensity 8), and simultaneous tones and flashes, and comprised the three experimental conditions, presented in that order, respectively. Stimuli were separated by a regular 4-second interval. Eyes were closed throughout. Additional conditions were presented to older and younger groups which involved simple motor presses to each type of stimulations, and a go-no go contingency situation. From 60 to 80 stimulus presentations were administered for each condition and averages based on 25 to 35 trials free from eye movement artifact composed each average. Signal processing was performed on a Nicolet MED-80 system.

Typical ERP responses for these conditions are contrasted for an old (74 yrs) and young (25 yrs) subject in Figure 5. In the young, the mean latency of the prominent negative peak for tones ranged between 123 to 125 msec at frontal sites and between 119 to 126 msec at parietal locations; response latencies for the negative peak for flashes ranged between 181 to 183 **msec at frontal sites and approx-** imately 168 msec at both parietal locations. Older subjects showed response latencies for the negative peak for tones between 132 to 133 msec at frontal sites and 145 to 150 msec at parietal sites; response latencies for the negative peak to flashes ranged between 191 to 193 msec at frontal sites and between 178 and 179 msec at parietal locations. The combined tone and flash conditions resemble the separate tone and flash conditions for both young and old subjects. While the cerebrovascular cases showed significantly greater variability in latencies, the mean values for the prominent negative peaks were similar to the old subject group.

If the separate responses to tones and flashes are added together and normalized, the composite waveform can be compared with the condition in which the tones and flashes were actually paired. Figure 6 illustrates this process and shows that the prominent negative peak observed in the tones and the prominent negative peak in the flashes are maintained in the young subject (age = 25 yrs). The time interval between these negative peaks for tones and the negative peaks for flashes was approximately 50 msec, disregarding anterior-posterior differences. This procedure has been carried out for our different subject groups, and Figure 7 depicts selected composite and tone-flash presentations for a young (age = 28 yrs), old (age = 77 yrs), and left hemisphere damaged patient (expressive aphasia with right hemiparesis, age = 60 yrs) across electrode sites. In the young subject a good correspondence between the composite waveform and the actual waveform for tones and flashes can be observed for all of the electrode sites. This was also true for the normal healthy older individual at frontal sites, but less so at parietal locations. In the cerebrovascular case with left hemisphere damage, less of a correspondence can be seen between the composite and actual waveform at F_3 than at the F_4 location. The form of both the composite and actual waveforms are altered in parietal areas when compared to either the younger or older subjects' responses.

This pattern of differential negative peaks (or, in some instances, one negative peak accompanied by a readily identifiable flexion point during bimodal **stimulation) consistently displayed latencies for the waveforms that correspond** with the latencies of the negative peaks in the polyphasic waveforms for the tone and flash conditions alone. While this complex waveform was routinely observed in the community subjects, it frequently was missing in recordings from both hemispheres in the patient group and always in the damaged hemisphere. Although these are small alterations within the ERP waveform when compared to other methods (which may more easily demonstrate behavioral deficits or pathology),

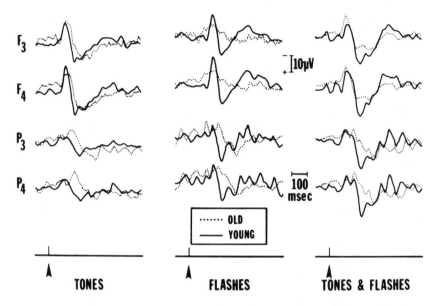

Fig. 5. Event related potentials to tone, flash, and tone-flash combinations for a young (age = 25) and old (age = 74) community volunteer.

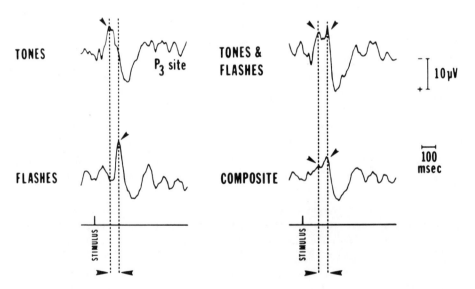

Fig. 6. Comparison of event related potentials to tones, flashes, and tone-flash combination. The composite waveform was obtained by adding and normalizing the separate responses to tones and flashes. Note the similarity in latencies for the prominent negative peaks.

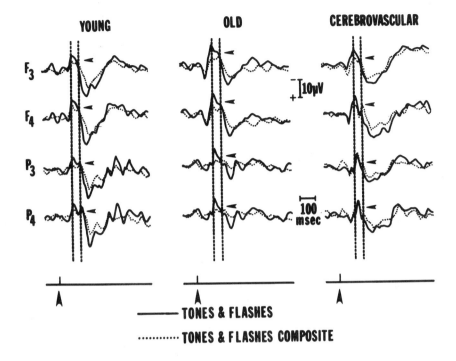

Fig. 7. Comparison of ERP waveforms from the combined tone-flash condition to the generated composite waveform for a young (age = 25), and old (age = 77) community volunteer, and cerebrovascular patient with left hemisphere damage (age = 60, aphasic with right hemiparesis). Note that in the young subject a close correspondence between the actual tone-flash combination and composite can be observed. Similarly, the old subject showed a close correspondence at frontal sites, but less so at parietal locations. The vascular patient demonstrated less similarity over the damaged left hemisphere at the left frontal site than for the right hemisphere site.

the modality comparisons offer the opportunity to examine separately and together the individual's unique responses through different sensory pathways. In a sense, the differential transmission times apparent in the cross modal comparisons may provide a basis for precise predictions of the time sequence of complex waveforms. If this is the case, deviations from this pattern then could conceivably take on added significance in making inferences regarding the functional integrity of the nervous system. This approach may be particularly useful in brain injured or cognitively impaired patients where latencies and amplitudes of the ERP may be aberrant, and for which no control or normative data are available.

151

ACKNOWLEDGEMENTS

This study was supported by HEW-NIA Grants AG 00088 and AG 00133. The Rancho Los Amigos Hospital (courtesy of Dr. Harry Fang) provided laboratory facilities and technical assistance.

REFERENCES

1. Liberson, W. T. Functional electroencephalography in mental disorders. Diseases of the Nervous System, 1944, 5, 357-364.

2. Wells, C. E. Response of alpha waves to light in neurologic disease. Archives of Neurology, 1962, 6, 478-491.

3. Wells, C. E. Alpha wave responsiveness to light in man. In G. H. Glaser (Ed.), EEG and behavior. New York: Basic Books, 1963.

4. Obrist, W. D. Electroencephalographic approach to age changes in response speed. In A. T. Welford & J. E. Birren (Eds.), Behavior, aging, and the nervous system. Springfield, Illinois: Charles C Thomas, 1965.

5. Thompson, L. W., & Wilson, S. Electrocortical reactivity and learning in the elderly. Journal of Gerontology, 1966, 21, 45-51.

6. Crighel, E., & Sterman-Marinchescu, C. Flash-evoked responses in acute cerebro-vascular diseases. The correlation with the clinical, electroencephalographic and rheoencephalographic course. Revue Roumaine de Neurologie, 1971, 8, 275-284.

7. Giblin, D. R. Somatosensory evoked potentials in healthy subjects and in patients with lesions of the nervous system. Annals New York Academy of Sciences, 1964, 112, 93-142.

8. Goya, T. Diagnostic significance of the evoked electrical responses in neurological diseases. I. Somatosensory evoked responses. Kumamoto Medical Journal, 1976, 29, 187-200.

9. Lee, R. G., & Blair, R. D. G. Evolution of EEG and visual evoked response changes in Jakob-Creutzfeldt disease. Electroencephalography and Clinical Neurophysiology, 1973, 35, 133-142.

10. Nakanishi, T., Shimada, Y., & Toyokura, Y. Somatosensory evoked responses to mechanical stimulation in normal subjects and in patients with neurological disorders. Journal of the Neurological Sciences, 1974, 21, 289-298.

11. Noël, P., & Desmedt, J. E. Somatosensory cerebral evoked potentials after vascular lesions of the brain-stem and diencephalon. Brain, 1975, 98, 113-128.

12. Schenkenberg, T., Dustman, R. E., & Beck, E. C. Cortical evoked responses of hospitalized geriatrics in three diagnostic categories. Proceedings, 80th Annual Convention, APA, 1972, 671-672.

13. Straumanis, J. J., Shagass, C., & Schwartz, M. Visually evoked cerebral response changes associated with chronic brain syndromes and aging. Journal of Gerontology, 1965, 20, 498-506.

14. Tsumoto, T., Hirose, N., Nonaka, S., & Takahashi, M. Cerebrovascular disease: Changes in somatosensory evoked potentials associated with unilateral lesions. Electroencephalography and Clinical Neurophysiology, 1973, 35, 463-473.

15. Visser, S. L., Stam, F. C., Van Tilburg, W., Op Den Velde, W., Blom, J. L., & De Rijke, W. Visual evoked response in senile and presenile dementia. Electroencephalography and Clinical Neurophysiology, 1976, 40, 385-392.

16. Williamson, P. D., Goff, W. R., & Allison, T. Somato-sensory evoked responses in patients with unilateral cerebral lesions. Electroencephalography and Clinical Neurophysiology, 1970, 28, 566-575.

17. Miyoshi, S., Lüders, H., Kato, M., & Kuroiwa, Y. The somatosensory evoked potential in patients with cerebrovascular diseases. Folia Psychiatrica et Neurologica Japonica, 1971, 25, 9-25.

18. Oosterhuis, H. J. G. H., Ponsen, L., Jonkman, E. J., & Magnus, O. The average visual response in patients with cerebrovascular disease. Electroencephalography and Clinical Neurophysiology, 1969, 27, 23-34.

19. Shibasaki, H. Movement-associated cortical potentials in unilateral cerebral lesions. Journal of Neurology, 1975, 209, 189-198.

20. Klorman, R., Thompson, L. W., & Ellingson, R. J. Event related brain potentials across the life span. In E. Callaway & S. Koslow (Eds.), Event related brain potentials. New York: Academic Press, in press.

21. Marsh, G. R., & Thompson, L. W. Psychophysiology of aging. In J. E. Birren & K. Warner Schaie (Eds.), The psychology of aging. New York: Van Nostrand Reinhold Company, 1977.

22. Ritter, W., Vaughan, H. G., Jr., & Costa, L. D. Orienting and habituation to auditory stimuli: A study of short term changes in average evoked responses. Electroencephalography and Clinical Neurophysiology, 1968, 25, 550-556.

23. Brent, G. A., Smith, D. B. D., Thompson, L. W., & Michalewski, H. J. Differences in the evoked potential in young and old subjects during habituation and dishabituation procedures. Paper presented at the 16th annual meeting of the Society for Psychophysiological Research, San Diego, California, October 20-23, 1976.

24. Smith, D. B. D., Brent, G. A., Michalewski, H. J., & Thompson, L. W. Age differences in the evoked potential for young and old subjects during attention, habituation, and orienting. Paper presented at the 57th annual meeting of the Western Psychological Association, Seattle, Washington, April 1977.

25. Smith, D. B. D., Tom, C. E., Brent, G. A., & Ohta, R. J. Attention, evoked potentials, and aging. Paper presented at the 56th annual meeting of the Western Psychological Association, Los Angeles, April 8-11, 1976.

26. Sutton, S., Braren, M., Zubin, J., & John, E. R. Evoked potential correlates of stimulus uncertainty. Science, 1965, 150, 1187-1188.

SLEEP PATTERNS IN DEMENTIA: ISSUES, EVIDENCE AND STRATEGIES

IRWIN FEINBERG, M.D.
Veterans Administration Hospital, San Francisco
University of California at San Francisco

ABSTRACT

The changes in physiological sleep patterns with normal aging and
in senile dementia are briefly reviewed. An attempt is made to define
the major questions at issue and a strategy of investigation to resolve
some of these questions is described.

INTRODUCTION

There does not yet exist a substantial body of literature describing
the sleep patterns of senile patients or those with multi-infarct
dementia. However, the changes in sleep between adulthood and normal
old age have been extensively investigated (1,2) and there exists
good agreement on both their general nature. Nevertheless, the health
and cognitive status of the normal elderly subjects (Ss) studied thus
far have not been fully documented. In this paper I shall first
outline what I believe to be the more important questions regarding
sleep in the elderly. The evidence bearing on these questions will
then be reviewed for both the normal and senile aged. I shall conclude
with a description of the strategies of our current investigations of
sleep in the elderly.

QUESTIONS AT ISSUE

The following seem to me to be the significant questions regarding
sleep in the aged:

(1) What sleep changes occur as a result of normal aging, i.e.,
independently of disease?

(2) Do the sleep patterns of the senile aged differ from those of
the normal elderly? If so, are these differences quantitative or
qualitative? Do senile patients simply show a more extreme degree of
the same changes in sleep pattern manifested by the normal elderly,
or do the sleep patterns of senile patients differ in certain unique
respects?

(3) Are sleep patterns correlated with cognitive impairment within
groups of normal and demented elderly subjects? I emphasize the

importance of establishing correlations between sleep and measures of psychometric function within groups of normal and pathological aged because, if the latter group simply show sleep abnormalities which are quantitatively greater than those produced by normal aging, significant correlations between cognitive function and sleep measures would necessarily occur in groups which contain a mixture of normal and senile individuals.

Of course, to establish that significant correlations exist between cognitive impairment and sleep measures does not in itself prove a causal relationship between these variables. However, the absence of such significant correlations would be a serious and perhaps decisive argument against the view that sleep patterns reflect the functional integrity of the brain.

(4) There is a fourth, more basic, issue which these rather clinical questions bear upon: What is the biological significance of the intimate link between sleep and aging? This association is manifest over the entire human life span, with especially dramatic changes occuring in infancy and adolescence as well as in old age.* I suspect that these later changes in sleep, which begin at the end of adolescence and accelerate in middle and old age, reflect a slight and then an increased rate of decline in the functional capacity of the brain. This view is by no means unanimous. Some consider that the main function of sleep in the elderly is to conserve energy (3); if this view were correct, changes in sleep in the elderly might simply be due to reduced energy requirements in the periphery. In this context, Dr. Villee's observations on progeria described elsewhere in this volume are relevant. In progeria, there is a premature aging of connective tissue associated with a marked increase in basal metabolic rate due to excessive heat loss. Nevertheless, the brain and intelligence are normal in progeria and in the one case studied, Karacan (4) found sleep patterns which were also entirely normal. If confirmed with additional cases, such results would argue against the hypothesis

*It seems clear that the changes in sleep patterns in infancy are related to brain maturation. However, changes in sleep during adolescence have received far less attention. I believe that these latter changes reflect a profound reorganization of brain function in which a substantial degree of brain plasticity is sacrificed for the ability to carry out extended and complex logical operations; a further discussion of this speculation would take us too far afield. These issues are touched upon in (1).

that sleep is a function of the rate of peripheral energy expenditure or that it is affected by the type of peripheral "aging" represented by progeria. Whatever the correct interpretation, it seems almost certain that a better understanding of the relationships between sleep and aging will shed light upon two unsolved questions in basic biology: the nature of aging in the central nervous system and the function of sleep in man.

CHANGES IN SLEEP WITH NORMAL AGING

The main electrophysiologic studies of sleep changes in the normal elderly were recently reviewed (5). Here we shall simply note the established findings without detailed citation of the literature; the interested reader is referred to our recent review for these references.

(1) Total Sleep Time (TST)

TST is not significantly reduced in normal old age, in spite of a marked increase in the amount of waking (see below). Elderly subjects compensate for their increased time awake by increasing the time they spend in bed. In the laboratory studies carried out thus far, subjects were permitted to spend their habitual amounts of time in bed. Some data suggest that sleep time in elderly females may be longer than in males (2,6). This question, which raises the possibility that sleep patterns reflect the differential rates of aging in men and women, requires more extensive investigation.

(2) Amount of Waking

The number of awakenings, the total time awake and the percentage of time in bed spent awake each provide somewhat different information. All studies agree that elderly normal subjects manifest significantly increased levels of awakening on each of these measures when compared to young adults. Between young adulthood and old age the number of awakenings increases linearly whereas the percentage of time spent in bed awake shows a curvilinear increase, the curve being positively accelerated after age 40 years (7).

(3) Sleep Spindles

Sleep spindles are bursts of sinusoidal waves - between 12 and 14 Hz - which are usually between .5 and 1.5 seconds in duration. They are characteristic of the NREM phase of human sleep. Spindle bursts are reduced in the elderly by 50% or more (8). Recent analyses of these earlier data suggest that decrements in spindle activity become apparent in late middle age rather than appearing for the first time after age 65 years (5).

(4) <u>Sleep Stage Changes</u>

(a) REM

The duration and proportion of TST made up of sleep with rapid eye movements (REM) do not show a mean reduction in the normal elderly. Neither is the mean density of eye movements or their total number significantly reduced in the elderly as compared with young adults. Nevertheless, within groups of elderly subjects, significant correlations have been obtained between age and both the duration of REM sleep per night, and total eye movement activity (8).

(b) Stages 3 and 4

Stage 4 sleep is characterized by dense high voltage slow waves. It is the EEG sleep stage most sensitive to age in man, showing a hyperbolic decline from infancy to old age with the asymptote being reached early in the 6th decade (7). Thus, the normal elderly show reduced stage 4 compared with young adults. However, they also show increased stage 3 sleep. Stage 3 sleep is characterized by an amount of delta activity intermediate between that found in stages 2 and 4. Part of the reduction of stage 4 sleep in the elderly can be attributed to a decline in delta wave amplitude. Thus, Agnew (10) found a reduction in integrated EEG amplitude (all frequencies) of about 36%; Smith et. al. (11) found a reduction of 60% in peak amplitude within the delta band in the first NREM period in small groups (N=5) of young adults and elderly. Computer techniques developed in our own laboratory have detected the decline in delta wave amplitude over the remarkably narrow age range of 18 to 22.5 years (9). These techniques are now being applied to studies of the elderly (see below). However, in addition to reduced amplitude, the elderly show a decreased density of delta waves. The effects of changes in amplitude, number and density of delta waves on alterations in amount of visually scored stage 4 can be determined with computer techniques which measure these variables separately (9).

(5) <u>Correlations Among Age, Sleep and Psychometric Variables</u>

The most extensive study on this question remains that reported in 1967 (8) in which correlation matrices which included age, sleep, and psychometric scores (Wechsler Adult Intelligence Scale, Wechsler Memory Scale and Raven's Progressive Matrices) were computed separately for groups of aged normal and elderly patients with chronic brain syndrome (CBS). These CBS subjects were of mixed etiologies including at least three with multi-infarct dementia, one with Korsakoff's psychosis and with the remainder presumably suffering from an

Alzheimer-type dementia. Table 1 shows the main results. In general, measures of REM sleep correlated positively and measures of waking correlated negatively with psychometric performance in both groups; amounts of spindling or stage 4 showed no significant correlations. However, both the sleep and psychometric variables which were significantly related were themselves correlated with age; with the age correlations partialed, the correlations between sleep and psychometric measures became statistically insignificant (8).

Kahn and co-workers (6,12) carried out a partial replication of these studies but with less adequate experimental controls. These investigators failed to demonstrate statistically significant correlations between sleep and psychometric variables, although the pattern of correlations that they found was similiar to that previously observed (see review by Feinberg (5)).

In the investigations cited thus far, the subjects' current level of cognitive function was measured to obtain an index of degree of cognitive impairment. While such measures of current level are affected by age-related impairment they also reflect variations in original endowment, education, degree of social activity and other variables. Only in a longitudinal study can impairment (i.e., a decrement from a previous level of function) be measured directly. Prinz (13) employed such data available from Ss participating in longitudinal studies at the Duke University Center for the Study of Aging and Human Development. She studied sleep in three male and nine female healthy elderly volunteers; these Ss had been selected from a group of fifty who had received regular evaluations of social, psychological, and physical functioning over the previous 18 years. Ss were between 76 and 90 years of age (mean= 82 years) and their sleep was recorded for three or four consecutive nights in their own homes using a portable polygraph. Prinz found correlations of rho = .76 between duration of REM sleep and current WAIS Performance score. In addition, the slope of the decline in WAIS Performance scores showed a significant negative correlation with REM sleep duration (rho = .841). These results are consistent with those previously reported by Feinberg et al (8). Prinz found no significant correlations between sleep stages other than REM sleep and psychometric function. However, using a map distance measuring device to sum the time spent in delta, Prinz obtained a score which was highly correlated with both REM sleep and WAIS Performance scores.

In spite of these strongly suggestive findings, it is our view that the question of whether EEG sleep patterns are related to cognitive

TABLE 1

Selected Correlations of Sleep Variables with Age and
Psychometric Test Scores (from Feinberg et. al. (8))

	Age	WAIS		Wechsler Memory Scale	Progressive Matrices
		Verbal	Performance		
(N)			(14)+		
Aged Normal					
Age	-	.06	-.58*	-.59*	-.45
Total Sleep Time	-.03	.33	.13	.28	.55*
% Time Awake	.54*	-.27	-.44	-.31	-.62*
REM Duration	-.69**	.09	.72**	.67**	.46
EM Activity	-.61*	-.03	.68**	.56*	.41
% Stage 4	.15	-.37	-.13	-.08	-.21
(N)		(13)	(10)	(12)	-
CBS					
Age	-	.02	-.46	-.11	++-
Total Sleep Time	-.41	.70**	.74**	.48	-
% Time Awake	.61*	-.45	-.64*	-.41	-
REM Duration	-.35	.63*	.72*	.43	-
EM Activity	.27	.55	.50	.02	-
% Stage 4	-.05	-.24	-.54	.17	-

++ N = 15 for all other correlations in aged normal group

+ Progressive Matrices test was too difficult for CBS Ss.

* p <.05   ** p <.01

impairment within groups of healthy elderly normal subjects has not yet been definitively resolved. Further investigations are needed with larger numbers of well-characterized normal subjects tested on a wide range of cognitive functions.

OTHER OBSERVATIONS

The threshold for arousal from sleep, while not systematically measured, was observed to be remarkably low in the normal elderly by Feinberg, et al (8). These elderly subjects seemed able to awaken almost instantly, even from their deepest (delta) sleep stages and immediately appeared in almost complete possession of their waking faculties.

A different kind of arousal phenomenon was noted in a small number of CBS patients. These subjects awoke repeatedly from REM sleep in states resembling acute delirium (although all of the patients were considered clinically stable at the time of testing). The subjects would awaken abruptly, appearing extremely agitated and often with a fixed idea on which they attempted to act, eg. "I must get to work", or "I must meet my daughter's train". Their agitation and confusion would last 5 to 10 minutes after which they would return quietly to bed. Feinberg and co-workers (8) suggested that such behavior at home might produce nocturnal wandering, a problem which often necessitates hospitalization of geriatric patients. A recent analysis of data from these normal and CBS groups revealed that the tendency of CBS patients as a group to awaken more frequently from REM sleep was statistically reliable (14). This difference in frequency of REM awakenings in normal and CBS elderly groups was statistically significant for each of the first four REM periods of the night.

MORE RECENT STUDIES IN SLEEP AND DEMENTIA

In the studies of Feinberg, et al (8) the sleep patterns of patients with chronic brain syndrome showed both quantitative and qualitative differences, as well as some similiarities, to those of aged normal Ss. The CBS patients showed more extensive awakenings leading to a reduction in total sleep time. They also showed an increased rate of awakening from REM sleep and a few Ss awoke repeatedly from REM in states resembling acute delirium. However, the CBS and elderly normal Ss did not differ significantly with respect to amount of spindling or EEG stages 3 and 4. The CBS subjects showed a reduction in percentage of stage REM which was directly attributable to their reduced total sleep time. As noted above, the amount of waking in the

CBS group was negatively correlated and the amount of REM sleep positively correlated with psychometric test scores.

A review of the literature since 1967 reveals additional studies of interest. It may be worth emphasizing that we are concerned here only with intellectual impairment due to chronic brain disease. Subjects with acute brain syndrome (delirium) show quite different sleep patterns and sometimes manifest high levels of REM sleep (7,8,9)

The most extensive recent study that we have found of patients with brain impairment is that of Harada et al (20). They studied sleep in 105 patients with severe brain damage. They observed two general types of altered sleep. In the "functionally abnormal" type, differences from normal were mainly quantitative, with increased awakening, decreased total sleep and deep sleep, and altered cycle patterns. In the "degenerative" type, there was a disappearance of vertex sharp waves and sleep spindles and the appearance of abnormal EEG wave forms. Patients with degenerative sleep profiles had a poor prognosis. Harada and co-workers did not present detailed quantitative results on total sleep time and awakenings because "those findings were affected considerably by the environment or conditions of examination". However, Harada et al noted that some patients with brain impairment showed high rather than low proportions of REM sleep. They found no association between the type of sleep pattern and the etiology of the brain disease. Ten patients in this study showed nocturnal delirium. Eight of these ten manifested an EEG pattern during sleep which was difficult to distinguish from waking. Since the delirium occurred more frequently during the latter part of the sleep cycle (when REM sleep would be proportionately greater) "some relation with REM was suspected to exist".

Popoviciu and co-workers (16) studied sleep for a single night in twenty patients with vascular brain disorder: 17 had lesions in the distribution of the vertebral-basilar system and 3 in the distribution of the carotids. In general, REM sleep was reduced, but high proportions of REM (up to 65%) were found in several patients. However, these high proportions were associated with low total sleep times. Popoviciu et al noted that, in some patients with normal waking EEGs, abnormal foci appeared during sleep which correctly indicated the localization of the lesion. They also noted an abnormal phase of REM sleep in which the rapid, low voltage EEG was associated with extremely sparse eye movements.

Schneider et al (5) studied 30 patients with angiographically verified ischemic lesions of the cerebral hemispheres for seven hours on two to three nights each. The Ss were studied about 45 days after the onset of the illness. Complex reaction time measures were obtained in addition to thorough assessment of neurological and mental status. These stroke patients showed delayed sleep onset, increased awakening and a reduction of delta sleep. Higher levels of awakening were associated with longer reaction times and "euphoric state of mind which can be considered as a sign of psycho-organic impairment". Neurologic symptoms were less clearly associated with sleep pattern than they were with measures of mental function.

A recent study by Hachinski et al (21), while dealing with acute rather than chronic cerebro-vascular lesions, may be of interest to the readers of this volume. These investigators studied 33 patients with acute strokes. They found that all patients who displayed a stage 2 sleep pattern had a favorable prognosis and they noted that all-night sleep recordings were particularly helpful in predicting prognoses of patients who suffered from a hemispheric infarct and severe neurological deficit.

The present review has been restricted to studies of sleep in relation to aging and brain impairment in humans. However, it should be noted that investigators are beginning to direct their attention to the effects of age on sleep in animals (22,23), effects which seem similiar to those in man. It may also prove of interest to attempt to develop animal models for the study of sleep after vascular and anoxic brain lesions.

Thus, there is increasing interest in the relation of sleep patterns to neurological disorder and there is ample evidence that the sleep EEG is altered with brain disease. However, the question of whether the degree of change in sleep pattern is quantitatively related to the magnitude of impairment in patients with dementia has not yet been resolved. It is such quantitative studies, rather than further qualitative descriptions, which are now required to advance our under-standing of sleep in senile dementia.

ASSUMPTIONS AND STRATEGIES OF CURRENT STUDIES OF SLEEP IN THE ELDERLY

It is our view that senile dementia is probably the end result of a variety of different pathological conditions. We would also assume that at least one of the causal pathological processes is an accelera-tion of normal age changes. To the extent that changes in sleep are related to changes in brain function, one would therefore expect a subgroup of demented subjects to show quantitatively more extreme changes from young adult levels than are manifested by the normal elderly. For this reason, we thought it essential to define in greater detail the changes in sleep found in normal elderly subjects and to determine whether these changes are, in fact, substantially correlated with cognitive impairment. These initial studies will be followed by investigations in smaller numbers of carefully selected patients with clinically-defined classical syndromes of Alzheimer's and multi-infarct dementia.

There are several methodological advantages in initial study of the normal elderly:

(a) One has a much larger population to select from, making possible for control for socioeconomic status, education and other variables which affect intellectual and health status, thus avoiding contamination by many possible confounding variables.

(b) One can carry out more effective and meaningful psychometric assessments in normal subjects.

(c) One can also obtain better cooperation in a physiological recording (avoidance of naps, etc.).

Thus, in terms of the issues stated above, our initial goals are to determine the nature of sleep changes in the healthy normal elderly and to investigate the relation of these changes to the degree of cognitive impairment measured within this group. We indicated above that, in the absence of longitudinal study, one cannot measure age-associated cognitive decrement directly. We have attempted to deal with this problem by the selection of a group of subjects - retired school teachers - who are relatively homogeneous with respect to education, life experiences, and socio-economic status. In such a group, marked variations in current level of cognitive function could reasonably be interpreted as reflecting, to a larger extent than would be the case with a more heterogeneous group of subjects, variations in the effects of age on cognition.

In seeking relations between cognitive impairment and sleep variables our underlying assumption is that variations in the severity of aging of the brain will be associated with variations in sleep patterns. However, many other changes occur with chronological age and it is important to attempt to rule out the contribution of the multitude of other concomitants of aging to changes in both sleep patterns and cognition. Stated differently, one wishes to determine whether variations in degree of cognitive impairment produced by variations in rate of brain aging are correlated with degree of change in sleep patterns. To control for the contribution of other changes associated with chronological age one could study subjects in a wide age range and employ statistical techniques (partial correlation, analysis of

covariance) or, instead, simply hold chronological age relatively
constant. We have chosen the latter approach, restricting our
subjects to the ages of 70 to 75 years. If chronological age proves
correlated with sleep and psychometric variables even within this
narrow age range, our N (50 subjects) should be sufficiently large
to permit statistical control of this variable.

Four general classes of data are being collected on these subjects:

I. Psychiatric, medical and neurological status:
    (a) Psychiatric and medical histories
    (b) Physical and neurological examinations
    (c) Laboratory screening tests including EKG
    (d) CAT Scans with computer analysis (24)

II. Sleep Recordings
    (a) Five nights of sleep including one night of extended sleep
and one night of recovery from extended sleep
    (b) Visual sleep stage analysis of these sleep records
    (c) Computer analysis of sleep EEG wave forms (9)

III. Waking Psychophysiology
    (a) Waking EEG (Clinical reading and spectral analysis)
    (b) Cortical evoked potentials (basal auditory, visual, and
auditory-visual combined)

IV. Psychometric Assessment
    (a) Rey Auditory Verbal Learning Test (25)
    (b) Design Learning (SFVA, unpublished)
    (c) Trials A & B (26)
    (d) Finger Oscillation (27)
    (e) Perceptual Apperception (27)
    (f) Wechsler Adult Intelligence Scale (28)
    (g) Famous Faces (M. Albert and N. Butters, personal communica-
tion)
    (h) Long Term Memory Retrieval and Recognition (M. Albert and
N. Butters, personal communication)
    (i) Memory for Cartoons (SFVA, unpublished)
    (j) Face Recognition (SFVA, unpublished)
    (k) Paired Associate Learning
    (l) Block Tapping Test (29)
    (m) Memory, recognition and temporal sequence for abstract
art and words (29)
    (n) Controlled Word Fluency Test (30)
    (o) Token Test (31)
    (p) Raven's Advanced Progressive Matrices (32)

(q) Tactual Performance Test

(r) Self-Assessment Questionnaire (SFVA, unpublished)

It is our view that the validity of this study depends critically upon the validity of our measurements of cognitive function and upon the degree to which the measurements obtained reflect impairment produced by aging. It is for this reason that we have included such extensive psychological testing. Nevertheless, we are impressed by the difficulty in measuring with objective techniques the changes in cognitive function - particularly in memory - of which our subjects are themselves so keenly aware. It is for this reason that we devised and are applying a self-assessment questionnaire. However, this questionnaire is untested and may be greatly affected by response bias. We must await the analysis of the complete set of data to learn whether our efforts will be successful. In any event, we shall obtain, in a single group of subjects, a set of measures - health status, sleep EEG, waking clinical EEG, evoked potentials, and CAT Scans - which are each sensitive to the brain changes produced by aging and we should be able to define, for the first time, their interrelations.

REFERENCES

1. Feinberg, I. (1974) J. Psychiat. Res. 10, 283-306.

2. Williams, R. L., Karacan, I. and Hursch, C. J. (1974) Electroencephalography (EEG) of Human Sleep, Clinical Applications, Wiley, New York.

3. Berger, R. J. (1975) Fed. Proc. 34, 97-102.

4. Rosenbloom, A. L., Karacan, I. and Busk, F. L. (1970) J. of Pediatrics 77, 692-695.

5. Feinberg, I. (1976) in Neurobiology of Aging; Gershon, S. and Terry, R. D. eds., Ravens Press, New York, pp. 23-41.

6. Kahn, E., Fisher, C. and Lieberman, L. (1970) Compr. Psychiatry 11(3), 274-278.

7. Feinberg, I. and Carlson, V. R. (1968) Arch. Gen. Psychiat. 18, 239-250.

8. Feinberg, I., Koresko, R. L. and Heller, N. (1967) J. Psychiat. Res. 5, 107-144.

9. Feinberg, I., March, J. D., Fein, G., Floyd, T. C., Walker, J. M. and Price, L. (1978) EEG and Clinical Neurophysiol. 44, 202-213.

10. Agnew, H. W., Jr. (1973) EEG and Clinical Neurophysiol. 34, 391-397.

11. Smith, J. R., Karacan, I. and Yang, M. (1977) EEG and Clinical Neurophysiol. 43, 229-237.

12. Kahn, E. and Fisher, C. (1969) J. Nerv. Ment. Dis. 148(5), 495-505.

13. Prinz, P. N. (1977) Gerontol. 32(2), 179-186.

14. Floyd, T. C., Fein, G. and Feinberg, I. (1978) Sleep Research, in press.

15. Schneider, E., Ziegler, B., Jacobi, P. and Maxion, H. (1977) Arch. Psychiat. Nervenkr. 223, 131-138.

16. Popoviciu, L., Pasco, I., Asgian, B. and Sipos, C. (1970) Rev. Roum. Neurol. 7, 153-172.

17. Feinberg, I., Koresko, R. L., Heller, N. and Steinberg, H. R. (1965) Am. J. Psychiat. 121, 1018-1020.

18. Greenberg, R. and Pearlman, C. (1967) Amer. J. Psychiat. 124, 133-142.

19. Gross, M. M., et. al. (1966) J. Nerv. Ment. Dis. 142, 493-514

20. Harada, M., Minami, R., Hattori, E., Nakamura, K., Kabashima, K., Shikai, I. and Sakai, Y. (1976) Kumamoto Med. J. 29, 110-127.

21. Hachinski, V., Mamelak, M. and Norris, J. (1978) Sleep Morphology and Prognosis in Acute Cerebrovascular Lesions, In Cerebral Vascular Disease (Proceeding of 8th Salzburg Conference), Meyer, J.S., Lechner, H. and Reivich, M. eds., George Thieme Publishers, in press.

22. Eleftheriou, B. E., Zolovick, A. J. and Elias, M. F. (1975) Gerontologia 21, 21-30.

23. Zepelin, H., Whitehead, W. E. and Rechtschaffen, A. (1972) Behav. Biol. 7, 65-74.

24. Jernigan, T. and Naeser, M. (1977) The CT Scanner - Minicomputer System in Neuropsychological Research in International Neuro-psychology Society, European Conference, St. Catherine College, Oxford, pp. 39.

25. Rey, A. (1964) L'examen Clinique en Psychologie, Presses Universitaires de France.

26. Reitan, R. M. (1958) Percep. Mot. Skills 8, 271-276.

27. Halstead, W. C. (1947) Brain and Intelligence, Univ. of Chicago Press, Chicago, Ill.

28. Wechsler, D. (1958) The Measurement and Appraisal of Adult Intelligence, 4th ed., Williams & Wilkins, Baltimore.

29. Milner, B. (1971) Brit. Med. Bull., 27(3), 272-277.

30. Benton, A. L. (1973) in Aspectos Pathologicos del Lengage, Velasquez, A. C. ed., Centro Neuropsicologico, Lima.

31. Boller, F. and Vignolo, L. A. (1966) Brain, 89, 815-831.

32. Foulds, G. A. and Raven, J. C. (1950) Brit. J. Educ. Psych. 20, 104-110.

SECTION II

DIAGNOSIS AND TREATMENT

CLINICAL MANIFESTATIONS OF SENILE DEMENTIA

ERIC PFEIFFER, M.D.

Professor of Psychiatry, University of Colorado School of Medicine,
Denver, Colorado

INTRODUCTION

The presenting signs and symptoms of senile dementia are of primary concern to persons afflicted with this disorder, to their families, and to their health-care providers. They are also of central concern to investigators seeking to understand the biomedical basis of the disorder. For it is only through a clear delineation of the clinical manifestations of senile dementia that we can delineate the type of index case to be studied through a variety of diagnostic and investigative techniques. A full understanding of these manifestations can also provide some of the necessary leads for scientific inquiry into etiological and treatment aspects.

NORMAL NEURONAL DEPOPULATION AND SUSCEPTIBILITY TO DELIRIUM

The brain is the organ of adaptation. Its cells, once destroyed, from whatever cause, cannot be replaced. Brain cell destruction goes on throughout adult life, at a rate of a fraction of one percent per year.[1] This neuronal depopulation of itself does not lead to clinical manifestations, even in the sixth, seventh, or eighth decade of life. It does, however, lead to a greater vulnerability of the remaining brain tissue in later life to noxious, toxic, or substrate-reducing influences. As excess reserve capacity is slowly eroded, delirium occurs easily. That is, in old age the disease-free brain functions normally under optimal nutritional, internal and external environmental circumstances. But even small changes in such factors as cardiac output, electrolyte balance, level of internally generated toxins or externally supplied toxins, including medications, can alter brain function temporarily, leading to clinically significant manifestations of brain impairment, also known as delirium or reversible organic brain syndrome. In other words, the healthy older brain is like a man walking along the edge of a cliff: he remains quite safe and intact in the absence of any disturbing influences.

MANIFESTATIONS OF ORGANIC BRAIN SYNDROMES, INCLUDING DELIRIUM AND DEMENTIA

The core clinical manifestations of both delirium (reversible organic brain syndrome) and dementia (irreversible organic brain syndrome) are similar to the extent that like cognitive functions are impaired in each. Without specific understanding of the etiology involved it is not always possible to distinguish between delirium and dementia. History and certain physiological measurements generally contribute to differential diagnosis.

Commonly, however, delirium is characterized by rapid onset of core and of associated symptoms, by the coexistence of medical disease, medical procedures and/or medications. On the other hand, dementia is more commonly characterized by a gradual onset of core symptoms, with or without associated symptoms; the absence of significant medical diseases; and the absence of recent treatment and/or present medications.

Rapidity of onset, extent of brain tissue death or impairment, diffuse versus localized brain involvement, environmental and pre-existing personality factors tend to shape the specific clinical manifestations of delirium and dementia, both their core symptoms and their associated symptoms.

CORE SYMPTOMS AND ASSOCIATED SYMPTOMS OF ORGANIC BRAIN DISEASE

Core symptoms of organic brain disease, both delirium and dementia, are those symptoms directly attributable to either temporarily malfunctioning or permanently destroyed brain tissue. Associated symptoms constitute the individual's various mechanisms for coping with the awareness of impaired brain function. The former symptoms are primarily in the cognitive sphere; the latter are primarily in the affective sphere, including various transformations of anxiety, as into paranoid delusional ideas.

The core symptoms of organic brain syndromes are diagnostic of either dementia or delirium. The associated symptoms are not diagnostic of either delirium or dementia. They are significant, however, in determining the treatment approach to the patient's disorder.

The Core Symptoms of Organic Brain Disease

The core symptoms of organic brain disease include the following, briefly stated:

> disorientation
> decreased recent memory
> decreased memory for spatial relationships
> decreased capacity for correct sequencing of events
> decreased capacity to perform serial cognitive tasks
> decreased remote memory

Depending on the recency and severity of onset of the brain impairment, there also may be rapid changes in levels of consciousness or awareness, ranging from differing levels of orientation to drowsiness to unconsciousness, all the way to coma.

The assessment of the presence and degree of this particular constellation of symptoms requires sophistication on the part of the person carrying out the assessment. If changes are minimal, rather extensive psychological testing needs to be carried out, including subtests of the Wechsler Adult Intelligence Scale (WAIS), the Reitan-Halstead battery of tests for organicity, and such tests of spatial memory capacity as the Bender Gestalt Test. However, these tests tend to be useful only in the discovery of early manifestations of organic brain disease, either localized or diffuse. They tend to be too complex and demanding for patients with serious degrees of organic impairment. In such cases, only a few of the subtests of the WAIS can be utilized. This author has developed a still more simple test of organicity*, the Short Portable Mental Status Questionnaire, a ten-item test measuring the presence and degree of organic deficit, especially in older persons, applicable either in an office setting or at the bedside in the hospital.[2] This test is sensitive to educational attainment, and can be quickly administered by any health-care professional. Serial measurements are possible, either to follow the course of delirium over a matter of days or the course of dementia over a period of months or years. Schuckit[3] has verified the usefulness and simplicity of this test in comparison with other available test procedures, and it is now widely used as a bedside and screening procedure. It consists of ten questions which tap into the various categories of cognitive performance outlined above. Assuming a high-school level of education, a score of 0-2 errors implies that the person is cognitively intact. A score of 3-4 errors raises the question of borderline intellectual impairment. Errors in the range of 5-7 imply definite organic

---

*See Appendix A

173

impairment to the point where the patient cannot be expected to manage his own medications or finances and needs assistance with major but not with routine decisions. Error scores between 8-10 imply the need for continuous supervision by another responsible adult. While this test is only a rough indication of intellectual impairment, and while it is not capable of detecting the earliest signs of organic impairment, its simplicity and broad applicability recommend it for widespread clinical and for limited research use. The test has now been translated into both German and French for clinical and research protocol use.[4]

Symptoms Associated with Organic Brain Disease

A plethora of secondary, largely affective or affect-derived symptoms, is frequently but not invariably associated with organic brain disease, both acute and chronic, reversible and irreversible. These symptoms are not at all specific for organic brain disease. They may also be seen in purely functional disorders. They may also be present at one phase of the disorder but not in others. Such symptoms include depression, loss of interest, joviality, emotional lability, perplexedness, bewilderment, panic, or other manifestations of anxiety such as pacing and/or agitation. There may be outbursts of hostility, with both destructive and self-destructive activities. There may be well or ill-formed delusions, both visual and auditory. Suspiciousness not yet organized into a delusional system may also be observed.

As already indicated, these symptoms are largely dependent on rapidity of onset, degree of tissue affected, and environmental and personality factors. Rapid onset, large deficits, rapidly changing environments tend to produce rather florid associated symptoms, as does an emotionally unstable personality. Slow onset, mild to moderate involvement, a stable environment and a stable personality tend to lead to relatively uncomplicated cognitive deficits only. The coexistence of these associated symptoms often requires environmental manipulation, psychotherapy and counseling, and when appropriate, psychoactive medication. Caution should be taken, however, that the use of such medication does not lead to further cognitive impairment. For this reason minimal effective doses for the shortest period of time are desirable.

SPECIFIC CLINICAL MANIFESTATIONS OF SENILE BRAIN DISEASE

While some general symptoms of and associated with organic brain disease have thus far been outlined, the more characteristic manifestations of senile brain disease will now be presented. These tend to be somewhat phase-specific, related to the degree of neuronal loss which has occurred. (It is assumed that the specific neuropathology of senile brain disease of the Alzheimer's type is already known to the reader.)

Early Dementia

Early manifestations of dementia are often quite subtle, and their onset is quite gradual, over a period of several months and sometimes even short years. Initial presenting features may not be any obvious intellectual deficit, but rather a constellation of subtle personality and emotional changes. Depression, listlessness, loss of interest, easy fatiguability, lack of concentration, anxiety or agitation, are often seen in early stages of dementia. These symptoms may initially result in a tentative diagnosis of functional neurosis or psychosis. Irritability, social withdrawal, emotional outburst, inconsiderateness, petulance, unaccustomed moral laxity or irregular work attendance are frequent in the history of early dementia. Even at this stage, however, careful mental status examination or psychological evaluation will reveal impairments of orientation, abstraction capacity, recent and remote memory, and particularly, retention and reproduction of geometric designs involving memory and visual-motor recognition, such as is required in the Bender Gestalt Test.

At this stage some patients are aware at a conscious level that "something is wrong" without being able to specifically identify intellectual or memory difficulties. Other persons seem to be aware of these changes only at a subconscious level, nevertheless responding as though some decline or loss were occurring. Somatic concerns may emerge for which no particular organic basis can be identified. Patients may begin to blame their difficulties on their job, their relatives or friends, minority groups, or other persons in their environment. At points when individuals are suddenly confronted with evidence of some intellectual deficit, they may suddenly be overcome with massive anxiety (Goldstein reaction)[5] which they themselves cannot explain, but which is related to an unexpected awareness of intellectual deficit. At this point already the individual's repertoire of coping mechanisms can come into play. He may deny that anything is wrong; he may try especially hard to make a favorable impression. Almost as important as the individual's own reactions to his vague awareness of "something wrong" is the reaction of those around him - family members, employers, fellow employees. If he is rejected by them because of his changed condition or behavior, his self-esteem will be further eroded, necessitating further adaptive (or maladaptive) mechanisms that may be additionally alienating or self-defeating.

Fully Developed Dementia

Fully developed dementia does not appear overnight. It takes months and sometimes years to develop. But it may be _noticed_ suddenly by those around the dementing patient, because something in his behavior alerts them to make further inquiries or to set up test situations which demonstrate for the first time considerable intellectual deficits that have been developing over an extended period of time. When fully developed, there is usually little difficulty in recognizing this syndrome. A study by Babigian et al.[6] of diagnoses made in a large psychiatric register program showed that dementia could be diagnosed more reliably (consistently) than any other psychiatric disorder. Different psychiatrists, examining the patient at different points in time, will reach the same conclusion regarding diagnosis more often than with any other psychiatric diagnosis.

In fully developed dementia, disorentiation to time and place are very common. Since orientation to time is something that must be continually updated, orientation to time is poorly maintained. Orientation to place is less vulnerable if place of residence is held constant; if the patient is moved around at all, orientation to place is also difficult to maintain. Orientation to one's own person is extremely well maintained: one's own name is probably the single most overlearned item of information. However, identification of other persons in the environment suffers, with both mistaking the unfamiliar with the familiar[7] occurring (in which the patient identifies strangers as persons whom he has knwon, such as one's wife, sister, brother, minister) as well as failing to recognize familiar persons correctly

176

("Who are you? What are you doing here?"). The patient may himself complain of difficulty with memory, but this is not a constant observation. (Incidentally, depressed patients will also complain of memory deficit, but in their instance no memory deficit can be demonstrated objectively.) Observation, however, indicates that the patient does not remember events which have recurred recently; that he asks the same questions repeatedly although answers to them have only just been supplied; and that instructions are quickly forgotten. Such patients may wander away from their home, or if hospitalized, from their assigned room, without necessarily becoming aware that they are lost. When such patients are asked to give medical history, they will generally comply and respond to most questions asked, giving plausible answers. However, a check of collateral information shows that the information is either incorrect altogether or is misplaced in time. A person may correctly report that he has a gall bladder operation or was widowed " a couple of months ago" when the actual events may have taken place fifteen and five years ago, respectively. Telephone numbers are no longer remembered correctly, and gross errors are made in check writing and in keeping checkbook balances, another task requiring serial intellectual operations. Medications which have been prescribed may be taken grossly incorrectly, with both omission and added dosages not infrequent. Personal appearance, such as grooming and cleanliness, may begin to suffer, with zippers left undone, buttons incorrectly buttoned, and signs of spilled food or cigarette ashes appearing on clothing and furniture.

Sleep paterns become seriously altered, with several major episodes of daytime drowsiness and irregular sleep at night, in some patients only. Occasionally complete reversal of sleep pattern occurs with daytime sleep and nighttime wakefulness. The sleep pattern of older patients with and without dementia is more fully characterized by Feinberg (this volume).

Only the simple or core symptoms of dementia have been outlined above. We shall now discuss some of the common associated symptoms that occur in some demented patients. It is also important to note what functions, intellectual or otherwise, remain intact in the substantially demented patient. Social graces and manners, standard social niceties and speech patterns that actually make up a good part of the day to day

social interactions ("How are you doing today?" "Oh, just fine. How are you?")
are often very well maintained giving the casual observer the impression that no
deficit exists. It is only when the person is thrown into unfamiliar circumstances,
or when specific cognitive demands are made on him, that deficit is clearly apparent.

Indicators of Chronicity in Dementia

Certain behaviors, basically adaptive in nature, when present, indicate that
the cognitive deficit has existed for upward of six months and that the patient has
made a valiant attempt to cover up the deficit both from himself and from others.
These mechanisms are adaptive in that they shield the individual from anxiety
concerning his deficit and they are somewhat successful in covering up the deficit
in front of other people. They are maladaptive, however, in that they may lead to
errors, represent a break with reality to a major degree, and significantly
narrow the range of activities the patient can engage in. The list of such mechanisms
includes prominently: denial, especially denial of any memory deficit; confabulation;
avoidance; negativism; jocularity; various kinds of diversionary maneuvers; bantering;
and perseveration.[8] The maneuvers are employed primarily in unfamiliar and hence threat-
ening situations in which the patient's cognitive intactness is likely to be challenged
or tested.

Denial is among the most common of these mechanisms. The person simply says
there is nothing wrong. His memory is fine. He has no difficulty. He does not
understand why anyone is concerned. Why don't people just leave him alone.

Confabulation is probably the best known of these mechanisms. The patient is faced
by an intellectually challenging situation. Some stranger asks him about his present
situation. The patient is likely to "fill in the blank spaces in his cognitive map"
and to make up a plausible but, if need be, constantly changes set of responses that
do not necessarily have any relationship to reality but which never leave the patient
at a loss for an answer. Historically this symptom has been most frequently associated
with dementia due to chronic alcoholism, but it may occur in any of the dementias,
including senile dementia. It may be simply that the alcoholic individual is more

accustomed to banter and repartee and has always been filling in blank spaces with rather tall stories or approximations to the truth.

Perseveration is another interesting phenomenon characteristic of long-standing cognitive deficit. Perseveration may be observed in any sphere of psychomotor activity: speech, writing, drawing locomotion. It is a graphic demonstration of a demented person's difficulty in changing set or frame or reference. Examples might include the retelling of the same story in full detail over and over again; giving the same answer to all questions asked, usually a correct or nearly correct answer to the first question asked. Thus one patient who was first asked about the date, subsequently answered all other questions with the partial answer to the first question ("Nineteen..." standing for ninteenhundred, the beginning of the correct year). An illustration of perseveration in writing would be the patient who began to write the sentence "Now is the time..."; his version looked like this: Now is the time time t t t t; the t's finally trailed off the page. Another illustration was a demented patient who had been given a Rorschach Test. She identified the first inkblot as a "Christmas tree decoration" and responded to every other card with the identical response, simply "Christmas tree".

Avoidance is rather cleverly practiced by some demented patients with good record of social skills. When asked a question they do not know the answer to, they may respond that it is a foolish question, or that they don't bother about such things anymore, or turn around and ask the examiner the same question: "Now I'd like to know that too. You tell me the answer to that." One dignified lady who was severely demented was inventive in the answers she gave regarding her own age. At one time she would break out into laughter, slap her knee and say, "Why, I am a hundred and fifty years old." On another occasion, responding to a stimulus in her room, she looked over at a bouquet of flowers on her nightstand and said, smiling: "Why I am as young as that rose over there."

The presence of such defensive maneuvers indicates two things: the intellectual deficit has been present for some considerable period of time, six months at a minimum, more likely a year or longer; the ego is not overwhelmed by the deficit but is still trying to cope with it.

Deterioration in Dementia

If the dementing process continues (and it should not be assumed that there will
be progression - see below), the patient will gradually enter into a period of
deterioration that will affect not only intellectual adaptive capacity but physiological
adaptive capacity as well. Social control over urination is lost, and later control
over defecation both in terms of appropriate time and place. Speech becomes
either monosyllabic, peseverative, or unintelligible. Thus the patient's needs
cannot be verbally communicated any longer and he may now require constant attention
and supervision. Motor control falters too. The patient may no longer be able to
feed himself and may require assistance with most activities of daily living, including
dressing, bathing, and grooming. Finally, the patient may become so weak and uncoordin-
ated that he becomes bedridden. When this occurs, the end is generally near. Recumbency
may lead to decubitus ulcer formation with resultant infection, including septicemia.
The most common cause of death is bronchopneumonia resulting from decreased responsivity
of the breathing mechanism and decreased reflex activity in clearing sputum from the
bronchial tree. The brain, the organ of adaptation, has ceased to adapt.

Arrest and Stabilization of the Dementing Process

While it was previously assumed that senile dementia as well as presenile dementia
of the Alzheimer's type was a clearly progressive disorder that generally led to
deterioration, this assumption is no longer supported by longitudinal clinical data.
Whereas it is true that those patients with symptom onset in their fifties and very
early sixties do follow a fairly rapid course that may result in death from two to ten
years after onset, some newer observations on patients with senile dementia whose onset
is somewhat later modify this picture and open up new avenues for research. These
observations relate to the fact that some persons develop quite serious degrees of
dementia, over extended periods of time, but then seem to clearly stabilize, without any
further progression of the clinical manifestations of dementia. Whether the death of
brain cells has simultaneuously slowed or ceased cannot be said, but such patients
either maintain stable intellectual functioning, or sometimes even improve over a matter
of years, and may eventually die from unrelated causes. This gives hope to the idea that

if something is able to arrest the progress of the disease spontaneously, then research into this arresting process ought to turn up techniques for arresting the disease intentionally. It is very likely that answers to this intriguing question will come from one of the disciplines represented at this conference. But it would be impossible to predict which of these disciplines will be able to provide this critical answer.

The magnitude of the problem involved in senile dementia, however, should be clear to everyone. Very nearly half of all persons currently in chronic care institutions for the aged reside there with senile dementia as either a primary or secondary diagnosis. The dollar figures involved in the long-term care industry for these patients alone are truly staggering. It should be clear that a major nationally coordinated research program needs to be undertaken to discover the root causes of the disease rather than trying only to improve the quality of care by small steps through incremental legislation and regulation.

MULTIPLE INFARCT DISEASE

Distinctions need to be drawn between the clinical manifestations of senile dementia of the Alzheimer's type and the clinical manifestations of multiple infarct disease. They are both organic brain diseases evidencing core and associated symptoms. The course and development of these symptoms, however, is quite different. The development of symptomatology in multiple infarct disease is generally stepwise with a sudden worsening of intellectual performance, clouding of consciousness, disorientation, confusion, and sometimes associated symptoms of hallucinations and delusions. Gradually over a period of weeks or months, but especially when there are deliberate efforts at intellectual retraining and relearning of the environmental situation, improvements result that may lead to near-normal or even normal functioning. With repeated insults, however, new episodes of disorientation and clouding of consciousness occur from which recovery tends to be less complete. After several years of such episodes the clinical picture, where adequate history is not available, may in fact be quite similar, because the cumulative effect has been a significant reduction of total brain mass to which the patient has been able to make some adaptation.

SUMMARY

In conclusion, senile dementia of the Alzheimer's type is part and parcel of the
organic brain disorders in general. It shares with them the characteristic core
symptoms of organic brain disease, specifically certain cognitive deficits which have
been detailed. It may also share with these other disorders certain associated or
secondary symptoms that are the result of interaction of the underlying brain deficit
and the personality of the individual and his environment. It is the gradually
developing core of these clinical manifestations that allows the physician to
suspect, in the absence of other defineable or diagnosable disorders, the presence of
senile dementia. Recent observations that the degree of intellectual deficit seems
to stabilize in substantial numbers of patients gives hope that research efforts will
be successful in understanding and arresting the progress of this devastating disorder.

REFERENCES

1. Vogel, F.S. The Brain and Time. In Busse and Pfeiffer, Behavior and Adaptation
   in Late Life, second edition. Boston: Little, Brown, 1977, pp. 228.-239.

2. Pfeiffer, E. A short portable mental status questionnaire for the assessment
   of organic brain deficit in elderly patients. J. Amer. Geriat. Soc. 23: 433-441,
   1975.

3. Hagland, R.M.J. and Schuckit, M.A. A clinical comparison of tests of organicity
   in elderly patients. J. Gerontol. 31: 654-659, 1976.

4. McDonald, R.J. Personal Communication (Translation by G. Junkers), 1976.

5. Goldstein, K. Functional Disturbances in Brain Damage in Arieti, Handbook
   of Psychiatry. New York: Basic Books, 1959, pp. 770-794.

6. Babigan, H.M. et al. Diagnostic consistency and change in a follow-up of 1215
   patients. Amer. J. Psychiatr. 121: 895-901, 1965.

7. Levin, M. Delerious disorientation, the law of the unfamiliar mistaken for the
   familiar. J. Ment. Sci. 91: 447-453, 1945.

8. Weinstein, E. and Kahn, R. The Denial of Illness. Springfield,Ill.: Charles
   C. Thomas, 1955.

APPENDIX A: Short Portable Mental Status Questionnaire (SPMSQ)

Eric Pfeiffer, M.D.

Instructions: Ask questions 1-10 in this list and record all answers. Ask question 4A only if patient does not have a telephone. Record total number of errors based on ten questions.

+	−

1. What is the date today? _____
   Month   Day   Year
2. What day of the week is it? _____

3. What is the name of this place? _____

4. What is your telephone number? _____

4A. What is your street address? _____
    (Ask only if the patient does not have a telephone)
5. How old are you? _____

6. When were you born? _____

7. Who is the President of the U.S. now? _____

8. Who was President just before him? _____

9. What was your mother's maiden name? _____

10. Subtract 3 from 20 and keep subtracting 3 from each new
    number, all the way down.

_____   Total Number of Errors

To Be Completed by Interviewer

Patient's Name: _____ Date _____

Sex: 1. Male   Race: 1. White
     2. Female   2. Black
                              3. Other

Years of Education: _____ 1. Grade School
                                              2. High School
                                              3. Beyond High School

Interviewer's Name: _____

NEUROPSYCHOLOGICAL ASPECTS OF ALZHEIMER'S DISEASE AND MULTI-INFARCT DEMENTIA

FRANCISCO I. PEREZ, JOE R. A. GAY, AND NORMA A. COOKE
Neuropsychology Laboratory - Department of Neurology, Baylor College of Medicine,
Houston, Texas 77030

INTRODUCTION

Aging may be defined as a decline in physiologic competence that inevitably increases the incidence and intensifies the effects of accidents, disease, and other forms of environmental stress[1]. Presently it is not clear whether there is a specific cause of aging, whether several potential causes operate together, or even if aging is simply an accumulation of physiologic deficits[2]. Research has been unable to determine whether aging results from an evolutionary necessity related to the survival of the species, from the accumulated effects of "wear and tear", or from the natural process of physiological change. In general, aging leads to a growing inability of the organism to adapt to the environment and thus to survive. It is very difficult to separate the physiological, social, and psychological effects of aging from the effects of disease since aging and disease are highly correlated. That is, as individuals age they generally become more troubled by chronic diseases and the effects of aging and disease compound one another. Nonetheless, it is important to attempt to distinguish between the changes that result from aging per se and from disease. Otherwise, we are easily misled into equating aging with disease.

The relationship between organic dementia and normal aging is one of the main problems facing the behavioral gerontological researcher. The issue is whether dementia is the ultimate outcome of cerebral aging or is it a disease process which is independent of aging although most frequently found in the aged individual. Recent studies indicate that old age and dementia are far from synonymous[3,4]. Kral[3] indicates that dementia is not the final outcome of normal cerebral aging but seems to be a disease process which is different from normal aging. It appears that many of the psychological changes usually attributed to aging are better seen as the result of disease and even in the absence of disease there are changes in physiological and psychological functioning with age. Intensified research and refined methodology can provide significant information regarding the crucial distinction between the physiological and psychological changes resulting from aging and changes resulting from disease. The present report will summarize the neuropsychological aspects of Alzheimer's disease and multi-infarct dementia emphasizing the studies being carried out at the Baylor Neuropsychology Laboratory.

DEFINITION OF DEMENTIA

One good definition for dementia is not available. Dementia is a disruption of behavior with impairment in the ability to learn new responses and thus to adapt to a changing environment[5]. Psychological and intellectual changes are the essential elements for a diagnosis of dementia. Most authors agree that a consistent feature in dementia is overall neuropsychological deterioration. However, dementia is not a disease but is a syndrome of behavioral and cognitive reduction which may be produced by a wide variety of etiologies. The clinical and behavioral pattern may vary according to the nature of the cause, the localization of the etiologic process within the central nervous system, the rate of progression, the age of onset and environmental factors.

Current thinking proposes two main underlying diseases accounting for dementia. These are Alzheimer's disease (AD) which is considered a primary degenerative disease of the central nervous system, particularly the cerebrum, and multi-infarct dementia (MID) which is a primary disease of the brain vasculature with secondary degenerative changes in the brain. These two conditions are the primary subject of the present communication.

Alzheimer's disease (AD). Terry[6] reports that AD is the most common type of dementia. It is now generally accepted that both "presenile" and "senile" dementia are forms of Alzheimer's disease with the same clinical manifestations and histopathological findings. The brain is shrunken in size and weight, with lessened cortex and white matter and enlarged lateral ventricles.

Alzheimer's disease patients usually present with a history of chronic progressive dementing process without risk factors or evidence of cerebrovascular disease. The clinical course in these patients is not characterized by episodic worsening of mentation as typically occurs in patients with cerebrovascular disease. There is usually no history of transient cerebral ischemic attacks. The signs of cerebral dysfunction are diffuse and bilateral. Grasp, sucking, and glabellar reflexes are usually prominent. Computerized axial tomography (CAT) usually shows cortical atrophy predominantly in the frontal and parietal regions with enlarged ventricles.

Multi-infarct dementia (MID). Hachinski et al.[4] indicate that multiple infarcts can produce a condition in which dementia may be the dominant symptom. Besides dementia there are focal neurological signs and symptoms, a stepwise deterioration and quite often hypertension. They[4] claim that multi-infarct dementia is a relatively small group and the early diagnosis and identification is important since hypertension can be controlled. A patchy and irregular reduction of cerebral blood flow is seen in the zones of ischemia and infarction[7].

The dementing process in MID patients is usually associated with documented risk factors for cerebrovascular disease, particularly a long-standing history of hypertension. The clinical course of the dementia is characterized by episodic strokes with cumulative worsening of mentation plus associated transient cerebral ischemic episodes. The neurological exam usually shows multiple signs of diffusely represented cerebral deficits attributable to multiple vascular lesions such as hemiplegia,

186

dysphasia, hemianopia, or cortical sensory loss confined to segmental zones of half
the body. The CAT scan usually shows patchy zones of cerebral infarction.

NEUROPSYCHOLOGICAL EVALUATION OF DEMENTIA

   Since psychological and intellectual changes are the essential elements for a
diagnosis of dementia it is useful to follow up the initial clinical neurological
examination with a more detailed neuropsychological evaluation. This evaluation is
a systematic assessment of brain-behavior relationships. It includes detailed
measurement of: 1 - Intellectual and cognitive functioning; 2 - Memory functioning;
3 - Language functioning; 4 - Perceptual-motor functioning; and if necessary 5 -
Personality functioning.

   The primary aim of the neuropsychological evaluation is to describe and identify
in detail the nature of the psychological disturbances of a given patient. The first
step is to establish that there is a true mental deterioration[4]. It can help in the
differential diagnosis since different dementing diseases produce distinct patterns
of neuropsychological performance[5]. Depression, systemic illness, and overmedication
are all common conditions that can mimic dementia in the elderly. The evaluation
can also provide a baseline for the assessment of medical and environmental therapeutic interventions. Hachinski et al.[4] indicate that only the establishment of
reliable psychological measures and longitudinal study will test the validity of pur-
ported general treatments of dementia including pharmachological agents. However,
this requires more refined and precise behavioral measures than those currently used
including conventional psychometric procedures. The Baylor Neuropsychology Laboratory
is currently engaged in the systematic development of a computerized Automated
Behavioral Assessment System (ABAS) in order to more precisely define the individual
behavioral performance of demented and normal elderly patients[8].

PATTERNS OF BEHAVIORAL PERFORMANCE IN DEMENTIA

   Research in our laboratory has shown different patterns of intellectual and memory
performance in patients with multi-infarct dementia (MID) and Alzheimer's disease
(AD)[5,9,10]. Perez et al.[5] found significant differences in cognitive and intellectual performance on the Wechsler Adult Intelligence Scale (WAIS) between MID and AD.
The AD group performed significantly and consistently lower on all intellectual measures. A discriminant function analysis classified 74% of the patients correctly
based on the individual WAIS scores. The discrimination was more easily made when
tasks measuring visual motor coordination and abstract reasoning were included in the
analysis. The data also suggested that the MID group was less homogeneous than the
AD group as might be predicted from the patchy nature of the disease process. The
degree and pattern of intellectual deficit varied with each MID patient depending on
the sites, location, extent and number of cerebral infarctions.

   Different patterns of memory performance using the Wechsler Memory Scale (WMS) were found by Perez et al.[9] in patients with AD and MID. Univariate statistical procedures revealed that the AD group again performed significantly and consistently poorer on all memory measures. A discriminant function analysis classified 100% of the patients correctly based on the individual WMS scores. The discrimination was primarily based on the Memory Quotient (MQ) score and the individual performance on the pair-associate subtest measuring the ability to learn new verbal information.

These two studies[5,9], even though preliminary in nature, provide support for the potential clinical and practical application of neuropsychological and behavioral procedures in identifying the patterns of psychological changes associated with the various diseases producing dementia. If these findings are consistently replicated, it might be possible to develop an "early behavioral warning system" in order to detect a dementing process in the elderly at its onset and possibly institute remedial or preventive measures.

REPLICATION STUDIES

This section presents the comparison of three independent samples of patients with the clinical diagnosis of AD and MID[7,9]. These samples consist of carefully diagnosed demented patients seen clinically in our laboratory in the last three years. Each independent sample is composed of patients seen in a given year. The first sample is composed of 26 patients (10 AD - 16 MID) seen during 1975. To arrive at this sample, two independent neurologists evaluated the medical records of over 100 demented patients and only those who met the criteria previously presented for identifying MID and AD were included. The second sample consisted of 31 patients (17 AD - 14 MID) seen during 1976. The third sample consisted of 29 patients (19 AD - 10 MID) seen during 1977. Again, independent neurologists reviewed the medical records of numerous demented patients and only those with a convincing clinical diagnosis were included. The psychological measures were not included in the medical evaluation. These measures are the Verbal IQ (VIQ), Performance IQ (PIQ) and Full IQ (FIQ) from the WAIS and the Memory Quotient (MQ) from the WMS.

Table 1 shows the mean comparison between AD and MID - 1975 - first sample for each measurement obtained. Statistical differences were found between the groups for Performance IQ and Memory Quotient with the AD group performing significantly poorer. In this sample it is interesting to note that significant differences were found for the education variable with the AD group having on the average 3 more years of formal education.

Table 2 shows the mean comparison for the - 1976 - second independent sample. Even though the AD group was better educated and consistently performed lower on all the psychological measures, significant statistical difference was only found for the MQ measure.

TABLE 1

MEAN COMPARISON BETWEEN AD AND MID - 1975 - FIRST SAMPLE

Variables	Multi-infarct Mean	Alzheimer's Mean	p<
Age	69.3	62.2	n.s.
Education	10.3	13.7	.05
Verbal IQ	86.8	75.0	n.s.
Performance IQ	85.3	71.6	.05
Full IQ	85.6	72.3	n.s.
Memory Quotient	80.4	62.9	.05

TABLE 2

MEAN COMPARISON BETWEEN AD AND MID - 1976 - SECOND SAMPLE

Variables	Multi-infarct Mean	Alzheimer's Mean	p<
Age	63.9	64.1	n.s.
Education	10.9	12.7	n.s.
Verbal IQ	89.5	83.5	n.s.
Performance IQ	87.9	77.3	n.s.
Full IQ	88.3	79.7	n.s.
Memory Quotient	84.5	66.5	.001

A closer inspection of the data indicates that the two independent MID samples were similar but there were obvious quantitative differences between the two AD groups. The second AD sample performed consistently better. This sample's performance appears to be similar to the two MID groups. In order to analyze this quantitative difference between the two AD samples, we carefully inspected the clinical records of each AD patient. We found that the average reported time since the first symptoms were noted and the neuropsychological evaluation for the first sample was 4.2 years and for the second sample was 3.2 years. This difference of one year progression of the disease might account for the quantitative difference since AD is associated with progressive behavioral deterioration. Future behavioral studies should carefully control this relevant variable. Serial behavioral measures on AD patients over time are necessary in evaluating the nature as well as natural course of the psychological disturbances associated with AD.

An additional important implication is that the AD group on these two samples had on the average, three years more formal education. Careful inspection of the clinical records of each patient included in the two studies, revealed that the chief complaint at the time of admission for every AD patient was memory or psychological problems. The typical MID patient presented with a primary physical disorder (i.e., hemiparesis or history of strokes) and psychological concerns were secondary. This difference in presenting symptoms might lead to sampling biases in the behavioral study of dementia. Educational and socioeconomic factors might select the patient with AD who is admitted for medical services. The MID patient will tend to seek medical treatment for his physical condition. However, the AD patient might tend to seek help for his memory and psychological problems primarily because of a higher previous level of functioning which makes subtle changes detectable by himself or members of the family. It is possible that in lower educational and socio-economic levels, the psychological changes associated with AD go unnoticed longer and/or these cases tend to be admitted to state psychiatric institutions with the unfortunate diagnosis of "organic brain syndrome". These considerations indicate the importance of collecting a detailed social, psychological and medical history in patients with dementia. Demographic and epidemiological studies are urgently needed in the light of the present hypotheses.

Recently, we have completed the comparison of the - 1977 - third sample of AD and MID patients seen in our laboratory. Table 3 shows the results. The two previous studies have shown that the memory deficit in AD was consistent and in relation to cognition memory was more impaired. The present results replicate the previous findings indicating again a significant difference in Memory Quotient performance with the AD group having a greater memory disorder. Since the WMS Memory Quotient and the WAIS Full Scale IQ correlate highly, we were interested in evaluating the hypothesis that in AD the memory impairment was more severe than the cognitive impairment and that in MID the cognitive and memory performance did not differ. The difference between the Full IQ and Memory Quotient (FIQ - MQ) was computed and analyzed statistically. The hypothesis was confirmed indicating in general, that in AD the dementing disorder affects memory performance significantly more than cognition even though cognition is also impaired. The Hard Paired Associates learning task of the WMS was also compared. This task measures primarily the ability to learn and remember new verbal information. Again, the AD group showed a greater memory impairment.

The last variable analyzed involved the finger-tapping test with each hand. This test compares the fine finger motor dexterity of the preferred hand to the non-preferred hand. This test is highly sensitive to unilateral cerebral disease with decrements on the opposite hand. Since the analysis of the individual clinical records for the two previous samples suggested a difference in the presenting symptomatology for AD and MID, we were interested in evaluating the motor performance for both groups. The hypothesis was that in MID we expected a greater percent difference between right and left hand performance than in AD since MID was more susceptible to discrete focal cerebral lesions. The results confirmed this hypothesis.

TABLE 3

MEAN COMPARISON BETWEEN AD AND MID - 1977 - THIRD SAMPLE

Variables	Multi-infarct Mean	Alzheimer's Mean	p<
Age	69.5	63.5	n.s.
Education	12.9	12.0	n.s.
Verbal IQ	98.0	90.1	n.s.
Performance IQ	87.0	80.7	n.s.
Full IQ	93.3	85.3	n.s.
Memory Quotient	89.9	72.0	.05
FIQ - MQ	1.8	13.3	.005
Hard Paired Associates	3.6	.6	.002
R-L Finger Tapping (% difference)	24.9	12.7	.05

Disorders of memory are a characteristic and often a prominent feature of dementia. Karp[11] considers memory loss as a logical focal point for the clinical analysis of disorders of mental functioning in the elderly. The present psychological findings demonstrate that the MQ was consistently reduced in both groups and particularly in the AD group when compared to the MID. This finding was replicated in three independent samples. Previous studies from our laboratory[10] have demonstrated that it was possible to discriminate the two dementia groups by the MQ. Recent studies have reported that the concentration of neurofibrillary tangles and neuritic or senile plaques found at postmortem examination in AD corresponded with the degree of psychometric impairment[12]. Terry and Wisniewski[13] report that in AD the neurofibrillary tangles and the granulovacular changes are most obvious in the hippocampus-limbic system. Milner[14] has shown the relationship of lesions in the hippocampal area and material-specific memory disorders. The severe memory deficit presently demonstrated in the three independent AD samples corroborates the pathological findings.

LONGITUDINAL STUDIES

Intellectual processes in particular, and all systems of the organism in general, are affected by the physiological changes of senescence. However, there is a crucial distinction between the physiological and psychological changes resulting from aging

and changes resulting from disease. Longitudinal studies[15,16] have demonstrated
that psychological performance of a very healthy and a mild diseases group of aged
individual, differed with consistent poorer performance on the mild diseases group.
Re-evaluation eleven years later[16] showed that the mild degree of disease that differentiated these two groups was important in terms of eventual mortality. The
behavioral differences initially found were related to survival. In addition, they
found that among the surviving subjects there was a remarkably limited amount of
change. There is accumulating evidence for the existance of a discontinuous and
abrupt drop in performance on ability tests in the periods ranging from a few months
to about five years or more prior to death[17]. It appears that measures of intellectual functioning in the aged are important predictors of mortality and health.

Presently we are analyzing the longitudinal data on serial neuropsychological
evaluations of 10 patients with AD and 10 patients with MID. The variables are WAIS
Verbal IQ, Performance IQ and WMS Memory Quotient. Preliminary analysis suggests
that the initial level of performance was predictive of the subsequent trend of performance. Patients with higher scores tended to maintain their level of performance.
In contrast, fewer patients with poorer scores remained fairly stable and most tended
to deteriorate over time. The AD patients tended to be over-represented in the
lower scores group. The Memory Quotient, and to a lesser extent, the Performance
IQ, seemed to be more sensitive than the Verbal IQ to declines in the level of performance in the group with higher scores. It was not possible to determine, on the
basis of the brief preliminary analysis, whether or not the declines observed were
reflective of meaningful changes in the general level of adaptive functioning of a
given patient nor associated with the natural course of the given dementing disorder.

CEREBRAL BLOOD FLOW PATTERNS IN DEMENTIA

Reduction of cerebral blood flow (CBF) in organic dementias has long been recognized[18]. Research studies have also established that this reduction is not attributed solely to normal aging[19,20]. Regional cerebral blood flow (rCBF) studies in
dementia report a selective regional reduction of blood flow[18]. Ingvar[21] applying
a 20% reduction from the patient's CBF value as a criterion for regional decrease,
found a fronto-temporal pattern of reduction in "senile dementia". Obrist et al.[18]
have similarly found consistent focal reduction in the fronto-temporal region in a
similar group of patients. Hachinski et al.[22] analyzed patients with primary degenerative dementia and MID and found that the relative weight of the gray matter (Wg)
was reduced in both groups when compared to a control group. They[22] interpreted
this as indicating a considerable loss of functioning gray matter relative to white
matter in both MID and primary degenerative dementia.

In our laboratory we have applied multivariate data analysis statistical procedures in order to identify rCBF patterns in patients with AD and MID when compared
to a control group[7,23]. A fronto-temporal-parietal pattern was identified for the

AD group. The MID group demonstrated a predominant temporal-parietal or sylvian pattern corresponding with the distribution of the middle cerebral artery. In addition, we found a significant reduction of mean hemispheric blood flow for both AD and MID groups when compared to a control group. This reduction was more significant for the MID group. It was also found that relative weight of the gray matter (Wg) was reduced in both AD and MID, but to a greater extent in MID. These results are consistent with those previously reported[18,21,22]. It appears that the different underlying pathological processes for AD and MID produce distinct rCBF patterns. Our study was performed using the 133-Xenon intracarotid injection method. Studies are needed, however, using the now popular Xenon[133] inhalation technique in order to assess the utility of this non-invasive procedure in the evaluation of the demented patient and the normal aged individual.

CEREBRAL BLOOD FLOW AND NEUROPSYCHOLOGICAL CORRELATES

A correlation between the severity of psychological impairment in the dementias and reduction of CBF and metabolism have been reported[18,24]. Simard et al.[24] as well as Obrist et al.[18] found a positive correlation between the decrease in mean hemispheric CBF and the degree of psychological impairment in "senile dementia". However, Hachinski et al.[22] found no correlation between the degree of dementia and CBF reduction in a primary degenerative group.

Perez et al.[23] assessed the relationship of the degree of psychological impairment in AD and MID and rCBF reduction. A series of Spearman rank order correlations (Rho) were computed. The 13 CBF regions obtained with the intracarotid Xenon[133] injection method on the right hemisphere were grouped and averaged into frontal (7 regions), temporal (2 regions), parietal (2 regions) and occipital (2 regions) areas. Mean hemispheric CBF was obtained by averaging the values from the 13 regions. The psychological variables included age, Verbal IQ (VIQ), Performance IQ (PIQ) and the Memory Quotient (MQ). The patients included in this study were a subset of the patients included in the - 1976 - second sample replication study in which rCBF studies were performed.

Table 4 shows the Rho values between neuropsychological and rCBF data for MID. Significant correlations were found between advancing age and CBF reduction in the temporal and parietal regions as well as with mean hemispheric blood flow (HBF). The other significant correlation for MID was found between the degree of MQ impairment and CBF reduction in the temporal region. The more impaired the patient's memory performance the more reduced the temporal CBF.

Table 5 shows the Rho values between neuropsychological and CBF data for AD. The only correlation found was between CBF reduction in the frontal regions and age. The older the patient within the AD group, the more significantly reduced the frontal CBF.

TABLE 4

SPEARMAN RANK ORDER CORRELATION BETWEEN NEUROPSYCHOLOGICAL AND CEREBRAL BLOOD FLOW
DATA FOR MULTI-INFARCT DEMENTIA

Cortical Regions Blood Flow	Neuropsychological Variables			
	Age	VIQ	PIQ	MQ
Frontal	.3768	-.0150	-.3794	.0143
Temporal	.4759*	.0440	.3396	.6516**
Parietal	.6088**	-.2934	-.1240	.2055
Occipital	.3205	-.2932	-.1068	.4068
Mean HBF	.5072*	-.0830	-.0669	.2714

*p<.05
**p<.01

TABLE 5

SPEARMAN RANK ORDER CORRELATION BETWEEN NEUROPSYCHOLOGICAL AND CEREBRAL BLOOD FLOW
DATA FOR ALZHEIMER'S DISEASE

Cortical Regions Blood Flow	Neuropsychological Variables			
	Age	VIQ	PIQ	MQ
Frontal	.5310*	.1730	.0495	.2967
Temporal	.0375	.3893	.1902	.3214
Parietal	.0371	-.0385	.1044	.2692
Occipital	.4304	.1536	.0099	.1679
Mean HBF	.0375	-.3071	-.3455	-.1179

*p<.05

In summary, in MID the memory impairment correlates with the reduction of rCBF
in the temporal regions. This indicates that the degree of memory impairment in MID
is related to reduced blood flow and impaired energy production in the temporal area.
In addition, advancing age in MID corresponds to CBF reduction in the territory of
the middle cerebral artery distribution. In contrast, no actual psychological deficits correlated with rCBF reduction in AD except advancing age and frontal CBF reduction. It appears that different underlying pathological dementing processes produce
distinct rCBF patterns and only as expected in MID, this CBF reduction corresponds
with a specific behavioral impairment. The present results suggest that in AD the
specific behavioral deficits observed are not secondary to rCBF reduction.

AUTOMATED BEHAVIORAL ASSESSMENT SYSTEM (ABAS)

Knowledge about the behavioral status of the aged has been gained as a result of the development of experimental methods of assessment and the application of more precise conceptualization in the field of behavioral gerontology. Birren[25] proposes that laboratory research on the psychology of aging is a potential friend of the aging adult and that we ought to utilize the precise findings of the laboratory for the benefit of the aging population. However, in the behavioral study of dementia, some uncontrolled variables may lie outside the boundaries of immediate measurement and control in the clinical setting and cannot be identified and measured properly with current psychometric procedures. This is an important issue since the ultimate criterion of success or failure of a specific treatment approach, including pharmachological agents, in the organic dementias is behavioral in nature. Effective research on the treatment of demented patients is dependent on the existence of precise behavioral methods of assessing the effects of proposed, new forms of treatment. It is particularly important to be able to detect small, but significant improvements in a patient's condition so that potentially useful forms of treatment are not abandoned prematurely. In addition, correlations of morphologic brain changes and behavioral performance are exercises in futility if either set of observations is improperly controlled. The behavioral assessment must be as rigorous as the anatomic if the correlation is to be meaningful.

The Baylor Neuropsychology Laboratory has been performing preliminary work in developing a computerized Automated Behavioral Assessment System (ABAS)[8]. The primary objective is to develop a precise and direct behavioral measurement system that is sensitive to small changes in behavioral and psychological functioning of the healthy and diseased aged individual. Characteristics of this system include: a) The intensive study of individual subjects; b) Control of the assessment environment: c) Continuous observation and recording of behavior; and d) Automatic recording and programming.

A powerful advantage of the ABAS is that it permits the precise recording of response latencies (reaction time) as well as the precise timing of presentation of multi-modal stimuli, both of which are essential in tests of learning and memory in the aged.

The clinical studies in our laboratory have demonstrated that memory deficits are the logical focal point for the behavioral analysis in the dementias: Therefore, our initial efforts in the development of the ABAS has been the titration of short-term recognition memory in demented patients. We have accomplished titration of memory performance in over 60 demented patients. Two adjusting delayed visual-visual matching to sample tasks have been developed. ABAl involves random visual shapes used as a measure of visual memory. ABA2 involves nonsense syllable trigrams used as

195

a measure of verbal memory. Perez et al.[26] have reported that ABA1 is sensitive to right hemisphere strokes and ABA2 to left hemisphere strokes corresponding to hemispheric dominance. Each patient sits in front of a Human Test System (HTS) panel with a display screen. This screen is a rear-view projection window divided into four independent 3 x 2 inch sections arranged in a 2 x 2 matrix. The sample stimulus appears on the upper left window for one second. The delayed interval between stimulus appears on the upper left window for one second. The delayed interval between stimulus sample presentation and choices automatically increases or decreases by 7 seconds depending upon the performance of a patient on a given trial. An adjacent simultaneous simple color matching task is used as a distractor during the delay interval. The programming of the stimulus and responses as well as data acquisition and retrieval is computerized using an inexpensive IMSAI 8080 microcomputer. Titration of memory performance is then accomplished for each patient. A graphic report summarizing the individual memory performance for each task in 30 discrete trials is automatically printed.

Figure 1 shows the actual computer print-out for Control #756. The task is ABA2 - nonsense syllable trigram recognition task. This is a healthy 62 year old male with a high school education. His WAIS scores were: Full IQ 110; Verbal IQ 109; Performance IQ 112. His WMS Memory Quotient was 106. On the figure a "+" indicates correct recognition and a "-" indicates incorrect recognition on a given trial. The specific delay interval for a given trial is also presented. Summary statistics are presented at the bottom of the figure indicating the total percentage of correct and incorrect discriminations. Figure 1 shows that on ABA2 his accuracy was 80% with a ceiling delay interval of 108 seconds. On ABA1 (not shown) he obtained a 93% accuracy with a ceiling delay interval of 156.9. This performance is compatible with our series of normal controls.

Figure 2 shows the performance on ABA2 for a 59 year old male with a college education. He is a retired accountant. Medical records indicate that his problem started with memory difficulties which progressed and have become slowly worse. He is also described as becoming more irritable. No risk factors for cerebrovascular disease are present. The EEG showed marked diffuse slowing. Computerized axial tomography revealed moderate symmetrical enlargement of the bodies of the lateral ventricles and abnormally broad superficial cerebral sulci-changes which indicate the presence of bilateral cerebral atrophy. The patient was diagnosed as Alzheimer's disease. The neuropsychological results showed a Full WAIS IQ of 103; Verbal IQ 106; Performance IQ 91. His MQ was 86. Inspection of Figure 2 shows that his ABA2 performance is significantly impaired with 30% accuracy and a maximum delayed interval level of 20.7 seconds on trial 27. On ABA1 (not shown), he obtained an accuracy of 53% with a maximum delayed interval level of 39.40 seconds on trial 27.

NEUROPSYCHOLOGY LABORATORY - BAYLOR COLLEGE OF MEDICINE

[756]
RIGHTHANDED MALE 62 YRS*   TEST: IABA2   DATE: 18-NOV-76
DIAGNOSIS: NORMAL   EDU:

DELAY INTERVAL

Test Trials

```
 1  +                                                          1.00   1
 2  - ****                                                     8.00   2
 3  +                                                          1.00   3
 4  + ***                                                      7.90   4
 5  + ******                                                  14.20   5
 6  + *********                                               20.40   6
 7  + *************                                           26.80   7
 8  - ***************                                         32.90   8
 9  + *************                                           26.80   9
10  + ****************                                        32.80  10
11  + *******************                                     39.00  11
12  + ***********************                                 45.60  12
13  + **************************                              51.90  13
14  + *****************************                           57.90  14
15  - *******************************                         64.10  15
16  + ****************************                            57.90  16
17  + *******************************                         64.20  17
18  + ***********************************                     70.40  18
19  - **************************************                  76.70  19
20  + *************************************                   70.50  20
21  + **************************************                  76.60  21
22  + *****************************************               82.70  22
23  + *******************************************             89.00  23
24  + **********************************************          95.50  24
25  + ************************************************       101.20  25
26  - **************************************************     108.00  26
27  - *************************************************      101.60  27
28  - ***********************************************        108.00  28
29  + *********************************************          101.20  29
30  + ***********************************************        108.00  30
```

```
     10  20  30  40  50  60  70  80  90  100 110 120 130  Seconds

          TEST TRIALS        MEAN    S D     GREATEST
CORRECT   -    24/30(80%)    56.00   34.382   108.00 (30)
INCORRECT -    06/30(20%)    66.28   40.262   108.00 (26)
```

FIGURE 1.   ABA2 Titration for Normal Aged.

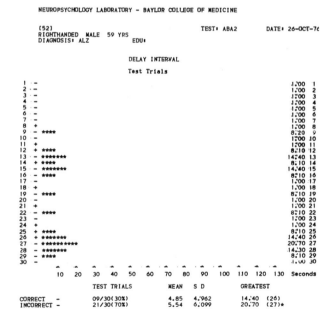

NEUROPSYCHOLOGY LABORATORY - BAYLOR COLLEGE OF MEDICINE

[52]
RIGHTHANDED MALE 59 YRS   TEST: ABA2   DATE: 26-OCT-76
DIAGNOSIS: ALZ   EDU:

DELAY INTERVAL

Test Trials

```
 1  - -                                                       1.00   1
 2  - -                                                       1.00   2
 3  - -                                                       1.00   3
 4  -                                                         1.00   4
 5  - -                                                       1.00   5
 6  -                                                         1.00   6
 7  -                                                         1.00   7
 8  +                                                         1.00   8
 9  - ****                                                    8.20   9
10  -                                                         1.00  10
11  +                                                         1.00  11
12  + ****                                                    8.10  12
13  - - ******                                               14.40  13
14  + ****                                                    8.10  14
15  - *******                                                14.40  15
16  - ****                                                    8.10  16
17  -                                                         1.00  17
18  +                                                         1.00  18
19  - ****                                                    8.10  19
20  -                                                         1.00  20
21  +                                                         1.00  21
22  - ****                                                    8.10  22
23  -                                                         1.00  23
24  +                                                         1.00  24
25  + ****                                                    8.10  25
26  - *******                                                14.40  26
27  - *********                                              20.70  27
28  - *******                                                14.30  28
29  - ****                                                    8.10  29
30  -                                                         1.00  30
```

```
     10  20  30  40  50  60  70  80  90  100 110 120 130  Seconds

          TEST TRIALS        MEAN    S D     GREATEST
CORRECT   -    09/30(30%)    4.85    4.962    14.40  (26)
INCORRECT -    21/30(70%)    5.54    6.099    20.70  (27)*
```

FIGURE 2.   ABA2 Titration for AD Patient.

The preliminary studies using the ABAS have demonstrated the sensitivity of the computerized memory assessment titration procedure to neurological disorders. Presently we are developing additional behavioral tasks using cross-modality matching to sample. These tasks include measures of language, learning and concept attainment. The ABAS methodology can provide the precision required for the study of molar and molecular behavioral changes associated with structural changes in the brain. Perhaps the most promising application is that it can afford the behavioral quantification necessary in order to evaluate promising therapeutic trials in the dementias.

FUTURE DIRECTIONS

With the gradual extension of the human life the field of gerontology is gaining increasing importance. The growing percentage of old people in society gives rise to a variety of health and social problems. Dementia is a major disorder afflicting the elderly. About 10% of old people are demented, half of them severely, and in the over-80's this proportion rises to more than one in five[27]. The financial burden in caring for such patients amounts to many billions of dollars per year. Despite their high incidence, the behavioral aspects of dementia have been of minimal interest to the psychologist. The relationship between dementia and normal aging is one of the main problems facing the behavioral gerontological researcher. However, the extent to which this problem can be usefully investigated is limited by the current state of behavioral technology. It is important to realize that psychology has a technical basis and it is hoped that new technological developments will lead to a more balanced approach to the technical basis of psychology than has usually prevailed in the past. A consideration of the psychological implications of these developments leads us, first, to ask to what extent psychologists in the past have looked at certain aspects of behavior, not so much because they were the most relevant things to look at, but because they were the only things they could look at and measure, given the then current state of behavioral technology, and, second, to a critical reappraisal of the psychology that has been inherited from previous generations. This re-evaluation could, in itself, make a significant contribution to the development of a science of behavior. Moreover, an increased awareness of the extent to which current practices are technically determined, allows us to appreciate the implications of future developments more readily than would otherwise be possible. This is particularly important in the field of gerontology since the behavior of the aged individual deserves precise and rigorous measurement.

Acknowledgements. This work was supported by Grants NS-09287 and NS-13708 from the National Institute of Neurological and Communicative Disorders and Stroke.

REFERENCES

1. Timiras, P. S. (1972) Developmental Physiology and Aging, New York, MacMillan.

2. Kimmel, D. C. (1973) Adulthood and Aging, New York, Wiley.

3. Kral, V. A. (1972) Canadian Psychiatric Association Journal, 17, 25-30.

4. Hachinski, V. C. et al. (1974) The Lancet, July 27th, pp. 207-209.

5. Perez, F. I. et al. (1975a) Journal of Neurology, Neurosurgery and Psychiatry, 38, 533-540.

6. Terry, R. D. (1976) Archives of Neurology, 33, 1-4.

7. Perez, F. I. et al. (1977) Le Journal Canadien Des Sciences Neurologiques. 4, 53-62.

8. Perez, F. I. et al. (1978) Le Journal Canadien Des Sciences Neurologiques, in press.

9. Perez, F. I. et al. (1976a) Le Journal Canadien Des Sciences Neurologiques, 3, 181-187.

10. Perez, F. I. et al. (1975b) Le Journal Canadien Des Sciences Neurologiques, 2, 347-355.

11. Karp, H. (1974) In A. B. Baker and L. H. Baker (Eds.) Clinical Neurology, Vol. 2, Chapter 27, Hagerstown, Maryland.

12. Tomlinson B. E. et al. (1970) Journal of Neurological Science, 11, 205-243.

13. Terry, R. D. and Wisniewski, H. (1970) In Alzheimer's Disease and Related Conditions, G. F. W., and O'Connor, M. (Eds.) London, J and A Churchill.

14. Milner, B. (1967) In F. L. Darley (Ed.) Brain Mechanisms Underlying Speech and Language, New York, Grune and Stratton.

15. Birren, J. E. et al. (1963) Publication No. (HSM) 71-9051, Washington, D.C., U.S. Govt. Printing Office.

16. Granick, S. and Patterson, R. D. (1971) Publication No. (HSM) 71-9037, Washington, D.C., U.S. Govt. Printing Office.

17. Riegel, K. F. and Riegel, R. M. (1972) Developmental Psychology, 6, 306-319.

18. Obrist, W. D. et al. (1970) Neurology, 20, 315-322.

19. Kety, S. S. (1956) Research Publication of the Association of Nervous and Mental Disorders, 31, 35.

20. Sokoloff, L. (1953) Journal of Gerontology, 8, 137-143.

21. Ingvar, D. H. (1970) In J. S. Meyer, M. Rievich, H. Lechner and O. Eichhorn (Eds) Research on the Cerebral Circulation, 4th International Salzburg Conference, Springfield, Illinois.

22. Hachinski, V. C. et al. (1975) Archives of Neurology, 32, 632-637.

23. Perez, F. I. et al. (1977) Cerebral Vascular Disease, Proceedings of the 8th International Salzburg Conference, Excerpta Medica, Amsterdam, pp. 35-39.

24. Simard, D. et al. (1971) Brain, 94, 273-288.

25. Birren, J. R. (1964) The Psychology of Aging, Englewood Cliffs, New Jersey.

26. Perez, F. I. et al. (1977a) Stroke, 8, 140.

27. Juel-Nielsen, N. (1975) In Modern Perspectives in the Psychiatry of Old Age, New York, Brunner/Matzel.

THE DIFFERENTIAL DIAGNOSIS OF DEMENTIA IN THE SENIUM

CHARLES P. HUGHES

Department of Neurology and Neurological Surgery (Neurology)
Washington University School of Medicine, 660 S. Euclid,
St. Louis, Mo 63110

ABSTRACT

The numerous potential causes of dementia occurring in patients
over age 65 are discussed with particular reference to those in which
some form of treatment may be effective. If these treatable causes
are excluded as well as patients with other neurologic diseases in
which dementia may be a secondary factor, there is left a group
consisting primarily (50%) of Alzheimer's disease - senile dementia.
While not as significant, multi-infarct dementia will also be involved
either alone (10-15%) or in combination with Alzheimer's disease
(10-15%).

DEFINITIONS

Dementia is usually defined as a global decline in intellectual
function from some previously attained level. This decline should
include both an impairment of memory and often orientation together
with a deterioration in some other intellectual functions resulting
in difficulties with judgement and problem solving ability. A usual
manifestation of these problems is a decreased ability to perform
customary functions outside the home and a withdrawal from personal
financial affairs and more complicated hobbies or recreational
activities. More severe cases may exhibit an inability to perform
even simple household chores, marginal personal care, and incontinence
of urine or feces.

This global decline must be established in the relative absence of
a impairment of consciousness or delirium and be more than could be
accounted for by a physical disability in motor performance, vision,
hearing, or somatic sensation. Moreover this state must be subacute
or gradual in onset, progressive, and maintained without a return to
the patient's usual state for a period of six months or more before
dementia can be safely diagnosed. Certain preexisting psychiatric
conditions make the diagnosis of dementia for neurological purposes
difficult or impossible. If the patient has a significant depression,
particularly if it is manifested by psychomotor retardation, or if

long standing schizophrenia is present, the diagnosis of dementia would be deferred.

The senium as a distinct period in life has been variously defined but usually suggests a person 65 years old or older and often retired from work. Even with the qualifications mentioned above, the problem of dementia in this period remains a formidable one. Numerous surveys in this country and elsewhere have attempted to measure the problem. In a well done study in a small British population, Kay et al[5] found a prevalence of senile dementia in persons over 65 of 5%. When a less restrictive diagnosis is cataloged (chronic brain syndrome), the accumulation of these patients in chronic facilities is much higher. Goldfarb[2] found between 20% and 80% of the occupants aged 65 and over of nursing homes, old age homes, and state hospitals to bear this label while in Syracuse, New York, the first admission rates to mental hospitals of patients diagnosed as 'chronic brain syndrome' approximated 112/100,000[6] population. These familiar figures point to the magnitude of the problem and indicate that many physicians will be faced with a large number of patients in older years who require an evaluation for their dementia. It is important in the course of this evaluation to focus particularly on treatable causes of this disorder and to be aware of the large number of conditions which may present in this fashion.

DIFFERENTIAL DIAGNOSIS

The causes of dementia in the adult will be considered under three categories. The first group (Table 1) are distinguished by the fact that they are potentially treatable and thus deserve primary attention. In Table 2 is grouped a set of neurologic entities in which dementia may be seen as a secondary or late phenomenon, often much less important than the presenting features of the disease. Finally, Table 3 outlines those diseases which may present primarily as dementia in adult life and for which no significant treatment is available at this time. It is particularly from this group of diseases that the majority of cases of dementia in the senium unfortunately arises.

POTENTIALLY TREATABLE CAUSES OF DEMENTIA

The sizeable listing of diseases and conditions in Table 1 does not, of course, exhaust the possibilities of treatable causes of dementia in the adult. Other toxic chemicals and drugs than those mentioned are probably involved here, for example, but those conditions listed appear to be the most important.

TABLE 1

POTENTIALLY TREATABLE CAUSES OF DEMENTIA

A. Failure of Organ Systems
   * heart failure, heart block
   * hepatic failure
   * uremia
   * pulmonary failure

B. Drugs
   * anticonvulsants (dilantin,
     phenobarbital, mysoline,
     tridione, etc)
   * sedatives (bromides,
     barbiturates, etc)
     stimulants (ritalin,
     amphetamine)
   * neuroleptics (major
     tranquillizers)
     phenothiazines,
     butyrophenones
     reserpine
     thioxanthines
   * antidepressants
     tricyclic antidepressants
     MAO inhibitors
     lithium salts
     psychodysleptics
     (hallucinogens)
     lysergide
     mescaline
     psilocybin
     tetrahydrocannabinol
   * alcohol
   * cardiac drugs, digitalis
   * antihistamines
   * analgesics
   * narcotics
     atropine, scopolamine

C. Infections
   * syphillis
     bacterial meningitis
   * encephalitis, acute and
     chronic
   * granulomatous meningitis
     (with and without
     hydrocephalus)
     cryptococcus
     tuberculosis
     protozoa
     sarcoid(?)
     Behcet's disease (?)
     Whipple's disease

D. Certain Mass Lesions
   * tumors of frontal and right
     temporal lobes (meningioma,
     glioma, etc)
   * subdural hematoma (unilateral,
     bilateral)

E. Nutritional Defeciencies
   * nicotinic acid (pellegra)
   * thiamine (Wernicke-Korsakoff)
   * vitamin B^{12} (combined systems
     disease)
     ? folate defeciency
     "concentration camp syndrome"
     ? Marchiafava-Bignami disease

F. Endocrine Disorders
   * hypothyroidism
   * hyperadrenalism
   * hyperparathyroidism

G. Vascular Disease
   * collagen vascular disease
   * giant cell arteritis -
     temporal arteritis
   * hypercoaguable states
     including thrombocytosis

H. Metabolic Conditions (ongoing)
   * hypoglycemia
   * hypoxia
     hyperthermia
     Wilson's disease
   * carcinoma - remote effect
     dialysis dementia
   * electrolyte imbalance
     hyperlipidemia

I. Heavy Metal Intoxication
   arsenic
   lead
   manganese
   mercury
   aluminum (?)

J. Hydrocephalus
   obstructive
   * communicating
   "idiopathic"
   secondary to subarachnoid
   hemorrhage or meningitis

K. Seizures
   psychomotor status epilepticus

L. Depression

* Of importance in patients over 65 years of age

Haase[3] has discussed the clinical features of many of these
diseases that may involve dementia and for many, the dementia may be
a minor component. Those physicians who first evaluate the patient
with intellectual deterioration, however, need to consider these
treatable causes.

While many of these entities represent quite rare findings, others
are more common. Because congestive heart failure, pulmonary failure
and uremia occur so commonly, they will account for a larger number
of cases of dementia, particularly in the senium. Invariably, however, the more usual manifestations of these conditions will be
present and make the diagnosis not difficult. In addition to this,
when these conditions are severe there is usually a delirium or other
altered state of consciousness that makes the diagnosis of dementia
difficult.

A detailed history of drug intake is of considerable importance in
older patients. While in general large doses are required to present
a picture of dementia, smaller amounts of hallucinogens and stimulants
may achieve the same end. In previous years, bromide ingestion ranked
high in this category and may still occur in older patients although
more modern and popular drugs now account for most cases.

Because of the ease of treatment and the often irreversible nature
of the dementia if treatment is delayed, vitamin deficiency states
require a high index of suspicion. With an impoverished dietary
intake, patients other than alcoholics may acquire Wernicke-Korsakoff
disease and pellegra is not yet a museum piece in this country.
Patients over 65 often have greatly reduced food intake for a variety
of reasons; poverty, depression, apathy, and the inability to acquire
and prepare food.

Computerized tomography is by now a standard part of the evaluation
of patients with dementia not easily explained by well established
metabolic causes. If large ventricles are identified then hydrocephalus must be considered. In old age hydrocephalus, if present,
is usually of the 'low pressure' or 'idiopathic' type and is at
times associated with a degenerative disease. This topic is more
fully discussed in a subsequent chapter. Computerized tomography
may, in most cases, also reveal large unilateral and bilateral
subdural hematomas. These hematomas, which may be frequently removed
with success and considerable improvement in the patient, can be
notoriously occult in older persons. Dementia may be the only significant finding without evidence of raised intracranial pressure, motor
or sensory signs, headache, or an impaired level of consciousness.

It should be noted that hypoglycemia, hypoxia, and hyperthermia are listed as potentially treatable metabolic conditions. While in many instances these represent single devastating events for the patient leaving behind a severe dementia, they may occur in a repetitive fashion, particularly hypoglycemia, causing further damage with each episode. Awareness of these possibilities, therefore, may lead to effective treatment before the patient is severely disabled.

DEMENTIA ASSOCIATED SECONDARILY WITH OTHER NEUROLOGIC ABNORMALITIES

A number of neurologic entities may include dementia as an intermediate or late finding in a course marked early by other more characteristic features. Table 2 lists many of these diseases. In a few cases, treatment of the condition may result in an arrest of a previously progressing dementia. Vascular disease that is amenable to surgical or medical treatment certainly falls in this category as do many brain tumors that may be successfully treated. Those tumors which are particularly likely to produce dementia while the patient is still alert include those in the frontal lobes, particularly the bilateral ones, those in the thalamus, and those in the posterior fossa producing hydrocephalus.

TABLE 2

DEMENTIA ASSOCIATED SECONDARILY WITH OTHER NEUROLOGIC ABNORMALITIES

A. Heredo-Degenerative
  * Parkinson's disease
  * Huntington's disease
    Hallervorden-Spatz disease
    myoclonic epilepsy (Lafora's disease)
  * multiple sclerosis
  * progressive supranuclear palsy
  * Shy-Drager syndrome
  * spinocerebellar degenerations
    parkinsonism-dementia (Guam)
    familial basal ganglia calcification

B. Vascular Disease
  * a pronounced, recognizable history of
    stroke preceeds the dementia

C. Tumor
  * in a wide variety of locations, with
    and without hydrocephalus

D. Infectious
    Kuru (New Guinea)
  * progressive multifocal leucoencephalopathy

E. Seizure Disorders
    frequent seizures over a prolonged period
    without definite hypoxia?

---

  * Of importance in patients over 65 years of age

For the rest of the conditions listed in Table 2 there is no effective treatment of the dementia that may be involved. In Parkinson's disease, for example, medical treatment may significantly improve the motor performance of the patient but it has never been shown to improve the dementia that usually accompanies the terminal stages of the disease.

DISEASES WHICH MAY PRESENT PRIMARILY AS DEMENTIA IN ADULT LIFE

It is with Table 3 that one comes to the major causes of dementia in older people once a careful medical and neurologic investigation has excluded other possibilities. In an autopsy study of demented persons[7] over age 65 in whom these other causes had been ruled out, more than 50% appeared to have Alzheimer's disease-senile dementia, the main focus of this symposium. These cases, therefore, represent more than half of that 5% of the population over 65 with dementia and certainly involves a much higher percentage of cases if older age groups are selected. Katzman[4] has both persuasively indicated the potential extent of this problem in the United States today and pointed out the manner in which it is officially ignored as a cause of death in vital statistics tables.

It has been increasingly recognized that if one excludes patients with a clear history of several past strokes, ischemic vascular disease plays only a minor role in dementia of old age. Tomlinson[7] further demonstrated that only 10-15% of such demented old people had significant (greater than 50cc of infarcted brain) degrees of vascular disease while another 15-20% had both significant degrees of vascular softening and significant Alzheimer's changes. While 'arteriosclerosis', therfore, is not as important as Alzheimer's disease in this regard, it still remains a significant finding at autopsy.

A few patients over age 65 will be seen with a rapidly progressive dementia, extrapyramidal signs, muscle wasting and fasciculations, an electroencephalogram which may show periodic bursts of sharp and slow 'triphasic' waves, and possibly cortical blindness. With the recognition that most cases of Jakob-Creutzfeldt disease or subacute spongioform encephalopathy that present in this fashion represent an infectious process it is now incumbent on the clinician to identify these patients clearly and institute certain precautions[1]. Those cases of what is now aptly termed 'transmissible viral dementia' are not common but represent a hazard to others who may be unwittingly innoculated.

206

TABLE 3

DISEASES WHICH MAY PRESENT PRIMARILY AS DEMENTIA IN ADULT LIFE

A. Heredo-Degenerative
    * Alzheimer's disease - senile dementia
    * Pick's disease
    associated with muscular dystrophy
    metachromatic leucodystrophy
    * "other" progressive dementias without
       characteristic pathology

B. Vascular Disease
    * multi-infarct dementia
    * Binswanger's disease?
    arteriovenous malformations
    * aortic arch syndrome

C. Infectious
    * transmissible viral dementia (Jakob-Creutzfeldt disease,
      'subacute spongioform encephalopathy')

D. Associated with:
    * alcoholism (apart from Wernicke-Korsakoff disease)
    head trauma (including punch-drunk syndrome)

E. Chronic Schizophrenia

---

* Of importance in patients over 65 years of age

CONCLUSION

In the evaluation of patients in the senium, therefore, who appear
to have dementia by the criteria indicated above several diagnostic
steps are indicated.   First and most importantly, the question must
be asked whether or not this patient has a treatable cause for the
dementing illness. A complete medical history and physical examination with particular attention to the intake of drugs and signs
of significant organ failure will identify a great majority of these
patients. Further laboratory procedures will be needed to exclude
endocrine disorders, intoxications, and certain metabolic processes.
Plain skull x-rays and computerized tomography would now be regarded
as essential in the investigation of hydrocephalus, tumors, and subdural hematomas. A study of the cerebrospinal fluid would be necessary
to exclude infections such as syphillis and the chronic meningitic
processes.   Cerebral arteriography carries a moderate risk in this
age group and should only be performed if surgically correctable
vascular disease seemed quite likely after these other investigations
are complete.

One is left, finally, with a group of older patients who in most
instances, will be found at autopsy to have Alzheimer's disease-senile

dementia, multi-infarct dementia, or elements of both. The management
of these patients requires the close cooperation of family, social,
and other supportive services together with medical management of
depression and behavioral disorders that may complicate the course
of the disease.

ACKNOWLEDGEMENTS

Appreciation is extended to the Dementia Study Group of
Washington University School of Medicine for their cooperation and
advice.

REFERENCES

1. Gajdusek, D. C., Gibbs, C. J., Asher, D. M., Brown, P., Diwan, A.,
    Hoffman, P., Nemo, G., Rohwer, R., White, L. (1977). Precautions
    in medical care of, and in handling materials from, patients
    with transmissible virus dementia (Creutzfeldt-Jakob disease).
    NEJM 297:1253-1258.

2. Goldfarb, A. I. (1962). Prevalence of psychiatric disorders in
    metropolitan old age and nursing homes. J. Am. Geriat. Soc.
    10:77-84.

3. Haase, G. R. (1977). Diseases presenting as dementia. In
    Wells, C. E. (Editor): Dementia. Philadelphia, F.A. Davis, 27-67.

4. Katzman, R. (1976). The prevalence and malignancy of Alzheimer
    disease. Arch. Neurol. 33:217-218.

5. Kay, D.W.K., Beamish, P. and Roth, M. (1964). Old age mental
    disorders in newcastle-upon-tyne, part 1: A study of prevalence.
    Brit. J. Psych. 110:146-158.

6. Riley, M.W. and Foner, A. (1968). Aging and Society. New York,
    Russell Sage Foundation, Vol 1, p.376.

7. Tomlinson, B. E., Henderson, G. (1976). Some quantitative
    cerebral findings in normal and demented old people. In Terry,
    R.D. and Gershon, S. (Editors): Neurobiology of Aging. New York,
    Raven Press, 183-204.

COMMUNICATING HYDROCEPHALUS IN THE ADULT

CHARLES P. HUGHES

Department of Neurology and Neurological Surgery (Neurology)
Washington University School of Medicine, 660 S. Euclid,
St. Louis, Mo 63110

ABSTRACT

The historical development of interest in adult idiopathic communicating hydrocephalus (ICH) is traced and the radiological and physiological methods of investigating these patients are presented here
together with their overall efficacy in predicting success in surgical
treatment with shunting procedures. Good results are often obtained in
patients with hydrocephalus due to well known predisposing causes of
meningeal inflammation (subarachnoid hemorrhage, purulent meningitis,
head trauma). In ICH, however, the rate of improvement after shunt is
probably less than 50% and must be considered together with the rate
of serious complications (15-30%) and the fact that a few patients may
remain stable or even improve without therapy. The clinical presentation in cases of ICH may be the most important factor in considering
surgical intervention.

INTRODUCTION

In 1964, McHugh[51] published a series of seven patients who were
discovered either in life or at autopsy to have an unsuspected hydrocephalus. One patient was treated but died a month later without
noticeable improvement. Prior to this time, the syndrome of hydrocephalus had been well recognized in the adult[63] and successful treatment of a subacute form subsequent to subarachnoid hemorrhage reported[25,71]. In 1965 Adams et al[3] published a series of three patients
whose hydrocephalus had been unsuspected and who responded dramatically
to surgical treatment with a ventriculoatrial shunt. Two of these were
true communicating hydrocephalus and all had normal cerebrospinal fluid
(CSF) pressures measured prior to surgery. Thus the notion of 'normal
pressure hydrocephalus' was born and excited considerable interest over
the following decade.

The numerous papers that appeared on this topic following 1965
attested to this interest. Long and short series of shunted patients
were presented; diagnostic techniques were evaluated; and summary
papers have appeared attempting to define what is and what is not
treatable communicating hydrocephalus in the adult. The best of

these[10,24,39] have focused on essentially the same clinical entity
(idiopathic communicating hydrocephalus, ICH) and the experience at
Washington University[35] is in accord with the concept that there is a
distinct, treatable form of hydrocephalus presenting with dementia,
gait disturbance, and incontinence in middle and later adult life.

In the years following the publication of Adams et al[3] patients
with a variety of clinical pictures, radiological findings, and
physiologic measurements were evaluated and shunted. Not surprisingly
a similarly wide range of results was obtained and in cases with ICH
the rate of success is probably under 50%. As this data gradually
became apparent and there was an increasing appreciation of the potential complications, enthusiasm for the shunting procedure waned and
patients were treated more selectively. In contrast to this it was
maintained at one point[64,65] that patients with large ventricles
associated with brain atrophy might respond to shunting as well as
those in whom there was a primary hydrocephalus.

TABLE 1

ETIOLOGIES OF HYDROCEPHALUS IN THE ADULT

I Non-communicating, Obstructive	II Communicating

A. Aqueductal Stenosis, Atresia	A. Meningitis
	  1. acute purulent meningitis
	  2. chronic meningitis
	    tuberculosis, crypto-
	    coccus, protozoa,
	    sarcoid, meningeal
	    carcinomatosis

B. Vascular Causes
  1. ectasia of basilar artery
  2. aneurysm of vein of galen
  3. arteriovenous malformations
    occluding 4th ventricle or
    foramina of Lushka and Magendie	

C. Tumors
  1. tumors of 3rd ventricle;
    colloid cyst
  2. tumors of 4th ventricle
  3. other tumors of posterior
    fossa blocking foramina
    of Lushka and Magendie
    bilaterally
	B. Subarachnoid hemorrhage
	  1. aneurysms
	  2. arterio-venous malforma-
	    tions
	  3. trauma
	
	C. Malformations at the Base of
	  the Skull
	  1. Arnold-Chiari malformation
	  2. platybasia
	  3. basilar impression

D. Bone Hypertrophy
  1. Paget's disease
  2. fibrous dysplasia
	D. Associated with Atrophic
	  Parenchymal Disease
	  1. Alzheimer's disease
	  2. hypertensive vascular
	    disease
	  3. Huntington's chorea
	  4. chronic epilepsy
	  5. Parkinson's disease
	E. "Idiopathic"

DIFFERENTIAL DIAGNOSIS

It seems clear that hydrocephalus following subarachnoid hemorrhage[25,39,41,66,71,82] responds very well to ventriculo-atrial and
other forms of shunting. This may be spontaneous subarachnoid hemorrhage from an aneurysm or arterio-venous malformation, secondary to a
surgical procedure, or associated with trauma. Typically there is some
improvement following the initial event with a secondary worsening and
clouding of consciousness from a few weeks to a few months following
the primary episode. This is now a well recognized complication and
these cases are often ignored in discussions of 'idiopathic' or 'normal
pressure' hydrocephalus. Although not as well documented in the adult,
such communicating hydrocephalus is also seen following acute purulent
meningitis as well as other entities listed in Table 1.

It can be easily seen that a careful study of the CSF and a radiologic evaluation is necessary to exclude many of these rarer causes of
hydrocephalus. In evaluating cases of dementia in the senium (age 65
and over) the most important problem is that of ICH which will be the
focus of the rest of this discussion.

CLINICAL FEATURES: GAIT DISORDER, DEMENTIA, URINARY INCONTINENCE

Occult hydrocephalus should be suspected whenever a patient is seen,
particularly in middle or later years, with complaints of abnormal gait
and failing intellectual function. The detailed studies of Fisher[24]
emphasize that if only dementia is present or if the dementia preceeds
a gait disorder and is much more severe, the patient is highly unlikely
to benefit from a shunt procedure. Such patients, often with prominent
vascular disease[22,42] or Alzheimer's disease[15,69] observed at autopsy
may have enlarged ventricles and meet other radiologic and physiologic
criteria for communicating hydrocephalus. The current experience
suggests, however, that either transient improvement or no benefit at
all would be obtained from a shunt procedure.

Fisher[24] points out that only one out of 16 patients in whom significant improvement occurred had a primary onset of dementia. In all
others the gait disorder preceeded and was more severe than the mental
change. Urinary incontinence, while prominent in discussions of
'normal pressure hydrocephalus', is not a universal finding and tends
to be a late phenomenon. Other authors[35,36,56,59] who have selected
patients on this basis have reported a high rate of success (60-70%)
among those who fulfill the criteria of an early and more severe gait
disorder, a later and milder dementia, and perhaps urinary incontinence.

The gait disorder that appears to be the most important component
of the clinical picture does not resemble other more clearly defined

211

neurologic gait problems (spasticity, cerebellar ataxia, the extra-pyramidal features of parkinsonism). In the early stages there may be no evidence of spasticity although increased tendon reflexes, increased muscle tone, and Babinski signs may be present later on. Cogwheel rigidity is rarely seen and the usual signs of cerebellar dysfunction (ataxia of the upper or lower extremities) are absent in most cases. In spite of a seemingly normal examination with the patient lying in bed, he may have a profound deficit on attempting to walk. The gait may be only slightly wide-based but with a marked tendency to fall, particularly backwards. At times the patients attempt to walk as if their feet were stuck to the floor and some of their difficulty has been attributed to a slowness in correcting for imbalance.

Yakovlev[81] drew attention to a 'spastic ataxia' frequently seen in children with hydrocephalus and explained that and the urinary incontinence on the increased stretching of upper motor neuron fibers related to leg and bladder around greatly distended ventricles relative to those fibers concerned with face and upper extremity movement. While there are elements of spasticity in severe cases of adult idio-pathic communicating hydrocephalus, the problem appears to be more one of slowness and balance.

Dementia has been a prime feature of this disorder but in most patients destined to improve with shunt therapy, it is a mild impair-ment confined at times to memory function only. If a severe memory loss, or other elements of dementia are present (impairment of judge-ment, problem solving, calculations, abstractions) then one suspects that a primary degenerative process may also be involved. If, moreover, evidence of aphasia or other evidence of focal cortical dysfunction exists, Alzheimer's disease or another degenerative disorder may be present and limit the response to therapy.

Urinary incontinence was present in only one half of Fisher's cases[24] and has been an inconstant finding in other series. When the process has advanced to a severe state, urinary and occasionally fecal incontinence may be present but this does not serve to differentiate it from some other degenerative process. Adams[2] used the term 'anosognosia of micturition' for the problem, emphasizing that unaware-ness or indifference played a more important role than bladder spasticity.

OTHER CLINICAL FEATURES

Any discussion of idiopathic communicating hydrocephalus must recog-nize the exceptions that have been published to the above description. Mention has already been made of the association of ICH with vascular and Alzheimer's disease. In 1966 Messert and his colleagues[53,54] published the case of a patient whose communicating hydrocephalus was accompanied by a progressive spastic ataxia and another whose obstructive hydrocephalus was marked by an akinetic mute state. To a certain extent these patients show an exaggeration of symptomatology that has been noted to a lesser extent in more typical cases of ICH. Many cases have been described in which an akinetic or mute state was noted either at the end of a protracted course[24,35] or immediately following pneumoencephalography.

Crowell et al[17] described 2 cases marked by aggressive tendencies and both of these showed improvement in this specific area with shunting. Features of Parkinson's disease was observed in a young man (27 years old) by Mazza et al[52] but only 'mild' improvement occurred after surgery. In more typical cases of ICH[24] and in communicating hydrocephalus following subarachnoid hemorrhage and surgery[73] features of parkinsonism have been described. The latter cases[73] showed distinct improvement after shunting suggesting that these extrapyramidal features might in part be due to a reversible lesion and not just a manifestation of latent classic parkinsonism. These relatively rare clinical syndromes do not seriously undermine the general clinical picture of ICH that will respond to treatment.

RADIOLOGICAL AND PHYSIOLOGICAL EVALUATION

Until the advent of computerized cranial tomography (CT) in 1974, pneumoencephalography (PEG) was the most important single tool in establishing the presence and nature of hydrocephalus. Most procedures have involved the fractional instillation of air and the removal of a concomitant amount of CSF. The latter practice was said to prevent the deterioration following PEG that marked a number of these cases. Some[24] have reported that an improvement may follow lumbar puncture and the removal of fluid alone although a failure to do so[58] does not necessarily indicate that the patient might not benefit from shunting.

The primary pneumoencephalographic features of ICH were well described by 1968[75] including enlargement of the ventricles and some failure of air to pass over the lateral convexities of the brain. These features suggested both a communicating hydrocephalus and the probable site of a block to reabsorption at the arachnoid villi along the saggital sinus or into subpial capillaries near the subarachnoid space over the convexity. For this latter concept there has been some pathological confirmation[2,18,20,39,69,78] but there has been no consistent pathology of the arachnoid villi identified. Indeed, the problem of whether CSF is reabsorbed at this level or via the capillaries around the Virchow-Robins spaces has never been fully resolved in these or other cases[39].

In searching for more precise pneumoencephalographic criteria that might predict success with shunting more accurately, several additional features have been described. Greitz and Grepe[29] emphasized the dilatation of the temporal horns of the lateral ventricles and the trigone, suggesting that if these features were not present, the enlargement of the frontal portions of the lateral ventricles only might suggest an atrophic process. Another aspect of the PEG that might differentiate an active hydrocephalus from primary brain atrophy was the 'callosal' angle[45]. While these features of the PEG are attractive when considering the supposed pathophysiology, they have not proved definitely predictive of therapeutic success[28,29,35,45,70,72,80].

In 1974 computerized cranial tomography (CT) was introduced into clinical neurology and immediately assumed a commanding position in the diagnosis and evaluation of ICH. In the first place this procedure demonstrated the size of the ventricles and to a certain extent, the cortical sulci, without significant risk to the patient. In addition to this there was the fact that neither the more detailed anatomy visualized via PEG nor the fact that air could or could not be visualized over the cerebral convexities proved definitely predictive of a success with shunt treatment. PEG or ventriculography, consequently, is little used now in the evaluation of these problems unless an obscure obstructive lesion within the ventricles or in the posterior fossa is strongly suspected.

CT has been discussed in relation to hydrocephalus and brain atrophy by a number of investigators[26,27,28,34,35,37,39,44,61]. The pertinent features include definitely enlarged ventricles, cortical sulci that are not particularly prominent, and no evidence of a mass lesion. Also felt to be of importance is the enlargement of the 3rd ventricle which can usually be seen clearly in this procedure.

Because air encephalography was not a perfectly physiological test of the patency of subarachnoid pathways[75], attention was turned early to radionuclide cisternography. Introduced by DiChiro[19] this procedure, which outlines the CSF pathways and appears to give some indication of flow patterns, was utilized in most subsequent clinical studies of ICH. From Bannister's[7] initial report to the present[35] certain criteria have remained firm[28,39,44,56,62,70,80]. The earliest and most popular material used in this fashion to outline the subarachnoid space was I^{125} labeled serum albumin (RISA). Subseqeuntly other isotopes (indium, technetium) conjugated to proteins have also been used as well as chelated compounds (^{111}In-DTPA). There have been a few reports of an aseptic meningitis following the instillation of this material[46] while one report[55] suggested that there might be frequent asymptomatic pleocytosis.

Currently it is felt that true ICH is marked by retention of the isotope in the ventricles for more than 48 hours and a block in the normally visualized progression of the radionuclide along the surface of the convexities to the midline. This block might be at the tentorial notch, midway along the convexities, or at the saggital sinus. The latter would be represented by a midline 'notch' in the radioactivity seen along the rim of the convexity of the brain. While compelling to many neurologists, this test has also failed to uniformly predict surgical success[28,35,39,74,80]. In some studies[1,8] the transfer of labeled albumin from CSF to plasma has been studied but it remains uncertain whether this can differentiate between those who will and who won't respond to a shunt.

Certain tests more directly related to the presumed physiological changes in ICH have been employed. Katzman[40] introduced the infusion manometric test in which saline or artificial CSF is infused at a constant rate and the CSF pressure measured. In cases of relatively acute hydrocephalus, a distinctly abnormal pressure curve was obtained[39] that did not plateau as in normal subjects. In patients suspected of having ICH, however, the results have been more variable. Some[76] have reported results consistent with the findings of PEG and cisternography while others[70,79] have reported a poor correlation. Because it did not appear useful enough to supplant cisternography, it is much less used now.

More prolonged monitoring of CSF pressure for periods lasting up to several days has been reported by several investigators[12,16,43,57,68,72]. This has been most easily accomplished via an extradural transducer[21] but direct intraventricular recordings have been made. It has been found that the 'normal' pressure recorded at a single lumbar puncture in many of these patients is not a consistent finding. There are frequent, transient elevations of pressure that may reach 300-400 mm H_2O or higher. Both rhythmic "B" waves and more protracted elevations ("A" waves) of Lundberg[48] have been noted. The presence of "A" waves and possibly "B" waves was felt to correlate most closely with shunt success. Since many of these elevations take place only in sleep[72], prolonged recording is necessary and as a diagnostic aid, this practice has not become widespread.

While easy to obtain, the electroencephalogram (EEG) has not proven very useful in the evaluation of patients with suspected ICH except to exclude the diagnosis of advanced Alzheimer's disease in which slowing of the EEG is frequent. Brown and Goldensohn[11] and most others have found the majority of patients to have a normal or near normal record. Hashi et al[32], on the other hand, found frequent frontal intermittent rhythmic delta activity (FIRDA) in patients with ICH and other experience[14] has confirmed that in a few cases this may exist.

Studies of <u>regional cerebral blood flow</u> (CBF) have been of some interest in that a decrease has been seen in many cases of ICH[30]. Raichle et al[60] have shown that in certain cases who benefited from shunting with ICH, a considerable increase in CBF was obtained by removing enough CSF to markedly lower the CSF pressure. Despite these tempting results the difficulty and risk of the procedure has limited its widespread application.

RESULTS OF TREATMENT

The treatment of communicating hydrocephalus in the adult has been largely confined to the placing of a shunt from the right lateral cerebral ventricle to the right atrium of the heart via the superior vena cava. The tube implanted in the ventricle is lead through a small skull defect, connected to a one-way valve, and thence to tubing leading subcutaneously to the superior vena cava in the neck. The valve at the point of exit from the skull can be palpated and its compressibility may be a partial affirmation of shunt patency in certain models. In one design there is a small reservoir attached at the cerebral side of the valve so that ostensibly intracerebral pressures can be measured percutaneously with a needle attached to a manometer and inserted at that point. The valves have been 'set to open' by the designers and manufacturers at pressures ranging from as low as 0 mm H_2O to nearly 200 mm H_2O.

For a brief period, medical management was attempted utilizing glycerol as an osmotic agent and acetazolamide to reduce CSF production at the choroid plexus. Three patients were given a trial of this therapy for periods up to 6 months at this institution without significant success.

Katzman[39] indicated the theoretical appeal of a lumbar-peritoneal shunt as opposed to that described above. In most cases, patency between the lumbar subarachnoid space and the ventricles can be demonstrated and it would be hoped[77] that fewer complications (see below) might result from avoiding an intracranial procedure. Too few of these shunts have been placed, however, to permit a comparison.

A large number of authors have published case material and series of cases related to shunt therapy for ICH. Table 2 lists the more important of these in which patients with ICH could be clearly iden-

TABLE 2

RESULTS OF TREATMENT

STUDY	YEAR	ICH PATIENTS TREATED	NUMBER IMPROVED	COMPLICATIONS (for entire series)
Adams et al[3]	1965	2	2	none
Bannister, R. et al[7]	1967	5	5	none reported
Ekbom et al[23]	1969	6	3	2 stroke; 1 shunt failure
Ojemann et al[59]	1969	13	8	none reported
Benson et al[10]	1970	9	7	2 pts. died 'shortly' after surgery
Heinz et al[33]	1970	6	4	1 died with complication
McCullough et al[50]	1970	2	2	none reported
Tator & Murray[74]	1971	7	2	1 death? cause; 2 shunt failure
Avant & Toole[4]	1972	7	3	1 died pulmonary embolus
Bannister, C.[6]	1972	8	0	none reported
Guidetti & Gagliardi[31]	1972	14	7	1 died immediately post-op
Nornes et al[57]	1973	1	0	none reported
Sypert et al[73]	1973	1	1	none
Chawla et al[12]	1974	12	4	none reported
Earnest et al[22]	1974	2	1	none
Lorenzo et al[47]	1974	3	2	seizures in 1 patient
Messert & Wannamaker[56]	1974	15	10	none
Stein & Langfitt[70]	1974	33	8	4 shunt malfunctions; 1 infection
Wood et al[80]	1974	13	11	43% total complications[77]
Lamas et al[43]	1975	1	1	none
Belloni et al[9]	1976	3	0	none reported
Hashi et al[32]	1976	2	0	none reported
Laws & Mokri[44]	1976	56	28	38% major and minor complications
Sincounas et al[67]	1976	2	2	none
Greenberg et al[28]	1977	73	33	11% disabling/39% total complication
Koto et al[42]	1977	1	1	none
Hughes et al[35]	In Prep	27	9	43% major complications
TOTAL		324	154	48% IMPROVED

tified. Many of the series contain cases of communicating hydrocephalus due to subarachnoid hemorrhage on the one hand, or cases of
primary cerebral atrophy on the other. An effort has been made to
select only those patients who probably had the idiopathic form of
adult communicating hydrocephalus in order to make a more valid comparison between groups. In some series it was not possible to identify
the patients with ICH so that only those who could be so identified by

case history are included. This may, therefore, represent an exaggerated rate of favorable response to shunt therapy if responders were selected more often for case presentation in a paper presenting a series of patients.

In this listing there were 325 patients with ICH treated and 154 showed a distinct improvement, an overall rate of 48%. This rate is similar to that obtained by Katzman[39] in his compilation and is a figure similar to the larger series listed here.

From a study of these cases together with those reported from this institution[35] it is clear that no one group of laboratory tests reliably predicts which patients will improve with shunt. Of course large ventricles, whether measured by CT or PEG, are a prerequisite and there is a tendency for cisternograms showing ventricular retention for greater than 48 hours to correlate with success. If one relies on the experience of Fisher[24], Katzman[35] and other larger series[28,35,44] it would appear that the best predictor of surgical success beyond the presence of enlarged ventricles is the clinical presentation. Those patients with a primary onset of a gait disturbance and in whom the severity of that disturbance exceeds the dementia are good candidates for a shunt procedure, particularly if the history is of a duration less than 1 year. Even in carefully selected cases, however, the rate of improvement will not be 100%.

Several groups[28,35,80] report a high rate of serious complications. Those include subdural hematomas[49], intracerebral hemorrhages, and ischemic infarctions that occur soon after surgery both in the hemisphere where the shunt is placed and contralaterally. Lesser complications have included shunt failure, seizures, and chronic headache, possibly due to excessively low CSF pressure when the patient is erect. The serious complications have often lead to death or greater disability than before surgery. In addition to this, some workers[5,35,79] have reported patients who were not operated upon and who remained stable or even showed a modest improvement on follow-up.

In summary, therefore, it would appear that while the diagnosis of hydrocephalus, if clinically suspected, is relatively easy now with the use of CT, the decision as to surgical intervention is much more difficult. If the patient has a recent history of subarachnoid hemorrhage, purulent meningitis, or head trauma then the likelihood of success is high. For the rest, the rate of significant improvement may not exceed 50% and there is a rate of serious complications that may approach 15-30%. For this group (ICH) the presenting clinical features of a moderate or severe gait disorder, a mild dementia, and possibly urinary incontinence combined with a relatively short course would seem to provide the best reason to consider shunt therapy.

ACKNOWLEDGEMENTS

The advice and experience of Dr. Leonard Berg and the other members of the Dementia Study Group of Washington University is appreciated. Patti Vessell was of considerable help in the preparation of the manuscript.

REFERENCES

1. Abbott, M. and Alksne, J.F. (1968). Transport of intrathecal I^{125} RISA to circulating plasma. Neurol. 18:870-874.

2. Adams, R.D. (1975). Recent observations on normal pressure hydrocephalus. Schweizer. Archiv. für Neurologie, Neurochirurgue, und Psychiatrie 116:7-15.

3. Adams, R.D., Fisher, C.M., Hakim, S., Ojemann, R.G., and Sweet, W.H. (1965). Symptomatic occult hydrocephalus with "normal" cerebrospinal fluid pressure. N. Eng. J. Med. 273:117-126.

4. Avant, W. S., and Toole, J.F. (1972). Diagnostic guidelines in hydrocephalic dementia. N. C. Med. J. 33:120-125.

5. Bachman, D.S. (1977). Spontaneous improvement in "normal" pressure hydrocephalus. Dis. Nerv. System 38:734-735.

6. Bannister, C.M. (1972). A report of eight patients with low pressure hydrocephalus treated by C. S. F. diversion with disappointing results. Acta Neurochirurgica 27:11-15.

7. Bannister, R., Gilford, E., and Kocen, R. (1967). Isotope encephalography in the diagnosis of dementia due to communicating hydrocephalus. Lancet 2:1014-1017.

8. Behrman, S., Cast, I., and O'Gorman, P. (1971). Two types of curves for transfer of RIHSA from cerebrospinal fluid to plasma in patients with normal pressure hydrocephalus. Neurosurg. 35:677-680.

9. Belloni, G., di Rocco, C., Focacci, C., Galli, G., Maira, G., and Rossi, G. F. (1976). Surgical indications in normotensive hydrocephalus. A retrospective analysis of the relations of some diagnostic findings to the results of surgical treatment. Acta Neurochirurgica 33:1-21.

10. Benson, D. F., LeMay, M., Patten, D. H., and Rubens, A. B. (1970). Diagnosis of normal pressure hydrocephalus. N. Eng. J. Med. 283:609-615.

11. Brown, D. G., and Goldensohn, E. S. (1973). The electroencephalogram in normal pressure hydrocephalus. Arch. Neurol. 29:70-71.

12. Chawla, J. C., Hulme, A., and Cooper, R. (1974). Intracranial pressure in patients with dementia and communicating hydrocephalus. J. Neurosurg. 40:376-380.

13. Co, B. T., Goodwin, D. W., Gado, M. H., Mikhael, M., and Hill, S. Y. (1977). Absence of cerebral atrophy in chronic cannabis users by computerized cranial tomography. JAMA 237:1229-1230.

14. Coben, L. Unpublished data.

15. Coblentz, M., Mattis, S., Zingesser, L. H., Kasoff, S., Wisniewski, H. M., and Katzman, R. (1973). Presenile dementia. Arch. Neurol. 29:299-308.

16. Crockard, H. A., Hanlon, K., Duda, E. E., and Mullan, J. F. (1977). Hydrocephalus as a cause of dementia· evaluation by computerized tomography and intracranial pressure monitoring. J. Neurol. Neurosurg. Psychiat. 40:736-740.

17. Crowell, R. M., Tew, J. M., and Mark, V. H. (1973). Aggressive dementia associated with normal pressure hydrocephalus. Neurol. 23:461-464.

18. DeLand, F. H., James, A. E. Jr., Ladd, D. J., and Konigsmark, B. W. (1972).

Normal pressure hydrocephalus: a histologic study. Am. J. Clin. Path. 58:58-63.

19. Di Chiro, G., Reames, P. M., and Matthews, W. B. (1964). RISA-ventriculography and RISA-cisternography. Neurol. 14:185-191.

20. Di Rocco, C., Di Trapani, G., Maira, G., Bentivoglio, M., Macchi, G., and Rossi, G. F. (1977). Anatomico-clinical correlations in normotensive hydro-cephalus. J. Neurol. Sci. 33:437-452.

21. Dorsch, N. W. C., and Symon, L. (1975). A practical technique for monitoring extradural pressure. J. Neurosurg. 42:249-257.

22. Earnest, M. P., Fahn, S., Karp, J. H., and Rowland, L. P. (1974). Normal pressure hydrocephalus and hypertensive cerebrovascular disease. Arch. Neurol. 31:262-266.

23. Ekbom, K., Greitz, T., and Kugelberg, E. (1969). Hydrocephalus due to ectasia of the basilar artery. J. Neurol. Sci. 8:465-477.

24. Fisher, C. M. (1976). The clinical picture in occult hydrocephalus. Clin. Neurosurg. 24:270-284.

25. Foltz, E. L. and Ward, A. A. (1956). Communicating hydrocephalus from subarachnoid hemorrhage. J. Neurosurg. 13:546-566.

26. Gado, M. H., Coleman, R. E., Lee, R. S., Mikhael, M. A., Alderson, P. O. and Archer, C. R. (1976). Correlation between computerized transaxial tomography and radionuclide cisternography in dementia. Neurol. 26:555-569.

27. Gawler, J., DuBoulay, G. H., Bull, J. W. D., et al (1976). Computerized tomography (The EMI scanner): a comparison with pneumoencephalography and ventriculography. J. Neurol. Neurosurg. Psychiat. 39:203-211.

28. Greenberg, J. O., Shenkin, H. A., and Adam, R. (1977). Idiopathic normal pressure hydrocephalus - a report of 73 patients. J. Neurol. Neurosurg. Psychiat. 40:336-341.

29. Greitz, T., and Grepe, A. (1971). Encephalography in the diagnosis of convexity block hydrocephalus. Acta. Radiol. (Diagn) (Stockholm) 11:232-242.

30. Greitz, T., Grepe, A., Kalmer, M., and Lopez, J. (1969). Pre and post-operative evaluation of cerebral blood flow in low pressure hydrocephalus. J. Neurosurg. 31:644-651.

31. Guidetti, B., and Gagliardi, F. M. (1972). Normal pressure hydrocephalus. Acta Neurochirurgica 27:1-9.

32. Hashi, K., Nishimura, S., Kondo, A., Nin, K., and Jae-Hone, S. (1976). EEG in normal pressure hydrocephalus. Acta Neurochirurgica 33:23-35.

33. Heinz, E. R., Davis, D. O., and Karp, H. R. (1970). Abnormal isotope cister-nography in symptomatic occult hydrocephalus. Radiol. 95:109-120.

34. Huckman, M. S., Fox, J., and Topel, J. (1975). The validity of criteria for the evaluation of cerebral atrophy by computed tomography. Radiol. 116:85-92.

35. Hughes, C. P., Berg, L., Siegel, B. A., Gado, M., Coxe, W. S., Grubb, R. L. and Coleman, R. E. (In prep). Adult idiopathic communicating hydrocephalus with and without shunting.

36. Jacobs, L., Conti, D., Kinkel, W. R., and Manning, E. J. (1976). "Normal pressure" hydrocephalus. Relationship of clinical and radiographic findings to improvement following shunt surgery. JAMA 235:510-512.

37. Jacobs, L., and Kinkel, W. (1976). Computerized axial transverse tomography in normal pressure hydrocephalus. Neurol. 26:501-507.

38. Katzman, R. (1976). Cerebrospinal fluid physiology and normal pressure hydro-cephalus. In Terry, R. D. and Gershon, S. (Editors): Neurobiology of Aging. New York, Raven Press, 139-153.

39. Katzman, R. (1977). Normal pressure hydrocephalus. In Wells, C. E. (Editor): Dementia. Philadelphia, F. A. Davis, 69-92.

40. Katzman, R., and Hussey, F. (1970). A simple constant-infusion test for measurement of CSF absorption: I Rationale and method. Neurol. 20:534-544.

41. Kibler, R. F., Couch, R.S.C., and Crompton, M. R. (1961). Hydrocephalus in the adult following spontaneous subarachnoid hemorrhage. Brain 84:45-60.

42. Koto, A., Rosenberg, G., Zingesser, L. H., Horoupian, D., and Katzman, R. (1977). Syndrome of normal pressure hydrocephalus: possible relation to hypertensive and arteriosclerotic vasculopathy. J. Neurol. Neurosurg. and Psychiat. 40:73-79.

43. Lamas, E., Esparza, J., and Diez Lobato, R. (1975). Intracranial pressure in adult non-tumoral hydrocephalus. J. Neurosurg. Sci. 9:226-233.

44. Laws, E. R. and Mokri, B. (1976). Occult hydrocephalus: results of shunting correlated with diagnostic tests. Clin. Neurosurg. 24:316-333.

45. Lemay, M., and New, P. F. (1970). Radiological diagnosis of occult normal-pressure hydrocephalus. Radiol. 96:347-358.

46. Levine, M. C., and Jayabalan, V. (1977). Complications of isotope cister-nography. Ann. Neurol. 1:172-176.

47. Lorenzo, A. V., Bresnan, M. J., Barlow, C. F. (1974). Cerebrospinal fluid absorption deficit in normal pressure hydrocephalus. Arch. Neurol. 30:387-393.

48. Lundberg, N. G. (1960). Continuous recording and control of ventricular fluid pressure in neurosurgical patients. Acta. Psychiat. Scand. 36:(suppl 149).

49. McCullough, D. C., and Fox, J. L. (1974). Negative intracranial pressure hydrocephalus in adults with shunts and its relationship to the production of subdural hematoma. J. Neurosurg. 40:372-375.

50. McCullough, D. C., Harbert, J. C., DiChiro, G., and Ommaya, A. K. (1970). Prognostic criteria for cerebrospinal fluid shunting from isotope cister-nography in communicating hydrocephalus. Neurol. 20:594-598.

51. McHugh, P. (1964). Occult hydrocephalus. Quarterly J. of Med. 33:297-312.

52. Mazza, S., Laudisio, A., and Bergonzi, P. (1976). Occult normal pressure hydrocephalus with parkinsonian symptomatology. Eur. Neurol. 14:39-42.

53. Messert, B., and Baker, N. H. (1966). Syndrome of progressive spastic ataxia and apraxia associated with occult hydrocephalus. Neurol. 16:440-452.

54. Messert, B., Henke, T. K., and Langheim, W. (1966). Syndrome of akinetic mutism associated with obstructive hydrocephalus. Neurol. 16:635-649.

55. Messert, B., and Reider, M. J. (1972). RISA cisternography: study of spinal fluid changes associated with intrathecal RISA injection. Neurol. 22:789-792.

56. Messert, B., and Wannamaker, B. B. (1974). Reappraisal of the adult occult hydrocephalus syndrome. Neurol. 24:224-231.

57. Nornes, H., Rootwelt, K., and Sjaastad, O. (1973). Normal pressure hydroceph-alus. Long term intracranial pressure recording. Eur. Neurol. 9:261-274.

58. Ojemann, R. G. (1971). Normal pressure hydrocephalus. Clin.Neurosurg. 19:337-370.

59. Ojemann, R. G., Fisher, C. M., Adams, R. D., Sweet, W. H., and New, P. F. J. (1969). Further experience with the syndrome of "normal" pressure hydro-cephalus. J. Neurosurg. 31:279-294.

60. Raichle, M. E., Eichling, J. O., Gado, M., Grubb, R. L., and TerPogossian. (1975). Cerebral blood volume in dementia. In Lundberg, N., Ponten, W., and Brock, M. (Editors): Intracranial pressure II. Proceeding of the Second International Symposium on Intracranial Pressure. New York, Springer-Verlag, 150.

61. Roberts, M. A., and Caird, F. I. (1976). Computerized tomography and intellect-ual impairment in the elderly. J. Neurol. Neurosurg. Psychiat. 39:986-989.

62. Rossi, G. F., Galli, G., DiRocco, C., Maira, G., Meglio, M., and Troncone, L. (1974). Normotensive hydrocephalus. The relations of pneumoencephalography and isotope cisternography to the results of surgical treatment. Acta Neurochirurgica 30:69-83.

63. Russell, D. S. (1949). Observations on the pathology of hydrocephalus. London. Medical Research Council Special Report Series #265, 1-138.

64. Salmon, J. H. (1972). Adult hydrocephalus; evaluation of shunt therapy in 80 patients. J. Neurosurg. 37:423-428.

65. Salmon, J. H. and Armitage, J. L. (1968). Surgical treatment of hydrocephalus ex-vacuo. Neurol. 18:1223-1226.

66. Shulman, K., Martin, B. F., Popoff, N., and Ransohoff, J. (1963). Recognition and treatment of hydrocephalus following spontaneous subarachnoid hemorrhage. J. Neurosurg. 20:1040-1049.

67. Singounas, E. G., Krasanakis, C. and Karvounis, P.C.(1976). Observations on the pathogenesis of low pressure hydrocephalus. Analysis of 25 cases. Neuro-chirurgia 19:22-25.

68. Sjaastad, O., and Nornes, H. (1976). Increased intracranial pressure in so-called 'normal pressure hydrocephalus'. Eur. Neurol. 14:161-177.

69. Sohn, R. S., Siegel, B. A., Gado, M., and Torack, R. M. (1973). Alzheimer's disease with abnormal cerebrospinal fluid flow. Neurol. 23:1058-1064

70. Stein, S. C., and Langfitt, T. W. (1974). Normal pressure hydrocephalus. Predicting the results of cerebrospinal fluid shunting. J. Neurosurg. 41:463-470.

71. Strain, R. E. and Perlmutter, I. (1954). Communicating hydrocephalus as a complicating factor in the surgical treatment of ruptured intra-cranial aneurysm. Bull. Jackson Mem. Hosp. 8:23-28.

72. Symon, L., and Hinzpeter, T. (1976). The enigma of normal pressure hydro-cephalus: tests to select patients for surgery and to predict shunt function. Clin. Neurosurg. 24:285-315.

73. Sypert, G. W., Leffman, H., and Ojemann, G. A. (1973). Occult normal pressure hydrocephalus manifested by parkinsonism dementia complex. Neurol. 23:234-238.

74. Tator, C. H., and Murray, S. (1971). A clinical, pneumoencephalographic and radioisotopic study of normal pressure communicating hydrocephalus. CMA Journ. 105:573-579.

75. Taveras, J. M. (1968). Low pressure hydrocephalus. Neuro-ophthalmology. 4:293-309.

76. Trotter, J. L., Luzecky, M., Siegel, B. A., and Gado, M. (1974). Cerebro-spinal infusion test. Identification of artifacts and correlation with cisternography and pneumoencephalography. Neurol. 24:181-186.

77. Udvarhelyi, G. B., Wood, J. H., James, A. E. Jr., and Bartelt, D. (1975). Results and complications in 55 shunted patients with normal pressure hydro-cephalus. Surg. Neurol. 3:271-275.

78. Vessal, K., Sperter, E. E., and James, A. E. Jr., (1974). Chronic communicating hydrocephalus with normal CSF pressures: a cisternographic - pathologic correlation. Ann. Radiol. (Paris) 17:785-793.

79. Wolinsky, J. S., Barnes, B. D., and Margolis, M. T. (1973). Diagnostic tests in normal pressure hydrocephalus. Neurol. 23:706-713.

80. Wood, J. H., Bartlet, D., James, A. E. Jr., and Udvarhelyi, G. B. (1974). Normal pressure hydrocephalus: diagnosis and patient selection for shunt surgery. Neurol. 24:517-525.

81. Yakovlev, P. (1947). Paraplegias of hydrocephalics (a clinical note and interpretation). Am. J. Ment. Def. 51:561-576.

82. Yasargil, M. G., Yonekawa, Y., Zumstein, B., and Stahl, H. J. (1973). Hydrocephalus following spontaneous subarachnoid hemorrhage. J. Neurosurg. 39:474-479.

COMPUTERIZED TOMOGRAPHY SCAN IN THE DIAGNOSIS AND MANAGEMENT OF
SENILE DEMENTIA

MOHKTAR GADO; CHARLES P. HUGHES
Edward Mallinckrodt Institute of Radiology and the Department of
Neurology and Neurological Surgery (Neurology), Washington University
School of Medicine, 510 South Kingshighway, St. Louis, Mo 63110 (USA)

ABSTRACT

Computerized tomography (CT) has largely replaced pneumoencephalography as the primary screening test in the radiologic evaluation of
patients with dementia. The CT findings in hydrocephalus are distinct
from those in cerebral atrophy and differential points are discussed.
While CT may suggest either communicating hydrocephalus or aqueductal
stenosis, only a dynamic study using metrizamide or routine isotope
cisternography can resolve the question. The similarity between
congenital aqueductal stenosis and obstruction by a very small tumor
indicates the need for pantopaque or air studies in most cases so
diagnosed by CT. Currently the diagnosis of cerebral atrophy by CT
is nonspecific and the similarity between such atrophy and involution
due to aging precludes the drawing of functional predictions at this
time from the CT appearance.

INTRODUCTION

Computerized tomography (CT) is useful in the diagnosis of numerous
pathologic conditions that may lead to dementia such as hydrocephalus,
cerebral atrophy, tumors, and chronic subdural hematomas. The present
discussion deals only with the first two of these, however, which
constitute the majority of cases presenting primarily as dementia in
the adult.

Hydrocephalus and cerebral atrophy are two pathologic conditions
that share a common feature of enlargement of the cerebrospinal fluid
(CSF) spaces. A fundamental difference between these two conditions
is the nature of the primary morbid process. In cerebral atrophy the
primary morbid process involves the brain parenchyma resulting in loss
of volume. Consequently, there is secondary enlargement of the cerebral
ventricles and the cerebral sulci to take up the space. On the other
hand, the primary morbid process in hydrocephalus is a disturbance of
the dynamics of CSF circulation resulting in an accumulation of CSF

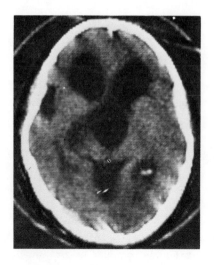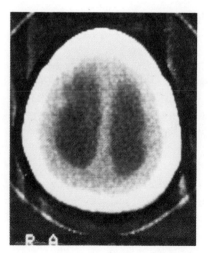

Fig. 1. Communicating hydrocephalus. Ventricles are severely dilated, sulci practically invisible.

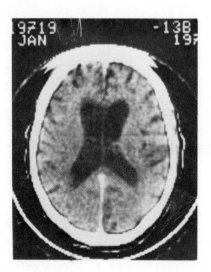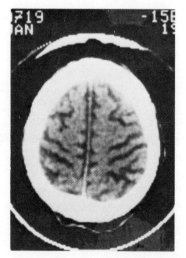

Fig. 2. Cerebral atrophy. There is dilatation of the ventricles and sulci.

in the ventricular system which in turn becomes dilated. The brain parenchyma then becomes compressed and secondarily undergoes a reduction in volume.

MORPHOLOGICAL AND PHYSIOLOGICAL CONSIDERATIONS

In hydrocephalus, the degree of dilatation of the ventricular system is out of proportion to the dilatation of the cerebral sulci so that in many cases, the ventricles are extremely dilated and the sulci practically invisible on CT (Figure 1). In cerebral atrophy, however, the cerebral sulci are involved as much or more than the ventricular system (Figure 2). Whether due to hydrocephalus or atrophy, the degree of ventricular dilatation shown by CT is a measure of the severity of the condition, the ventricular system tending to be larger in hydrocephalus than in atrophic conditions.

As an introduction to the application of CT in the diagnosis of hydrocephalus, and in order to understand its limitations, it is necessary to briefly review the dynamics of CSF circulation. The main bulk of CSF production occurs in the choroidal plexuses of the lateral ventricles[10] and flows into the third ventricle via the foramen of Monro. From the third ventricle it flows to the fourth ventricle via the aqueduct, leaves that ventricle via the foramina of Luschka and Magendie, and enters the cisterna magna. In the normal condition, therefore, there is free unidirectional flow of CSF from the ventricular system to the basal cisterns. The CSF in the cisterna magna is in free communication with that in the basal cisterns, the spinal subarachnoid space and the subarachnoid space over the convexities of the cerebral hemispheres. The flow over the convexities of the cerebral hemispheres is also unidirectional from the basal cisterns towards the presumed main absorption site at the superior sagittal sinus. On the other hand, there is a two-way flow between the basal cisterns and the spinal subarachnoid space[3].

A block in the CSF pathways leading to hydrocephalus may be caused by an obstruction inside or outside the ventricular system. If the obstruction is inside the ventricular system, the resulting hydrocephalus is termed internal or non-communicating hydrocephalus. If the obstruction is in the subarachnoid space over the convexity of the cerebral hemispheres or at the tentorial hiatus, the hydrocephalus is called external or communicating hydrocephalus. One therefore expects that in the case of external hydrocephalus the flow of CSF over the convexities of the cerebral hemispheres is impeded. As a result, there is "reflux" of CSF from the basal cisterns into the ventricular system which may be demonstrated only by diagnostic procedures entailing the injection of a tracer in the spinal subarachnoid space[4] and its detection in the ventricular system. Without such "dynamic" tests, one should not make a firm diagnosis of communicating hydrocephalus.

THE ROLE OF CT IN THE DIAGNOSIS OF HYDROCEPHALUS

Hydrocephalus is distinguished from cerebral atrophy by CT on the basis of the disproportionate enlargement of the lateral ventricles and the relative invisibility of the cerebral sulci. When these observations have been made, one should look for features that help differentiate internal (non-communicating) from external (communicating) hydrocephalus. The first of these features is the presence of a tumor obstructing the foramen of Monro, the posterior end of the third ventricle, the aqueduct, or the fourth ventricle (Figure 3). The detection of a mass depends on the difference in its tissue density, contrast enhancement, and its encroachment upon the CSF containing spaces. If no evidence of a mass is detected on CT, one should entertain the possibilities of communicating hydrocephalus and non-communicating hydrocephalus caused by an etiology such as aqueductal stenosis. As indicated above, the firm diagnosis of communicating hydrocephalus can only be made by a "dynamic" test based on introduction of material into the spinal subarachnoid space and observing its reflux into the ventricular system, usually achieved by isotope cisternography[4,6]. If ventricular "reflux" is not demonstrated on cisternography, then the hydrocephalus is not communicating and aqueduct stenosis is a major possibility. The firm diagnosis of aqueduct stenosis, however, should not be made before an air or pantopaque study since small tumors may cause obstruction of the aqueduct and may be invisible on CT.

Recently, with the use of metrizamide in conjunction with CT, information similar to cisternography has been obtained[7]. Metrizamide will opacify the CSF on CT because of its content of iodine and images taken after injection by lumbar puncture will demonstrate CSF flow. As with isotope cisternography it will indicate whether ventricular reflux occurred or CSF flowed normally over the convexities. There are, however, some limitations to this technique. Intraventricular reflux was demonstrated in normal individuals when precautions were not taken to keep the patient in the upright position for several hours after the lumbar injection. Owing to its higher specific gravity

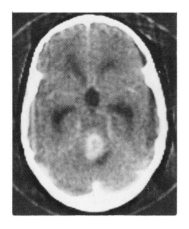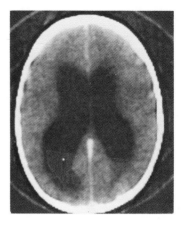

Fig. 3. CT of a patient with severe internal hydrocephalus (right) secondary to an ependymoma of the fourth ventricle (left).

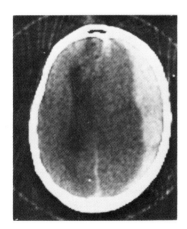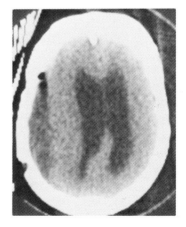

Fig. 4. CT in two cases of subdural hematoma. Left: Recent right subdural hematoma. Right: Old left subdural hematoma.

metrizamide may thus gravitate into the ventricular system and not be a true indicator of CSF flow.

The similarity between aqueductal stenosis and communicating hydrocephalus on plain CT (without metrizamide) cannot be over-emphasized. It has been claimed that the fourth ventricle is normal in aqueductal stenosis and dilated in communicating hydrocephalus. This, however, is not always correct and one may frequently see a small fourth ventricle in communicating hydrocephalus. This had been previously shown by pneumoencephalography and a review of 26 cases of communicating hydrocephalus proven by cisternography at this institution demonstrated dilatation of the fourth ventricle in only 33%. In some cases communicating hydrocephalus may be correctly suspected by the dilatation of the basal cisterns (Figure 1).

CT IN MANAGEMENT OF PATIENTS AFTER SHUNT PROCEDURE

Currently the primary treatment of communicating hydrocephalus is the placing of a one-way CSF diversion from the right lateral cerebral ventricle to the right atrium of the heart via the superior vena cava (VA shunt). There are two complications of this procedure which may be usefully investigated with CT; subdural hematoma and a malfunctioning shunt.

The detection of an acute subdural hematoma depends upon the high density of freshly extravasated blood. This appears on the CT image as a high density mass against the inner table of the skull with displacement of the cranial contents (Figure 4a). After a lapse of one to two weeks, the physical characteristics of the hematoma are altered and its density on the CT image is decreased so that the hematoma may be indistinguishable from the underlying brain. The ventricular system, however, will be displaced by the mass effect except in the cases where a bilateral hematoma is present. The balancing effect will cause no displacement but rather a compression of the ventricles. While an older subdural hematoma with a density equal to that of brain may be missed, the following clues may help make the diagnosis; obliteration of the cerebral sulci on the side of the hematoma, contrast enhancement of the subdural hematoma membrane, and layering of the hematoma if the patient is left in the supine position for an extended length of time. The dense component of the hematoma settles in the posterior part of the extra-cerebral space while the supernatant low-density component will contrast with the underlying brain. In some cases the difficulty is such that an isotope brain scan may be needed and carotid arteriography is the final method of confirmation if the above techniques are not definitive. In the chronic state (six weeks or more), subdural hematomas acquire CSF-density on the CT image (Figure 4b).

Evaluation of VA shunt malfunction may be possible by observing the size of the ventricles. It is expected that with a functioning valve, the ventricular size may decrease. While this is usually true in internal hydrocephalus and in communicating hydrocephalus of relatively short duration (due to post-traumatic, post-hemorrhagic and post-inflammatory causes), it may not occur in idiopathic communicating hydrocephalus (ICH). In ICH or "normal-pressure" hydrocephalus, the ventricular size has frequently been observed not to change after a VA shunt has been inserted. Since this may happen with a normally functioning valve, an atrophic element associated with ICH is presumed responsible. In this particular group of patients, therefore other methods of VA shunt evaluation such as isotope shuntography may be necessary when a clinical deterioration suggests shunt failure.

DIAGNOSIS OF CEREBRAL ATROPHY

For the purpose of CT, cerebral atrophy may be classified as focal or diffuse. Focal atrophy usually implies a restricted softening due to a particular insult to the brain. An isolated focal insult which may be ischemic, traumatic, or inflammatory is rarely implicated as a cause of dementia. In most instances of dementia due to a primary atrophic condition, diffuse atrophy is found. As discussed in more detail elsewhere in this volume this category contains various entities such as Alzheimer's disease - senile dementia, Pick's disease, Jakob-Creutzfeldt disease, Parkinson's disease and Huntington's disease. By far the most common of these in older patients is Alzheimer's disease - senile dementia while multi-infarct dementia with diffuse atrophy due to numerous areas of cerebral infarction is a distant second. The diagnosis of diffuse cerebral atrophy by CT is based on the demonstration of enlargement of the cerebral sulci and the ventricular system. From a descriptive point of view, one can classify cerebral atrophy into cortical and central. The first refers to involvement only of the cerebral cortex while the second refers to involvement of the deep white matter or the basal ganglia. In most cases a mixed type of atrophy is seen with predominance of either the cortical or the central component. When atrophy is of the mixed type, it is almost impossible to characterize the process with more precision. It has been stated

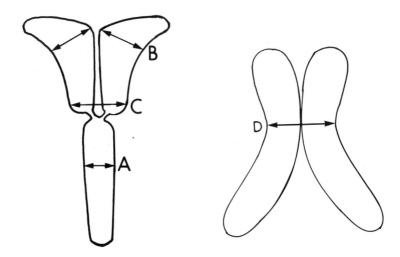

Fig. 5. The four linear measurements of the ventricular system obtained from CT. Three of these measurements are taken from the image at the level of the foramen of Monro (left). A: The width of the third ventricle. B: The sum of the shortest distance between the caudate nucleus and the anterior end of the septum pellucidum on both sides. C: The width of the lateral ventricles just anterior to the foramen of Monro. The fourth measurement D is taken from the image at the level of the bodies of the lateral ventricles (right). It is measured at the narrowest portion of the bodies. The score of the ventricular system in a given scan is obtained from the equation

$$\frac{A + B + C + D}{\text{the maximum biparietal distance.}}$$ Please see text.

that in Alzheimer's disease there is selective involvement of the mesial part of the temporal cortex both in its anterior and posterior parts[11] but this observation is rarely possible with CT. It has also been reported that the diagnosis of Huntington's disease may be made by a demonstration of loss of the indentation of the lateral margin of the lateral ventricle at the head of the caudate nucleus[9]. This finding is difficult to see in horizontal CT scans but in those obtained in the coronal plane, there may be a better chance for making this observation. The non-specificity of CT in the diagnosis of cerebral atrophy cannot be over-emphasized.

AGING AND ATROPHY

A more serious limitation than this non-specificity, however, is that "normal" elderly subjects may demonstrate volume loss in the brain resulting in a decrease in the thickness of the gyri, a widening of the cerebral sulci, and a dilatation of the ventricular system, a finding similar to that in Alzheimer's disease. The distinction between cerebral atrophy due to one of the morbid processes mentioned above and the "involution" due to aging is extremely difficult. Preliminary material from an on-going study at this institution illustrates and defines this problem.

Patients 65 years of age or more, for whom a CT scan was requested for any reason, were subjected to an evaluation of mental function. According to criteria selected by the Dementia Study Group at this institution, six parameters of intellectual and social function were assessed through patient and, where appropriate, family interview; memory, orientation, judgement and problem solving, function in community affairs, involvement in home and hobbies, and personal care. In this fashion the patient was assigned to one of five categories; 0 (no dementia), 0.5 (questionable dementia), 1.0 (mild dementia), 2.0 (moderate dementia), 3.0 (severe dementia).

The CT scans were evaluated for the size of the ventricles and of the cerebral sulci[5,7]. For the ventricular system, four linear measurements were obtained: A, the largest width of the third ventricle; B, the sum of the spans between the medial borders of the caudate nucleus and the anterior end of the septum pallucidum on both sides; C, the width of the lateral ventricles at the foramen of Monro; and D, the width of the bodies of the lateral ventricles in their narrowest central part. These measurements are shown in Figure 5. In order to correct for variations in ventricular size due to differences

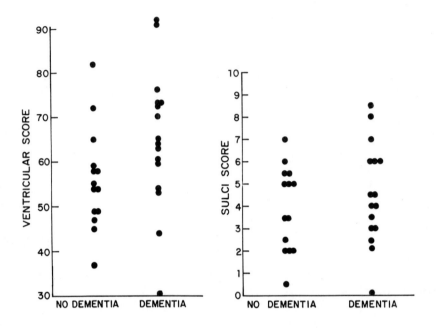

Fig. 6. Comparison of the CT measurements in the demented and the non demented groups of patients aged 65 years or more. The illustration on the left shows the ventricular score in these two groups of patients. Note the scatter indicating a wide range of variations in each group. There also appears to be little difference in the measurements between the two groups. The same findings are seen in comparing the measurements of the cerebral sulci in the two groups (right).

in cranium size, the widest inter-parietal distance was measured between the inner tables. This also corrected for any differences in the
minification factor of the image due to technical reasons. A score of
the ventricular size was obtained by the following equation:

$$\frac{A + B + C + D}{\text{inter-parietal distance}} \times 100$$

For the cerebral sulci we used the same score described by Huckman
et al[8], namely the sum of the maximum width of the largest four sulci
in the upper three slices.

Patients were included in this study randomly. We excluded patients
with neurologic deficits that interfere with the rating of the mental
status and those in whom distinctive focal lesions were present on CT.

At the present time we have collected data from 30 such patients;
there were 14 patients with no dementia and 16 patients with different
degrees of dementia. In an attempt to evaluate the aging process in
the non-demented group, we matched them with 16 patients ranging in
age from 30-45 who had CT scans performed in the same period of time
with no neurologic signs or history of trauma or surgery (young
normals). We also excluded patients with a history of epilepsy. The
results of the scoring of the ventricular system and the cerebral sulci
in all three groups are shown in Table I.

TABLE 1

COMPARISON OF CT SCORES OF THE VENTRICLES AND CEREBRAL SULCI IN
ALL GROUPS

GROUP STUDIED	N	VENTRICLES mean($\pm$S.D.)	SULCI mean (S.D.)
Demented elderly	16	65.06 ($\pm$15.8)	4.5 ($\pm$2.28)
Non-demented elderly	14	56.14 ($\pm$11.7)	3.89 ($\pm$1.98)
Young normals	16	42.44 ($\pm$6.03)	1.44 ($\pm$1.26)

There appears to be little difference between the size of the
ventricles or cerebral sulci in the demented compared with the non-
demented elderly. In order to determine the results of the aging
process, a comparison between the non-demented elderly and the young
normals is shown in the same table. In this small group there would
appear to be more of an effect with age than with the presence or

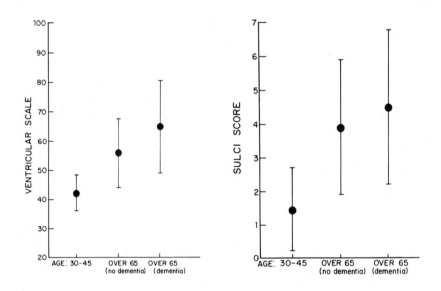

Fig. 7. The mean (and standard deviation) values of the ventricular (left) and sulcal (right) measurements in all three groups of patients (see Table I). There appears to be more of an effect with age than with the presence or absence of dementia.

absence of dementia. The results are also illustrated graphically in
Figures 6 and 7.

It seems, therefore, that an increase in ventricular size and in the
width of the cerebral sulci is manifest on CT in the senile (aged 65
and over) population as compared to those in the third and fourth
decades. These changes are close to those seen in the group with
senile dementia and the similarity warns against the validity of drawing any functional predictions at the time based upon these morphologic
CT changes in patients with suspected cerebral atrophy.

These preliminary results are not surprising in that a decline in
brain weight and in neuronal counts have been shown by post-mortem
studies[1,2]. It is hoped that more extensive future studies employing
different CT measures and more detailed psychometric tests will define
predictive features in this group of older patients.

REFERENCES

1. Appel, F. W., and Appel, E. M. (1942). Intracranial variation in the weight
   of the human brain. Human Biol. 14:48-68.

2. Brody, H. (1955). Organization of the cerebral cortex. J. Comp. Neurol.
   102:511-556.

3. DiChiro, G., Hammock, M. D., and Bleyer, W. A. (1976). Spinal descent of
   cerebrospinal fluid in man. Neurology 26:1-8.

4. DiChiro, G., Reames, P. M., and Matthews, W. B. (1964). RISA-ventriculography
   and RISA-cisternography. Neurology 14:185-191.

5. Gyldensted, C., and Kostejanetz, M. (1976). Measurements of the normal ventricular system with computer tomography of the brain. A preliminary study on
   44 adults. Neuroradiol. 10:205-213.

6. Harbert, J. C., McCullough, D. C., and Schellinger, D. (1977). Cranial computed
   tomography and radionuclide cisternography in hydrocephalus. Sem. in Nucl.
   Med. 7:197-200.

7. Hindmarsh, T., and Greitz, T. (1975). Computer cisternography in the diagnosis
   of communicating hydrocephalus. Acta Radiologica Suppl. 346:91-97.

8. Huckman, M. S., Fox, J., and Topel, J. (1975). The validity of criteria for the
   evaluation of cerebral atrophy by computed tomography. Radiology 116:85-92.

9. Menzer, L., Sabin, T., and Mark, V. H. (1975). Computerized axial tomography.
   JAMA 234:754-757.

10. Milhorat, T. H. (1972). Hydrocephalus and the Cerebrospinal Fluid. Baltimore,
    Maryland, Williams & Wilkins Company.

11. Tomlinson, B. E., Blessed, G., and Roth, M. (1970). Observations on the brains
    of demented old people. J. Neurol. Sci. 11:205-242.

THE ELECTROENCEPHALOGRAM IN SENILE DEMENTIA

HERBERT F. MÜLLER, M.D.

EEG Department, Douglas Hospital, Montreal (Canada), H4H 1R3; and McGill University

ABSTRACT

Despite a marked lability in its appearance which can be caused by various systemic influences, the geropsychiatric EEG is of great practical help in the diagnosis
of senile-Alzheimer's disease and related disorders. Deficiencies in homoeostatic
brain functions and excitatory counterreactions appear to be reflected in it. The
central feature of slowing and disorganisation of the EEG is related to the anatomical changes of the disorder, and distinguishes it from those of other conditions.

The slowing of the waking, resting electroencephalogram in senile dementia patients as contrasted with healthy old persons was first described 46 years ago by
Berger[1]. The subsequent development in this area has however been slow, compared
with the EEG investigation of epilepsy and other neurological disorders, mainly because interest in geriatrics has become more intense in recent years only. In consequence, there is still a widespread uncertainty about the value of electroencephalography in mental disorders of old age. That is unfortunate because it is one of
the areas of greatest practical usefulness of this method, for purposes of diagnostic evaluation, monitoring of changes in the clinical picture, of drug effects,
intercurrent illnesses, and for similar questions.

As studies by a number of investigators, notably those working at Duke University
over the past decades[2], have demonstrated, *healthy persons* show certain changes in
the EEG in their old age: a slowing of the background rhythm frequency, the appearance of slow waves in temporal regions (more commonly on the left side), changes in
fast frequency activity and a decrease of reactivity of the EEG to hyperventilation
and to stimulation. It was also noted that there is great variability in tracings
in this age group, so that while the mentioned changes are observed in many individuals, there are others in whom the EEG at age 80 and older is indistinguishable
from that of young adults. In institutionalized subjects a correlation was demonstrated between alpha frequency decline and decline of intelligence tests, but none
was seen in community volunteers, where both changes were less pronounced.

The presence of *fast activity* in old age is negatively related to EEG slowing, according to a number of investigators[2]. There is an increase of fast rhythms in mid-

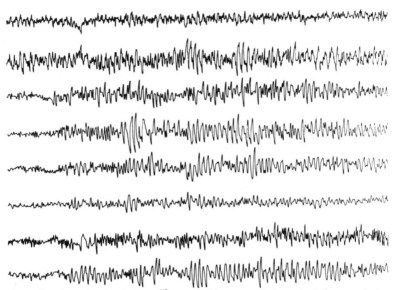

Fig. 1.   Tracing obtained in a 68 year old woman with marked fast and sharp
activity.   (First 6 channels: transverse bipolar run over central regions; last 2
channels: longitudinal derivations fronto-centro-parietal midline.   Paper speed
30 mm/sec, amplification 5 uV/mm).

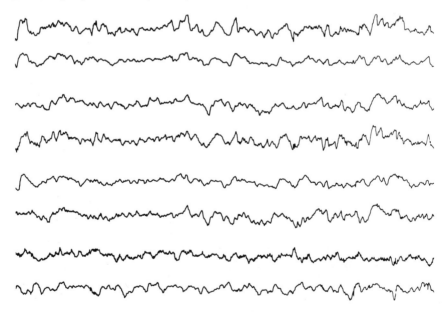

Fig. 2.   73 year old female patient with advanced senile brain disease, verified by
autopsy.   Severe slow wave disturbance and disorganization.   (First 6 channels:
fronto-occipital bipolar run over right and left parasagittal areas, 5 uV/mm; last 2
channels: transverse run right temporal-central vertex - left temporal, 10 uV/mm).

dle age, more marked in women than in men; generally, the presence of fast activity can be regarded as a favourable sign for intellectual function; it tends to disappear with senile deterioration[2]. With power spectrum analysis, Roubicek[3] found that the lower part of the beta band (with frequencies of 13 to 25 Hz) decreases with old age in the same way as the alpha activity does, while frequencies of 30 to 40 Hz increase. This may mean that different generators are responsible for the two types of activity[3]; however, the question of psychological concomitants has so far not been studied for the very fast activity.

In association with the increase of fast frequencies, the EEG background activity sometimes becomes rather *sharp* in appearance, both the spontaneous activity and particularly the photic driving effect. In one study[4] this was found in 41 of 510 geropsychiatric patients, or 8%. It is seen in all cortical regions though sometimes with emphasis on anterior or posterior areas. It is also observed in healthy old persons[5]. Psychological concomitants are better test performance[5], but also anxiety and irritability[5], as well as gross agitation[4]. If features of senile dementia are also present, the sharp and fast activity becomes intermingled with diffuse slow waves, and in serial tracings it is gradually replaced by slow activity and sharp-slow wave complexes[4]. It may be speculated that the sharp and fast activity are expressions of a biopsychological effort to counteract decreasing brain function[5], perhaps in terms of a more active search for structure, as Giannitrapani[6] has suggested, but which can also have certain side effects. Despite some similarity in the very intense examples of the EEG picture (Fig. 1) to the one seen at higher voltage during the tonic phase of Grand Mal seizures, clinical epileptic attacks are uncommon.

The central EEG feature of senile-Alzheimer's disease is progressive *diffuse slowing* followed by disorganization. This has been well documented by many investigators[2,7]. The slowing goes below the 7 Hz slow alpha activity which can also be observed in healthy old people. The correlation with the decline of mental function is quite strong[2]: depending upon the methods of assessment used and the populations studied, correlations between 0.2 and 0.8 were obtained[2]. Also, the EEG slowing distinguishes quite well between functional and organic patients[2,5,7]; and there is a strong predictive power concerning the chances of survival[8]: only few patients with a diffusely slow tracing survive beyond 5 years, while most of those with normal EEGs do (Table 1).

The *disorganization* of the EEG in the later stages of senile dementia is characterized by irregular theta and delta frequency slow activity which usually contains little well regulated rhythmic activity (Fig. 2). Not uncommonly one encounters at this stage an additional feature consisting of *sharp and slow wave complexes*[9], usually with a tendency to rhythmic occurrence at 1 to 1½ per second, (Fig. 3) which

TABLE 1. EEG Variables (Means ± Standard Deviations) Which Differentiate Between Those Who 5 Years Later Had Survived and Those Who Had Died (from (8))

Variables	Survivors N = 98	Deceased N = 82	t	p <
Occipital (P3-01) %-time theta (slow)	7.1 ± 9.8	21.0 ± 16.8	-6.92	.001
Occipital %-time alpha	55.2 ± 20.0	49.6 ± 17.2	1.99	.05
Occipital %-time beta (fast)	23.7 ± 17.7	15.1 ± 10.6	3.86	.001
Dominant occipital frequency (by inspection)	9.4 ± 2.5	7.8 ± 1.9	4.46	.001
Central (C3-Cz) %-time theta	5.1 ± 8.7	14.4 ± 14.7	-5.2	.001
Central %-time alpha	37.2 ± 15.1	41.9 ± 14.7	-2.1	.05
Central %-time beta	41.9 ± 23.9	30.0 ± 20.8	3.4	.001
Central peak frequency	12.7 ± 4.1	11.0 ± 4.0	2.7	.01
Flatness rating (1 to 4)	1.24 ± 0.6	1.04 ± 0.3	2.70	.01
Episodic slow waves, left hemisphere (1 to 4)	1.07 ± 0.3	1.32 ± 0.6	-3.7	.001
Episodic slow waves, generalized (1 to 4)	1.20 ± 0.5	1.55 ± 0.7	-3.82	.001
Triphasic waves (rating 1 to 4)	1.0 ± 0	1.14 ± 0.6	-2.53	.05
Photic flash rate with maximal response (1 to 4)	2.80 ± 0.9	2.18 ± 1.1	4.0	.001
Photic driving sharpness (1 to 4)	1.57 ± 0.7	1.28 ± 0.5	2.8	.01
Lack of reactivity to eye opening (1 to 4)	1.85 ± 0.7	2.41 ± 0.8	-4.88	.001

Source: H.F. Müller, B. Frad, and F. Engelsmann. "Biological and Psychological Predictors of Survival in a Psychogeriatric Population." Journal of Gerontology (1975): 30, 47-52. Reproduced with permission.

have some resemblance to the triphasic waves seen in hepatic coma[10] and to the tri-phasic or polyphasic complexes of Creutzfeldt-Jacob Disease[11], but usually with em-phasis on posterior rather than anterior head regions; and which have approximately equal amplitude over both hemispheres, in contrast to the periodic lateralized epileptiform discharges[12] seen in patients with lateralized brain lesions. (They are also different from the sinusoidal delta wave episodes of metabolic disorders with impairment of consciousness for which the term parenrhythmia has been proposed by Penin[13], although a correlation between bifrontal delta wave episodes and de-generative brain stem changes has now been reported as well[14]). The same subjects also tend to show abnormally large responses to light flashes which are presented at a very slow rate[9,15]. We have found[9] the spontaneous sharp and slow wave complexes in 38 of 331 (11.5%) unselected mental hospital patients over 60 years of age, of whom 37 had chronic degenerative brain disease and one an infectious hepatitis. This last one was the only patient whose confusional state subsequently improved, and her EEG returned to normal. She also was the only one who, at the time of the EEG, showed some impairment of consciousness, while the others did not, despite the presence of advanced senile symptomatology. Of the others, 23 (60.5%) died within $2\frac{1}{2}$ years, 14 actually within 6 months. For twelve of the deceased patients, complete autopsy re-ports became available: 10 showed findings typical for senile and Alzheimer's disease, 3 of them with additional infarcts, one showed multiple infarcts caused by arterio-sclerosis, and one exhibited neuronal loss of the mamillary bodies due to alcoholism. These results demonstrate an association between pathological changes of advanced senile-Alzheimer's disease and the appearance of the sharp and slow wave complexes (or triphasic waves) in most of our cases. It is, on the other hand, also true that metabolic (particularly hepatic) and other systemic disorders produce a similar pic-ture, and it has been suggested[7] that these disorders are more likely the causative factor than the brain disease. For this reason we have now reviewed 24 more recent cases with triphasic waves of varying intensity, with regard to this question. The results are as follows:

(a) 2 patients had liver disfunction

(b) 7 patients had other systemic disorders (pulmonary or abdominal infections)

(c) 6 patients had vascular cerebral disorders (often with a lateralization of the triphasic events)

(d) 2 cases were diagnostically unclear

(e) 7 patients suffered from uncomplicated severe senile-Alzheimer's brain disease

Autopsy results were available for only 2 patients, both in group (b) and were typical for senile brain disease. In all, 5 of the 7 patients in this group (b) were clinically diagnosed as senile dementia, one as depression, and one as acute brain syndrome. In some of these patients, the intensity of the triphasic waves varied

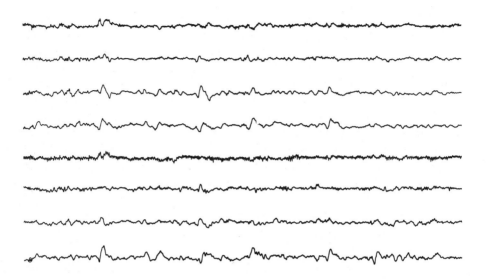

Fig. 3. 79 year old man with uncomplicated senile brain disease. Triphasic waves of moderate intensity, with emphasis over posterior head regions, showing some tendency to rhythmic appearance at about 1 per second. (Prefrontal-occipital bipolar run over left and right parasagittal regions, 5 uV/mm).

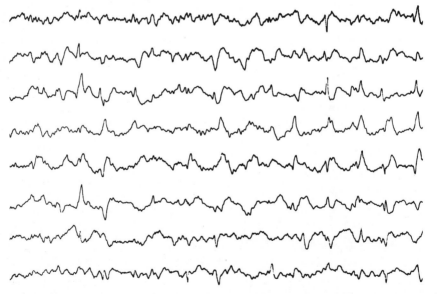

Fig. 4. Intense triphasic wave disturbance, with rhythmic recurrence at about 1½ per second. 77 year old woman with far advanced senile dementia and preterminal illness. Autopsy revealed in addition to senile atrophy an old contusion in the left frontal region. (Derivation as in Fig. 2).

with the intensity of the systemic disorder. The most intense examples of these discharges are indeed seen in such senile patients with infectious illness (Fig. 4). In 3 patients of groups (c) and (e), the triphasic waves disappeared during treatment with amantadine. - The results confirm that uncomplicated senile-Alzheimer's disease can result in the appearance of triphasic waves. It is furthermore suggested that this brain disorder contributes to their appearance if systemic illness is present. However, their presence alone does not allow the conclusion that senile-Alzheimer's disease exists.

Only few studies have correlated *EEG findings and autopsy results* in a larger representative sample of geropsychiatric patients. Leroy et al.[16] investigated 32 cases with autopsy and an EEG during the preceding 3 years, selected for clarity of anatomoelectrical relationships out of a total of 90. Their main finding was a significant relationship between presence of alpha activity and anatomical intactness of the subcortical gray nuclei, while anatomical structure of the cortex was not found to be important. - Constantinidis et al.[17] examined 102 cases where autopsies and EEG findings were both available; the time relationship was not specified. In 40 cases of senile-Alzheimer disease, the alpha rhythm was absent and replaced by slow activity in 70%, or else (in milder cases) it tended to be irregular with poor blocking response to eye opening, but alpha and slow activity were both symmetrical. Higher voltage slow wave episodes were commonly seen, with paroxysmal appearance in severe cases. When neurofibrillary lesions were most prominent in the anterior cerebral cortex, the alpha rhythm was more likely preserved than when the occipital cortex was maximally afflicted. In 25 cases with both senile and arteriosclerotic lesions the alpha rhythm tended to be better preserved, but paroxysmal activity was found in 90%. The authors concluded that, while the EEG alone could provide only probable clues with respect to the aetiology of the dementias, it was of fairly great usefulness when confronted with the clinical picture. - Some other studies, based on EEG-Pathology correlations, or on the EEG in relation to computerized tomography, have however reached opposite conclusions, namely that the EEG is of little value in this area. In studying these reports it becomes apparent that certain concepts are utilized in ambiguous ways, both in the EEG terminology and in the pathological results. One typical example is the term "psychosis associated with cerebral arteriosclerosis" (code 293.0, ICDA-8), which is commonly taken to mean pathology of the cerebral arteries, less often but more correctly to indicate brain lesions caused by artery disease, and less commonly in its real meaning, i.e., a psychopathological condition characterized by severe impairment of mental function, caused by brain artery disease. Ambiguities of this type do appear to interfere with endeavours to ask precise questions about EEG-pathology relationships, and it appears, on review of the literature, that they have sometimes contributed to the delay of the understanding of clinical-EEG relationships.

This situation became evident to us also in a recent study[18] of 100 autopsy reports in patients who had an EEG during the last 12 months of their lives. A severe methodological limitation was that we had to quantify autopsy reports of varying precision, written by a number of pathologists over a period of 15 years, and therefore our results are only tentative. With this limitation, it was found that there is a fairly close correlation between the two sets of data, which can however be obscured by a number of factors, notably the presence of severe physical illness (cerebral and systemic, including severe drug effects) at the time of the EEG. 22 Patients in this "sick" group had on the average more severe EEG disturbances than the others.

Severe diffuse EEG abnormality

	absent	present	
"sick"	7	15	N = 100 DF = 1
"not sick"	59	19	Chi^2 = 12.79 p = 0.0003

This result is entirely expected and in fact trivial as it is well known that systemic illness results in EEG slowing. However, some publications in this field do not mention that such illnesses can obscure EEG-pathology relations.

The main findings of our study were significant correlations between the degree of diffuse EEG slowing and the degree of pathology findings indicative of senile and Alzheimer's disease, for instance with plaque and tangle formation (r = .51, p <.001) cortical atrophy (r = .36, p <.001), and ventricular dilatation (r = .41, p <.001). With regard to the last 2 variables it must be remembered that changes in the state of hydration of brain tissue can influence the results[19]. We did not have sufficiently detailed histological data available to differentiate the results according to prevalent localization of plaques and tangles. However, the correlations tended to be less intense, and sometimes entirely absent, for the "sick" group. On the other hand, in the "non-sick" group the correlation between degree of plaque and tangle formation and degree of diffuse EEG slowness increased to r = .69 (p <.001) when only those subjects were included who were reported to demonstrate ventricular dilatation. The degree of cortical atrophy had a similar, but less intense, statistical "effect" upon the correlation between plaque and tangle formation and EEG slowness. The same EEG feature of diffuse slowness was on the other hand not significantly correlated with sclerosis of aorta, coronary, or brain arteries, nor with the presence of brain lesions due to the latter, or with brain weight.

Are there any normal EEGs in patients with senile or Alzheimer's disease? A detailed review showed that none of 5 patients with a combined clinical-pathological diagnosis of presenile Alzheimer's disease had normal tracings and that 4 of 32 with senile brain disease did. However, 2 of these 4 should in retrospect probably have

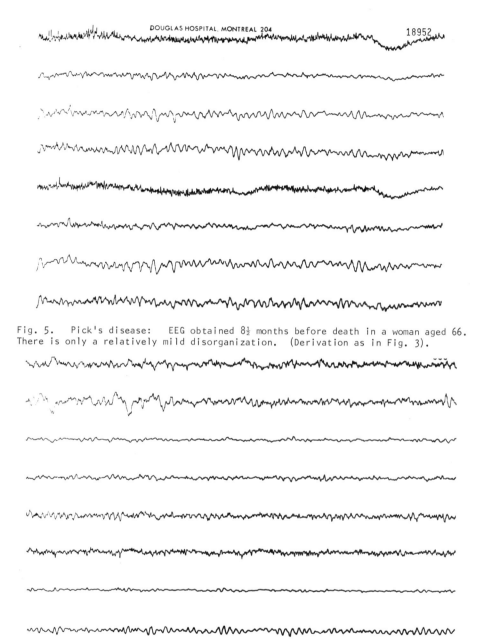

18952

Fig. 5. Pick's disease: EEG obtained 8½ months before death in a woman aged 66.
There is only a relatively mild disorganization. (Derivation as in Fig. 3).

Fig. 6. Left temporo-central intermittent slow wave disturbance, interrupting an
otherwise normal activity in this region. 75 year old woman with chronic alcoholism.
Autopsy: normal brain but sclerosis of cerebral arteries. (Derivation as in Fig. 1).

been labeled mild "nonspecific" atrophy (Hughes et al.[20]) because plaques and tangles were absent. One further case only showed a mild diffuse atrophy without ventricular dilatation and only mild plaque and tangle formation in the frontal cortex and hippocampus but no ventricular dilatation. Thus the EEG was normal in some patients with non-specific atrophy, and with mild senile changes; but no patient with both intense plaque and tangle formation and ventricular dilatation was among them.

Can there be diffuse EEG slowing in patients without pathological features of senile-Alzheimer's disease? Of 23 subjects without severe physical illness, without plaque and tangle formation, and without ventricular dilatation, 9 showed some slowing. Six of these 9 showed a 7 to 8 Hz sub-alpha frequency, another one mainly fast rhythms with some theta activity intermingled. Furthermore, 7 of these patients suffered from physical illness which at the time was not intense enough to include them in the "sick" group. In summary, in physically healthy patients, diffuse slowness was not found in the absence of plaque and tangle formation and ventricular dilatation.

Deisenhammer and Jellinger[21] have previously reported a significant correlation between the number of senile plaques and slowing of the alpha rhythm in dementia; and Leroy et al.[16] found a significant relationship between loss of alpha activity and the presence of degeneration of the central gray nuclei. It is thus not surprising that these two characteristic changes in senile brain disease potentiate each other statistically in their EEG correlate, as they did in our patient group. Pick's disease, in contrast, which has a different type of pathology, produces little diffuse slowing in the EEG, as has been reported by a number of investigators[17]. In our series[18] there was one case of Pick's disease with only a mild slow wave disturbance a few months before death (Fig. 5).

The EEG disturbances in *vascular brain disorders* are different from those seen in senile-Alzheimer's disease. The recent surge of interest in cerebrovascular function has helped to clarify a number of issues in this area. It is not possible here to discuss this topic fully, but the following are some of the important points. Vascular pathology, in particular atherosclerosis of the cerebral arteries, can result in insufficiency of blood supply to some areas of the brain; there are some reasons to believe that asymmetrical or focal intermittent slow wave disturbances (Fig. 6) are a consequence of intermittent vascular insufficiency[22]; in our autopsy series[18] we had results which are compatible with this view. For instance, in all cases where the EEG had shown lateralized episodic slow waves, there was sclerosis of the cerebral arteries. The occipital alpha activity was, in contrast, often well preserved, and in fact those with background slowing showed additional pathology evidence for senile brain disease. A different entity is constituted by those cases with brain

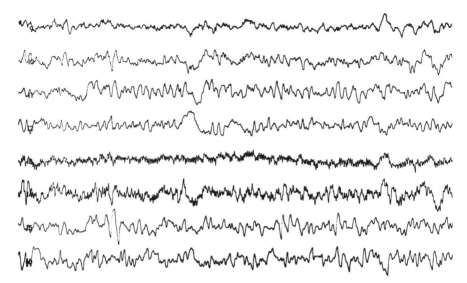

Fig. 7.   Lithium effect: 72 year old manic-depressive woman on Lithium 900 mg.
daily.   (Derivation as in Fig. 3).

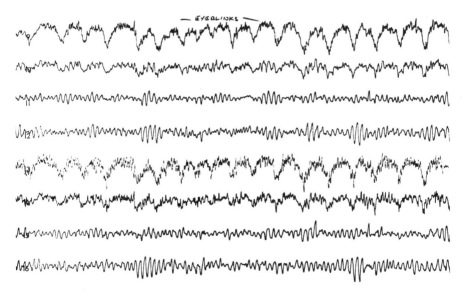

Fig. 8.   Same patient 4 weeks later without Lithium.(Derivations as in Fig. 3)

lesions of vascular origin, most commonly on the basis of thrombosis or embolism. Whether or not they result in EEG abnormalities depends on their size, proximity to the cortex, and acuteness. Small subcortical chronic lesions may have no influence on the EEG at all. If EEG changes result they can be expected to be asymmetrical but persistent. For these reasons it is somewhat misleading to lump both intermittent and persistent lateralized slow waves under the term "focal". - In summary, few types of EEG disturbance have to be distinguished in this area: (1) persistent lateralized abnormalities suggest brain damage; (2) intermittent lateralized slow waves, or slow waves alternating between the hemispheres, suggest artery disease with intermittent blood supply insufficiency; (3) additional background slowing suggests additional senile brain disease; and finally (4) symmetrical slow waves, particularly if they are sinusoidal or triphasic, are not usually caused by artery disease but by systemic disease and/or far advanced senile brain disease; the recent report by Jóhannesson et al.[14] which shows the importance of brain stem lesions for this, supports this contention.

As far as our own study[18] is concerned, these results are of a preliminary nature. They are however amenable, in principle, to testing, and one would hope for more definitive studies in this field. Of particular help would obviously be EEG investigations in conjunction with detailed quantitative macroscopic and histological studies of many brain regions, and assessments of short term blood flow changes, in the order of about ½-second intervals. Such primarily angiogenic blood flow changes are in contrast to those secondary to changes in neuronal tissue and neuronal function, which also have localizing and time-variant properties, as Ingvar[23] and co-workers have demonstrated.

Although the general correlations between EEG and brain pathology are reasonably close, it must again be emphasized that the geropsychiatric EEG can nevertheless show much *lability*, and sensitivity to many influences, which indicates a decreasing efficiency of homeostatic mechanisms. This amounts not to a contradiction but to a note of caution that one needs to be aware of these possibilities. Evidently, the same is true for the clinical picture. Both EEG and mental status can be strongly influenced by the various factors which are of course the same ones which were mentioned earlier as capable of obscuring EEG-pathology relationships. One example is the effect of drugs upon the EEG, among which lithium is among the most powerful (Figs. 7 and 8).

Other drugs can make a slow EEG more normal, for instance L-DOPA, or amantadine[24,25] (Figs. 9, 10 and 11) and sometimes antidepressants. Functional psychiatric disorders may also cause frequency shifts, such as a change from a depressed into a manic phase, and vice versa. Factors such as these have to be taken into account in the interpretation of the geropsychiatric EEG.

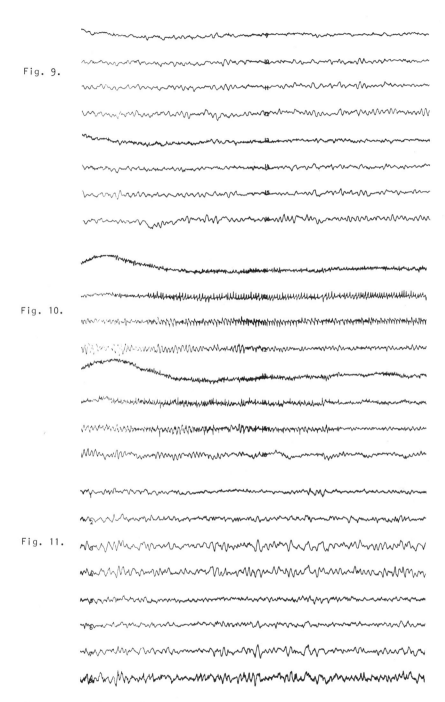

Fig. 9.

Fig. 10.

Fig. 11.

Fig. 9, 10, and 11.   81 year old woman with Parkinson syndrome and senile dementia; before, on, and after discontinuation of amantadine 200 mg. daily.   (Derivations as in Fig. 3).

REFERENCES

1. Berger, H. (1932) Translated into English in Gloor, P. transl. and ed. (1969), Hans Berger on the electroencephalogram in man. Electroenceph. clin. Neurophysiol. Suppl. 28, pp. 151-171.

2. Obrist, W.D. and Busse, W.E. (1965) In W.P. Wilson (ed.), Applications of Electroencephalography in Psychiatry. Duke University Press, Durham, pp. 185-205.

3. Roubicek, J. (1977) J. Amer. Geriatrics Soc., 25, 145-152.

4. Muller, H.F. (1969) J. Amer. Geriatrics Soc., 17, 337-359.

5. Muller, H.F. and Grad, B. (1974) J. Gerontol. 29, 28-38.

6. Giannitrapani, D. (1971) Electroenceph. clin. Neurophysiol. 30, 139-146.

7. Wilson, W.P., Musella, L. and Short, M.J. (1977) In Wells, C.E. ed. Dementia Edition 2, Contemporary Neurology Series, F.A. Davis Co., Philadelphia, pp. 205-221.

8. Muller, H.F., Grad, B. and Engelsmann, F. (1975) J. Gerontol., 30, 47-52.

9. Muller, H.F. and Kral, V.A. (1967) J. Amer. Geriatrics Soc. 15, 415-426.

10. Bickford, R.G. and Butt, H.R. (1955) J. Clin. Invest. 34, 790-799.

11. Abbott, J. (1959) Electroenceph. clin. Neurophysiol. 11, 184-185.

12. Chatrian, G.E., Shaw, C.M. and Leffman, H. (1964) Electroenceph. clin. Neurophysiol. 17, 177-193.

13. Penin, H. (1971) Nervenarzt, 42, 242-252.

14. Jóhannesson, G. Brun, A., Gustafson, I. and Ingvar, D.H. (1977) Acta Neurol. Scandinav. 56, 89-103.

15. Kooi, K.A., Eckman, H.G. and Thomas, M.H. (1957) Electroenceph. clin. Neurophysiol. 9, 239-250.

16. Leroy, C., Brion, S. and Soubrier, J.P. (1966) Rivista di Neurologia 36, 191-193.

17. Constantinidis, J., Krassoievitch, M. and Tissot, R. (1969) L'encéphale 58, 19-52.

18. Muller, H.F. and Schwartz, G. (1978) J. Gerontol. (in press)

19. Heinz, E.R., Martinez, J. and Haenggeli, A. (1977) J. Comput. Assisted Tomography, 1, 415-418.

20. Hughes, C.P., Meyers, F.K., Smith, K. and Torack, R.M. (1973) Neurology 23, 344-357.

21. Deisenhammer, E. and Jellinger, K. (1974) Electroenceph. clin. Neurophysiol. 36, 91.

22. Bruens, J.H., Gastaut, H. and Giove, G. (1960) Electroenceph. clin. Neurophysiol. 12, 283-295.

23. Ingvar, D.H. (1975) in Brain Work, Ingvar, D.H. and Lassen, N.A. eds,, Munksgaard, Copenhagen, pp. 478-497.

24. Muller, H.F. (1974) IRCS Med. Sci. 2, 1402.

25. Vardi, J. and Streifler, M. (1975) J. of Neurol. Transmission 37, 73-80.

DEMENTIA IN HUNTINGTON'S DISEASE AND COGNITIVE EFFECTS OF MUSCIMOL THERAPY

IRA SHOULSON, M.D.

Department of Neurology, University of Rochester School of Medicine, 601 Elmwood
Avenue, Rochester, New York 14642

ABSTRACT

The dementia in Huntington's disease (HD) was surveyed in a group of 30 patients.
Difficulties with attention, reasoning and memory operations were reported frequently;
moreover, the functional deterioration in HD patients was closely related to the extent of intellectual decline. Pharmacotherapeutic strategies in HD are reviewed with
emphasis on the gamma-aminobutyric acid (GABA) reductions found in investigations of
postmortem brain. Muscimol, a GABA-mimetic drug, failed to improve cognitive performance in 10 HD patients. The findings are examined in light of the present conception of the dementia in HD.

INTRODUCTION

Huntington's disease (HD) is an hereditary disorder wherein the central nervous
system bears the singular burden of genetic expression. The inheritance pattern is
autosomal dominant, penetrance is complete, and the mutation rate is negligible.
Dementia, psychiatric disturbances and extrapyramidal dysfunction are the cardinal
signs of HD. The onset and course of clinical manifestations vary considerably, but
the hereditary nature of HD affords a high degree of diagnostic precision. The no-
sologic clarity likewise provides an exceptional opportunity for clinical investigation[1,2].

The early therapeutic studies in HD focused on disordered movement with little
attention devoted to the assessment of intellectual performance. The pharmacologic
investigations were prompted largely by serendipitous observations of drug efficacy.
In recent years, a clinical conception of the dementia in HD has emerged. Moreover,
tactical strategies in pharmacotherapy have been nourished by the discoveries of
specific neurotransmitter alterations. These concurrent developments form the basis
of the present approach to the pharmacotherapy of dementia in HD.

DEMENTIA IN HD

In the qualitative sense, the dementia in HD is widespread but not global. The
idea is illustrated by comparison of HD to other recognized dementia syndromes. In
HD, the mental functions of memory, reasoning (judgment and interpretation), attention
and perception decay eventually; but, language remains unimpaired. The extent of intellectual failure may differ substantially in individual patients. In Korsakoff's

syndrome, the memory disturbance is prominent and perception may be somewhat impaired, but other mental operations are typically intact. In Alzheimer's dementia, more global intellectual failure is observed; language, memory, perception, attention and reasoning are all involved. While admittedly broad, this conception of the dementia in HD is useful in the evaluation and care of patients. Furthermore, it conforms with the empirically derived data of clinical investigations[3,4].

The dementia in HD was examined initially from the patient's perspective. In the past two years, 30 patients with HD have been evaluated at the HD Clinic of the University of Rochester. A family history of HD was confirmed in all patients. Ages at onset of symptoms ranged from 9 to 68 years (43 ± 2.6 years, mean ± sem).

TABLE I

INITIAL SYMPTOMS REPORTED BY HD PATIENTS

General Categories	Number of Patients (N = 30)
None	5
Motor	18
Cognitive	14
Other (somatic, psychiatric)	11
Cognitive Symptoms	Number of Patients (N = 14)
Attention	9
Reasoning	6
Memory	5
Perception/Language	0

The number of patients in each group exceeds N because some individuals reported more than one symptom.

For the entire group of patients, the number of initial symptoms referable to motor problems slightly exceeded the number of cognitive complaints. Of the 14 patients reporting cognitive symptoms, nine felt the problems were related to poor concentration, six described difficulties in reasoning and problem solving, and five admitted to memory disturbances. None reported problems suggesting dysfunctions in language or perception.

Difficulties in problem solving and in coping with novelty were frequently encountered themes in our patients' histories. Routine work or accustomed behavior tended to delay the recognition of cognitive deficits. The clinical observations are in close accord with those of other investigators who have emphasized the impairment in organizational, planning and sequencing skills of HD patients[5,6]. Although anamnestic deficits were easiest to quantify, memory impairment did not appear out of proportion to disturbances in other mental operations. Central language disorders have not developed in any patients.

The intellectual decline attending HD is a manifest source of disability and concern to patients and family. All patients were evaluated independently for motor signs, cognitive deficits and overall functional capacities[2]. In 20 of the 30 patients, the degree of cognitive disturbance exceeded the extent of motor involvement. Motor deficits were judged slightly more severe than intellectual disturbances only in those few patients requiring total domiciliary care. The foregoing survey supports our clinical sense that the functional deterioration in HD is closely related to extent of intellectual impairment.

Affective disorders and delusionary-hallucinatory states, as termed by McHugh and Folstein, constitute the major psychiatric disturbances in HD[3]. The distinction between psychiatric disorders and dementia is dictated largely by pragmatic considerations. Recognition of specific psychiatric disorders conveys implications for particular therapeutic approaches. The distinction is also in keeping with current dementia nosology whereby "genuine" intellectual decline is separated from the functional disorders or pseudodementias. In our HD population, depressive mood disorders were identified clinically in 40% patients. Improvement in daily functional capacity occurred in more than half of the depressed patients treated with tricyclic antidepressants. Moreover, four of the treated patients have shown an appreciable gain in performance on the Wechsler Memory Scale. The findings suggest that the psychiatric disorders in HD may contribute substantially to the cognitive disruptions. This is not surprising since improvement in memory performance has been verified in depressed patients following treatment with antidepressants[7]. A systematic evaluation of the cognitive and functional effects of antidepressant therapy in HD is clearly needed in order to verify the therapeutic significance of these observations.

COGNITIVE EFFECTS OF MUSCIMOL THERAPY

There is a glaring lack of information concerning the cognitive effects of drugs considered to be therapeutic in HD. On the basis of accumulated clinical experience, the antipsychotic drugs appear to exert a modest antichoreic effect. However, the mental influence and long term efficacy of these medications have not been evaluated in any systematic fashion. A more well-ordered scheme in the pharmacotherapy of neurologic disorders has developed through the advent and application of neurochemical techniques[8]. This rational approach to pharmacotherapy is premised on the contention that impaired synaptic transmission contributes to the genesis of some neuropsychiatric disorders, and that drugs which restore the chemical derangement will ameliorate signs and symptoms. In Parkinson's disease the achievements of this strategy are well recognized. As applied to HD, the approach offers therapeutic promise and also provides an opportunity to examine the cognitive effects of drugs which influence selective neurotransmitter functions.

Considerable investigative attention has been accorded to the neurochemical alterations attending HD. By analyzing selected regions of postmortem brain tissue from HD patients, several investigators have reported and confirmed a reduction in gamma-aminobutyric acid (GABA) and in its synthesizing enzyme, glutamic acid decarboxylase (GAD)[9-13]. The diminution in GABA and GAD activity is rather uniform in the neostriatum, globus pallidus and substantia nigra, the subcortical sites where major neuronal loss is found. The postmortem findings are supported by studies in HD patients demonstrating reductions in the cerebrospinal fluid concentration of GABA[14,15]. The foregoing observations suggest that alterations in GABA mediated neurotransmission may produce some of the clinical features of HD. Presently, there are insufficient data from clinical and postmortem correlations to determine the extent to which the GABA reductions relate to motor or mental disturbances. The assumption that restricted disease of the basal ganglia leads exclusively to motor dysfunction is not supported by recent investigations[16,17].

The effort to enhance GABA-ergic neurotransmission in HD has been the focus of several pharmacologic studies. Previous attempts to treat HD patients with oral GABA, either alone or in combination with a presumed GABA transaminase inhibitor, produced negligible clinical results[18]. Both oral and intravenous administration of imidazole acetic acid, a drug possessing GABA-mimetic properties, failed to exert any beneficial effects in HD patients[19]. The realization that imidazole acetic acid may not penetrate adequately into the brain when administered systemically prompted a search for more specific and active pharmacologic agents.

Muscimol (5-aminomethyl-3-isoxazol), a derivative from the mushroom Amanita muscaria, is a cyclic structural analogue of GABA. Several preclinical studies have demonstrated that muscimol exerts potent agonist activity at the sites of GABA postsynaptic receptors[20,21]. The clinical experience with muscimol has been limited. Theobald and co-workers found alterations in memory and attention performance following 7.5-10 mg. doses of muscimol to human volunteers[22]. Waser described a series of experiments in which he ingested the drug under medical supervision; a single, 5 mg. dose of muscimol was reported to improve performance on concentration tests[23].

The pharmacologic strategy of enhancing GABA-ergic neurotransmission depends in large part on the capacity of postsynaptic GABA receptors to respond to agonist drugs. By the use of radiolabeled techniques, Enna et al, demonstrated that GABA binding at neostriatal receptor sites of postmortem HD brains was not significantly different from that found in control specimens[13]. The postmortem findings and the pharmacologic profile of muscimol were persuasive reasons to conduct a trial of muscimol in HD patients. In addition to the therapeutic intent of the study, it was hoped that the

mental effects of muscimol administration could be better defined. The detailed
design of the study and the overall findings of muscimol therapy are described in
a separate report[24].

Ten HD patients agreed to participate in this study after discussion of potential
risks and benefits. All patients were hospitalized on our clinical research center
during the four week, double-blind, cross-over study comparing the effects of muscimol
to placebo. Parameters of motor and mental functions and EEG recordings were evaluated by independent observers. Tests selected to measure cognitive performance included: 1) sequential digit recall, forward and backwards, 2) word list recall following auditory presentation and 3) the Trail Making Test[25]. The digit and word recall
tests were selected because they could be administered to patients with relative ease
and because they had been helpful previously in surveying memory disorders. The
Trail Making Test was chosen because of its reported validity as an indicator of organic brain damage and because of the sequencing and organizing difficulties found
in HD patients.

TABLE II

EFFECT OF MUSCIMOL ON COGNITIVE TEST PERFORMANCES

	Placebo (N = 10)	Muscimol (5mg/day)
Forward Digit Recall	5.8 ± 0.34	5.6 ± 0.44
Backward Digit Recall	3.4 ± 0.24	3.3 ± 0.38
Word List Recall	5.3 ± 0.40	5.6 ± 0.58
Trail Making Test	9.1 ± 0.74	9.1 ± 1.20

For the recall tests, scores indicate the numbers of items (mean ± sem) recalled
correctly after one trial. The Trail Making Test scores include the total
credits (mean ± sem) obtained in parts A and B of the test.

In comparing placebo to muscimol 5 mg/day treatment, none of the test scores in
Table II were significantly different. Even at 10 mg/day of muscimol, a dose administered to 7 patients, cognitive test scores did not differ significantly from placebo
values.

A constellation of untoward symptoms developed in four patients who were receiving
muscimol 9 ± 0.8 mg/day (mean ± sem). All of these patients complained of difficulties in concentration, loss of interest and sleeplessness. The independent observers
commented that lethargy, irritability and restlessness were present in three of the
four symptomatic patients. In two patients, the onset of adverse effects coincided
with the appearance of paroxysmal EEG activity. The untoward symptoms and EEG changes
disappeared promptly following reduction in the dose of muscimol. EEG recordings

remained normal in the other two symptomatic patients. We sensed that disturbances in attention and perception were occuring in these patients, but we were unprepared to verify this contention by objective measure.

The failure to demonstrate a therapeutic effect of muscimol in HD was disappointing in terms of the persuasive neurochemical and pharmacologic data which prompted this study. Furthermore, consistent findings were not demonstrated in the selected battery of cognitive tests. It could be reasonably assumed that muscimol therapy does not produce discernable cognitive changes in HD patients. However, the appearance of untoward mental symptoms in four patients, the objective clinical recognition of altered behavior in three symptomatic subjects, and the appearance of EEG changes in two individuals suggest that the drug exerts psychoactive effects. It is possible that the observed mental changes represented non-specific, toxic effects of muscimol and were thereby inconsequential to any presumed cognitive action of the drug. There is presently insufficient clinical experience with chronic muscimol administration to exclude this alternative. Finally, it should be considered that the tests employed to measure cognitive performance were insufficiently sensitive to register drug related effects. The development and proper selection of cognitive tests for neuro-pharmacologic studies is clearly needed.

The dementia in HD has been typified by widespread cognitive decline, language failure excluded, and coextensive psychiatric disturbances. Admittedly, the conception is unrefined and provisional. Systematic clinical examination and a well-ordered approach to pharmacotherapy will be useful methods in unraveling the complexities of this dementia. The compelling care needs of patients and the diagnostic clarity in HD should stimulate investigations in this area.

ACKNOWLEDGMENTS

The studies were funded by a grant from the Hereditary Disease Foundation, Beverly Hills, California. The University of Rochester Clinical Research Center is supported by PHS Research Grant RR-00044, Division of Research Facilities and Resources, NIH.

REFERENCES

1. Shoulson, I. and Chase, T.N. (1975) Annal. Rev. Med. 26: 419-426.
2. Shoulson, I. and Fahn, S. (1978) Neurology, in press.
3. McHugh, P.R. and Folstein, M.F. (1975) in Psychiatric Aspects of Neurological Disease, Benson, D.F. and Blumer, D. eds. Grune & Stratton, N.Y. pp. 267-286.
4. Bruyn, G.W. (1968) in Handbook of Clinical Neurology, Vol. 6, Vinken, P.J. and Bruyn, G.W. eds. Amsterdam, North-Holland, pp. 298-378.
5. Caine, E.D., Ebert, M.H. and Weingartner, H. (1977) Neurology 27: 1087-1092.
6. Butters, N. and Grady, M. (1977) Neuropsychologia 15: 701-706.

7. Sternberg, D.E. and Jarvik, M.E. (1976) Arch. Gen. Psychiat. 33: 219-224.

8. Chase, T.N. (1976) in The Basal Ganglia, Yahr, M.D. ed. Raven Press, N.Y., pp. 337-350.

9. Perry, T.L., Hansen, S. and Kloster, M. (1973), N. Engl. J. Med. 288: 337-342.

10. McGeer, P.L., McGeer, E.G. and Fibiger, H.C. (1973) Neurology 23: 912-917.

11. Bird, E.D. and Iversen, L.L. (1974) Brain 97: 457-472.

12. Stahl, W.L. and Swanson, P.D. (1974) Neurology 24: 813-819.

13. Enna, S.J., et al (1976) N. Engl. J. Med. 294: 1305-1309.

14. Glaeser, B.S., et al (1975) N. Engl. J. Med. 292: 1029-1030.

15. Enna, S.J., et al (1977) Arch. Neurol. 34: 683-685.

16. Teuber, H.L. (1976) in The Basal Ganglia, Yahr, M.D. ed. Raven Press, N.Y., pp. 151-168.

17. Bowen, F.P. (1976) in The Basal Ganglia, Yahr, M.D. ed. Raven Press, N.Y., pp. 169-180.

18. Shoulson, I., Kartzinel, R. and Chase, T.N. (1976) Neurology 26: 61-63.

19. Shoulson, I., et al (1975) N. Engl. J. Med. 293: 504-505.

20. Johnston, G.A., et al (1968) Biochem. Pharmacol. 17: 2488-2489.

21. Krogsgaard-Larsen, P., et al (1975) J. Neurochem. 25: 803-809.

22. Theobald, W.V. et al (1968) Arzneimittel-Forsch 18: 311-315.

23. Waser, P.G. (1967) in Ethnopharmacological Search for Psychoactive Drugs, Efron, D.H. ed. USPHS Publication No. 1645, pp. 419-439.

24. Shoulson, I., et al (1978) Annals Neurol., in press.

25. Reitan, R.M. (1958) Percept. and Motor Skills 8: 271-276.

PROGERIA: A MODEL FOR THE STUDY OF AGING

DOROTHY B. VILLEE, M.D. and M. LINDA POWERS, M.S.

Department of Pediatrics, Harvard Medical School, Endocrine Division, Children's

Hospital Medical Center, Boston, Massachusetts

ABSTRACT

Progeria may serve as a useful model of certain facets of the aging process.

Particularly striking clinically are: 1) massive atherosclerosis involving primarily

the coronary arteries and aorta; 2) hair loss and dystrophic skin, nails, and joints;

3) growth retardation; 4) an aged appearance; and 5) a short lifespan. Tissues

and cells from such patients demonstrate: 1) decreased growth potential with

decreased DNA chain elongation and fidelity of DNA polymerase; 2) abnormal proteins

including increased heat labile enzymes and altered HLA antigens; 3) relative

insulin resistance; 4) deposition of lipofuscin; and 5) highly cross-linked collagen.

The biochemical and clinical findings are similar to those observed in aged indivi-

duals.

INTRODUCTION

In order to understand the process of human aging investigators have sought

models of the aging process. Ideally one would like a model as close to the human

as possible with characteristics of accelerated aging. The anthropomorphic appear-

ance of the aged is mimicked by a disorder first described by Hutchinson in 1886[1]

and called progeria by Gilford shortly thereafter[2,3]. This disorder is characterized

by stunted growth and the appearance of premature senility. The disease first

manifests itself at the end of the first year of life with a decline in growth rate

and the loss of hair and subcutaneous fat. Subsequently skeletal changes occur

including thin bones, small clavicles, defective ossification of the skull and coxa

valga. The joints become enlarged in relation to the shafts of the long bones and

flexion deformities are common. The hands with their flexed fingers and enlarged

joints simulate the hands of an old person; however, there is minimal, if any, osteoarthritis. The joint changes consist primarily of periarticular fibrosis.

A prominent aspect of progeria is the extensive atherosclerosis which develops in the coronary arteries, the aorta and in many of the major vessels serving the abdominal organs. The carotid arteries may be atherosclerotic also; however, the vessels of the brain, for the most part, are spared. The heart valves may have atherosclerotic plaques with calcification. Several patients have died of myocardial infarction secondary to coronary occlusion. It is common for patients with progeria to develop congestive heart failure and cardiac murmurs, but not before age 5 years. Not all patients with progeria show evidence of myocardial infarction at autopsy. Reichel[4] has described multifocal interstitial myocardial fibrosis and necrosis. This patchy and focal fibrosis has been described also by Gabr et al[5] and Makous et al[6]. Myocardial fibrosis has been described in senescent rats[7]. These focal changes in the heart may not be circulatory in origin since myocardial disease was present without significant coronary artery occlusion in two patients.

Cardiac fibrosis may be part of a generalized disorder of connective tissue metabolism. Subintimal fibrosis of coronary arteries, periarticular fibrosis, and hyaline fibrosis of the skin have all been noted in patients with progeria. Some years ago we studied skin biopsy material from two patients with progeria[8]. Dr. Melvin Glimcher at Children's Hospital Medical Center extracted the collagen from progeric skin and studied the solubility properties and shrinkage temperature of this collagen. In each case he compared these properties with collagen extracted from skin of age-matched controls, adults, and one boy with hypopituitarism who had virtually ceased growing. Progeric collagen had a higher percentage of insoluble collagen than had collagen of age-matched controls[8]. The amount of insoluble collagen found in the skin of progeric patients was similar to that in the skin of aged individuals and of a hypopituitary boy. The shrinkage temperature of progeric collagen is like that of older individuals and higher than that of age-matched controls. These physical parameters of collagen are considered to reflect the extent of cross-linking of the molecules, a property which is known to increase with age. Cross-linking is a post-translational, extracellular, time-dependent process.

Thus far we have evidence that in patients with progeria increased amounts of collagen are formed (fibrosis) and that this collagen, at least in the skin, rapidly becomes cross-linked. Another characteristic of progeric patients is the deposition of lipofuscin in various tissues. This pigment is known to accumulate as a function of age[9]. Pigment was found in the myocardium, brain, and other organs of two patients with progeria[4].

Despite the many characteristics of progeria which mimic the aging process there is no evidence that neurological function is impaired in most patients with this disorder. No sensory, motor, or mental deficits have been described, although one child with progeria had impaired hearing[10] and another had congenital cataracts[11]. Three patients had vascular accidents[12,13,14]. Pathological examination of the nervous system in patients with progeria has not revealed any striking abnormalities. No senile plaques, neurofibrillary tangles or granulovacuolar degeneration are seen[15]. The density of neurons is normal. The atherosclerotic process spares the brain in general.

Aging in vivo is a complicated process that is difficult to study because of the large number of hereditary and environmental variables involved. Many investigators have turned to isolated cells to investigate aging in vitro. Diploid human fibroblasts in culture have a limited replicative lifespan which is inversely correlated with the donor's age[16]. Fibroblasts from patients with progeria and Werner's syndrome show a decreased lifespan and growth potential in vitro[17,18,19]. Progeric patients themselves have a limited lifespan; the mean age at death is 16. With age, fibroblasts show an increase in the thermolability of certain enzymes[20]; progeric fibroblasts also manifest an increase in thermolabile enzymes[21]. Singal and Goldstein have demonstrated an altered expression of HLA antigens in progeric cells[22]. Some investigators have shown a decrease in DNA repair in progeric fibroblasts[23]; others have found the repair mechanism normal in these cells[24]. Senescent human diploid cells exhibit retarded rate of replicon elongation[25] and decreased fidelity of DNA polymerase activity[26]. Fujiwara et al[27] have shown that fibroblasts from patients with Werner's syndrome (the adult form of progeria) elongate newly synthesizing DNA more slowly than normal cells and yet repair DNA damage normally.

The impaired growth of progeric fibroblasts is particularly striking. These cells show decreased mitotic activity and decreased DNA synthesis and cloning efficiency compared to normals[19]. Fibroblasts from parents of progeric children (therefore heterozygous) show an intermediate growth potential. Using Sendai virus cell fusion technique it has been possible to hybridize progeric cells with other cell types. Human progeric-mouse cell hybrids showed a decrease in growth potential compared to normal cells; however, in those hybrids in which the human chromosomes were lost, growth was normal[28]. Thus, the impaired growth was dependent upon the presence of the human progeric chromosomes.

Our own interests in progeria have centered around alterations in sensitivity to insulin which we observed in vivo in progeric patients[8]. Along with the other changes ascribed to aging is an increased glucose intolerance[29]. In general, the one hour postprandial glucose concentration rises about 4 mg% per decade after the age of 30[29]. The fasting blood sugar level remains normal with age; however, the ability to respond rapidly to a load of glucose appears to be progressively impaired as one ages. It has been postulated that one cause of this glucose intolerance might be a progressive insensitivity to insulin with age[29]. We noted in our original study of two patients with progeria that it took a very much larger than normal dose of insulin to bring about a 50% fall in blood glucose in these children[8]. A normal child will respond to 0.05 or 0.1 unit/kg insulin with hypoglycemia. Our two progeric boys required 0.2-0.25 unit/kg for a 50% fall in blood glucose. This was of special interest in view of their lack of adipose tissue. We decided to pursue these in vivo findings by studying insulin sensitivity of progeric tissues in vitro.

Our two patients with progeria reported in 1969 died within a few years of that study. The present experiments utilized tissues from two other patients reported below.

Case Reports

Case I. A.K. (CHMC 65-19-90) was the 6 lb 9 oz product of an uncomplicated 36 week gestation with a normal delivery. At birth a prominent cephalic venous pattern was noted. By 8 months of age his rate of growth had decreased and by 1 year of age he was noted to have small facial features with trophic changes of the nails, hair, and skin. He subsequently developed the characteristic features of progeria and at 3 years of age that diagnosis was made. His developmental milestones were normal. At 5 6/12 years he sustained a skull fracture and subsequently had a cerebral arteriogram done which was normal. At 7 years of age he had a skin and muscle biopsy, the results of which are reported in this study. Chest x-ray at that age showed no cardiac enlargement. At age 12 1/2 years he first complained of fleeting chest pains and his EKG showed mild left ventricular hypertrophy. He had mildly elevated serum cholesterol (229 mg/dl) and triglycerides (176 mg/dl). Over the next year the patient had increased frequency of chest pains, occasionally radiating to his right arm. He had increased jugular venous pressure and a grade II/VI systolic murmur best heard in the aortic area. Echocardiogram showed a dilated left ventricle and right ventricle. Digoxin and diuretics were begun. He deteriorated progressively and died in congestive heart failure at age 14.

A postmortem examination revealed severe atherosclerotic coronary artery disease with occlusion of the left main coronary artery and severe narrowing of the proximal right coronary artery. There was marked calcification of the coronary arteries. Subendocardial and myocardial infarction, almost circumferential, of the left ventricle was noted. This infarct was probably weeks or months old. In addition, there was an old infarction of the septum and of the papillary muscles of the left ventricle. The anterior leaflet of the mitral valve was calcified. There was atherosclerosis of the aorta with one calcified plaque below the renal arteries. Subcutaneous fat was virtually absent. Pulmonary arteriosclerosis was evident. Diffuse macular hyperpigmentation of the skin was noted. The brain weighed 1410 g. There were no focal lesions noted grossly. The cranial nerves and vessels were unremarkable. The pituitary gland measured 1.2 x 0.5 x 0.4 cm. The cranial bones were thin, soft, and easy to cut.

Case II. S.K. (CHMC 87-56-92) was the product of a normal pregnancy, delivered
three weeks early and weighing 5 lb 1 1/4 oz. The head circumference was 30 cm.
She was thought to be an unusual looking child with a small head and was admitted
to the hospital at age 11 1/2 weeks. Positive findings included: an elevated
cholesterol (159 mg/dl) and x-rays showing decreased ossification of bones. On
physical examination she had alopecia, prominent venous pattern of the skull, thin
skin, and hypoplasia of the nails. She was diagnosed as probably having progeria
and has been seen biannually for measurement of growth and development. At 5 months
of age a punch biopsy of skin was performed and the results of studies with fibroblasts are reported here. The patient has had progressive decline in weight gain
with a lesser decrease in rate of linear growth. At 18 months she was 74 cm in
length (height age of 12 months), weighed 15 1/2 lb (weight age of 5 1/2 months),
and a head circumference of 44.4 cm (below the third percentile). At 10 months of
age (height age 7 months) she had a bone age of 11 months.

MATERIALS AND METHODS

Organ Culture. Portions of full thickness skin and muscle were surgically
removed from a 7 year old boy with classical progeria. Informed consent was
obtained from both parents prior to the biopsy. The tissues were placed in sterile
dishes and subsequently explanted on stainless steel rafts in small petri dishes[30].
Each explant weighed between 1 and 2 mg and 10 explants were placed in each petri
dish. The culture medium consisted of 4 ml of CMRL-1066, to which was added 0.1 ml
of uniformly ^{14}C-labeled amino acids (New England Nuclear - 10 mCi/mmol each amino
acid). One-half the dishes contained insulin (Lilly) at a concentration of
1 unit/ml. The cultures were maintained in 95% oxygen and 5% carbon dioxide for
24 hours at 37°C. Control tissues were obtained from aborted fetuses and two
normal children incidental to orthopedic surgery. Informed consent was obtained in
each case before surgery.

Tissues were removed from the petri dishes at the end of the culture period, rinsed in isotonic saline, weighed and then homogenized in 2 ml cold 10% trichloro-acetic acid (TCA). The homogenized material was centrifuged and the supernatant fluid discarded. The precipitate was rinsed twice in 1 ml cold 10% TCA followed by two ethanol (1 ml) and one ether (1 ml) rinse. After drying overnight in the cold the precipitate was dissolved in 0.3 ml 0.1N NaOH. The alkali treatment was contin-ued overnight after which the protein solution was brought to a known volume and aliquots removed for protein analysis[31] and for measuring total radioactivity. Samples for counting were solubilized in Hyamine and counted in a Packard liquid scintillation counter with corrections made for quenching. The results were expressed as CPM per μg protein. Samples from insulin exposed tissues were compared to paired control samples from dishes lacking insulin.

Tissue Culture. Skin from normal children and adults (obtained incidental to surgery) and from two patients with classical progeria were cultured as monolayers in our standard growth medium (minimum essential medium or MEM + 10% fetal calf serum) at 37°C in room air + 5% carbon dioxide. At confluency the cells were passaged. Cells were continually passaged; however, for the experiments to be reported only cells at confluency were used. In each case, cultures were passaged 7 to 10 days before the start of the experiment in order to allow for time to repair damaged cellular components caused by trypsinization. At the time of the experiment confluent cells were washed with serum-free MEM for 30 minutes to remove serum proteins. Cells were incubated 24 hours in serum-free MEM (plus 1% non-essential amino acids and 10 μg/ml bovine serum albumin). Glucose D-[^{14}C(U)] (New England Nuclear 200 mCi/mmol) was added to a specific activity of 0.3 μCi/ml. Insulin was added at 1 unit/ml to one-half of the dishes.

At the end of the incubation period the media were removed and the cells were hydrolyzed in 1N NaOH at 70°C for one hour or until they were dissolved. The material was cooled and duplicate aliquots were taken for protein determination[31]. Carrier glycogen was added (250 μl of 10 mg/ml solution) followed by ethanol to 66%. After precipitation in the cold the glycogen was centrifuged and the pellet dis-solved in 250 μl of water and used for glycogen determination[32]. Two 100 μl aliquots were absorbed on 1 x 2 cm Whatman 31 ET filters, then dipped into 66% ethanol and rinsed twice in ethanol and once in acetone. The filters were dried and counted in 4 ml of Instagel (Packard) for 10-20 minutes. The data are expressed as CPM/μg protein in each dish. The results from cells exposed to insulin were contrasted with those from paired controls lacking insulin.

RESULTS

Our studies with explants of normal human skin and muscle and with confluent normal fibroblasts show clearly that insulin can enhance the incorporation of amino acids and glucose into protein and glycogen, respectively (Tables 1 and 2).

TABLE 1

EFFECT OF INSULIN ON INCORPORATION OF AMINO ACIDS INTO PROTEIN IN EXPLANTS OF HUMAN SKIN AND MUSCLE

| Donor | Percent Increase in Specific Activity of Cell Protein in Cells Exposed to Insulin Relative to Control Cells | |
	Skin	Muscle
Fetus, crown-rump length		
5.5 cm	45	
6.5 cm	45	48
9.7 cm		36
11.5 cm (male)		67
12.4 cm (male)		85
15.3 cm (male	137	41
Child		
10 yr (female)	158	
11 yr (male)		137
Progeric		
7 yr (male) AK	0	0

Each value represents the average of three incubations.

TABLE 2

EFFECT OF INSULIN ON INCORPORATION OF LABELED GLUCOSE INTO GLYCOGEN IN HUMAN

FIBROBLASTS

Donor	Passage No.	Percent Increase in CPM in Glycogen/ug Cell Protein in Cells Exposed to Insulin Relative to Control Cells	
		Expt. 1	Expt. 2
4 day old male	7	216	170
4 day old male	21	79	78
60 yr old male	15		18
67 yr old male	16		25
14 yr old AK (male progeric)	6	15	48
5 mo. old SK (female progeric)	23		8

Each value represents the mean of 3 determinations

In contrast, progeric tissues and cells were relatively unresponsive to insulin in vitro, in agreement with our in vivo findings[8]. In general, cells from high passage numbered cultures were less responsive to insulin than comparable cells from low passage cultures. Thus, both in vivo and in vitro aging seems to influence cellular sensitivity to insulin. The number of experiments is small because of the difficulty of maintaining progeric fibroblasts in culture. We observed that fibroblasts from the older progeric patient grew very slowly in vitro, taking several weeks to reach confluency, in contrast to the 3 or 4 days required for the fibroblasts from young normal patients. The infant with progeria had fibroblasts which grow more rapidly but at a rate which was still less than normal.

SUMMARY

Many of the clinical aspects in progeria are similar to those found in aged individuals. In particular, the atherosclerotic and connective tissue changes are striking. The progeric patient is markedly underdeveloped, usually not exceeding the height of an average 5 year old and the weight of an average 3 year old. This growth failure, coupled with severe "aging" of connective tissue suggests that some regulatory process for growth and biosynthesis of proteins is amiss. The alteration of certain proteins, such as heat labile enzymes, HLA antigens, and possible insulin receptors would suggest increased errors in protein synthesis. Such errors could be secondary to activity of faulty DNA polymerase molecules. The increase in incorporation of non-homologous nucleotides into synthetic templates catalyzed by DNA polymerase from high passage ("old") human fibroblasts over that found in low passage ("young") cells is compatible with such an hypothesis[26].

We are particularly interested in possible alterations of the insulin receptor in these children which might explain the relative insulin resistance which we observed in vivo and in vitro. Fibroblasts are known to have insulin receptors[33]. Rosenbloom and Goldstein[34] have reported a positive correlation between age of fibroblast donor and amount of insulin bound to specific receptor sites. Cells from 3 children with progeria resembled those from chronologically old individuals[34]. Goldstein concludes that the increased affinity for insulin in aging and progeric cells may imply that more insulin molecules bind to achieve the same hormonal effect, which is consistent with greater insulin requirements in vivo with normal and precocious aging.

Insulin is a growth hormone as well as an important regulator of carbohydrate and lipid metabolism. Insulin is a lipogenic hormone and a relative insensitivity to its action could predispose to lipolysis (loss of subcutaneous fat) and high blood lipid. Many, but not all, patients with progeria have high levels of cholesterol and triglyceride in the serum. In turn, these excess lipids may predispose to atherosclerosis. Glucose tolerance tests are normal in progeric patients but the fasting levels of insulin are high normal[8].

Progeria serves as a model of many facets of the aging process. An elucidation of the basic pathophysiology of the disorder would aid in our comprehension of the sequence of events we call aging.

ACKNOWLEDGEMENTS

This research was supported by the National Foundation and by the Grant Foundation.

REFERENCES

1. Hutchinson, J. (1886) Medico-Chirugical Transactions, 69, 473.

2. Gilford, H. (1897) Medico-Chirugical Transactions, 80, 17.

3. Gilford, H. (1904) Practitioner, 73, 188.

4. Reichel, W. and Garcia-Bunuel, R. (1970) Amer. J. Clin. Path., 53, 243.

5. Gabr, M. et al.(1960) J. Pediatrics, 57, 70.

6. Makous, N. et al. (1962) Amer. Heart J., 64, 334.

7. Wexler, B.C. (1964) Circulation Research,14, 32.

8. Villee, D.B. et al. (1969) Pediatrics, 43, 207.

9. Reichel, W. (1968) J. Gerontology, 23, 145.

10. Nelson, M. (1962) Pediatrics, 79, 87.

11. Maehlig, R.C. (1946) JAMA, 132, 640.

12. Talbot, N.B. et al.(1945) Amer. J. Dis. Child., 69, 267.

13. Orrico, J. and Strada, F. (1927) Arch. Med. Enf., 30, 385.

14. Atkins, L. (1954) N. Engl. J. Med., 250, 1065.

15. Spence, A.M. and Herman, M.M. (1973) Mech. Aging and Devel., 2, 211.

16. Hayflick, L. (1965) Exp. Cell Res., 37, 614.

17. Martin, G.M. et al. (1970) Lab. Invest., 23, 86.

18. Goldstein, S. (1969) Lancet, 1, 424.

19. Danes, B.S. (1971) J. Clin. Invest., 50, 2000.

20. Holliday, R. and Tarrant, G.M. (1972) Nature, 238, 26.

21. Goldstein, S. and Moerman, E. (1975) N. Engl. J. Med., 292, 1305.

22. Singal, D.P. and Goldstein, S. (1973) J. Clin. Invest., 52, 2259.

23. Epstein, J. et al. (1974) Biochem. Biophys. Res. Comm., 59, 850.

24. Matthews, O.B. et al. (1976) Mutation Res., 37, 279.

25. Petes, T.D. et al .(1974) Nature, 251, 434.

26. Linn, S. et al. (1976) Proc. Natl. Acad. Sci. (US), 73, 2818.

27. Fujiwara Y. et al. (1977) J. Cell. Physiol., 92, 365.

28. Danes, B.S. (1974) Exp. Gerontology, 9, 169.

29. Reaven, G.M. (1977) Geriatrics, 32, 51.

30. Trowell, O.A. (1959) Exp. Cell. Res., 16, 118.

31. Lowry, O.H. et al. (1951) J. Biol. Chem., 193, 265.

32. Bernaert, D. et al. (1977) J. Cell. Biol., 74, 878.

33. Gavin, J.R. III et al. (1972) Proc. Natl. Acad. Sci. (US), 69, 747.

34. Rosenbloom, A.L. and Goldstein, S. (1976) Science, 193, 412.

THE THERAPEUTIC EFFICACY OF PSYCHOPHARMACOLOGIC AGENTS
IN SENILE ORGANIC BRAIN SYNDROME *

JONATHAN O. COLE, M.D.

McLean Hospital, 115 Mill Street, Belmont, Mass. 02178 (U.S.A.)

ROLAND BRANCONNIER

Research Director, Geriatric-Psychopharmacology Unit
Boston State Hospital, 591 Morton Street, Boston, Mass. 02124 (U.S.A.)

CLINICAL SYNDROME DEFINITIONS

In reviewing the literature of the effects of pharmacologic agents on senile

dementia, it is apparent that the vast majority of studies have subject samples

which would not comply with the proposed DSM-III[1] definition of senile dementia.

Under the draft version of DSM-III, senile dementia is a dementia with insidious

onset after age 65 and a uniformly progressive deteriorating course in a patient

for whom all other specific causes for dementia have been ruled out. Dementia,

to be diagnosed, requires a decrement in intellectual functioning after brain

maturation (age 15) of sufficient severity to interfere with social or occupational

functioning, or both. The changes must involve memory impairment plus either (a)

impairment in abstract thinking, (b) impairment in judgement, or (c) personality

change or impairment in impulse control.

Clearly, the subject samples employed should properly be called Senile Organic

Brain Syndrome (SOBS) since, in most cases, precise definitions of inclusion and

exclusion criteria are lacking. It must be assumed that the subject samples are

composed not only of true senile dementia, but also conditions which are masquerading

as senile dementia.

A variety of illnesses can produce dementia: major organ failure, post-traumatic

head injuries, heavy metal poisonings, post-anoxic and post-infective encephalo-

pathies, metabolic disturbances, vitamin deficiencies, and endocrine disorders as

---

*Portions of this paper appeared as an article in the McLean Hospital Journal,
Volume II, No. 4, pp 210-221, 1977.

well as a host of neurological diseases. Toxicities from a variety of medicinal
drugs as well as alcohol can also produce brain dysfunction. Treating the underlying medical problem, or withdrawing the offending drug can often return the
patient to his pre-illness status. Normal pressure hydrocephalus, usually manifested
by rather rapidly progressive dementia with ataxia and incontinence, can be treated
neurosurgically.[2] Dementia secondary to a small cerebral infarct will often clear
spontaneously; multiple infarct dementia (DSM-III's version of pschosis with
cerebral arteriosclerosis) often has an episodic, irregular course in contrast to
the slowly progressive course of senile dementia.

An equally important problem is the pseudodementia often seen with depressive
episodes in the elderly. This will respond nicely to antidepressant drugs or,
in more severe cases, electroconvulsive therapy. There is evidence that American
psychiatrists, in contrast to their British counterparts, tend to underdiagnose
depression when confronted with newly hospitalized elderly patients.[3]

A separate type of problem is posed by elderly patients living in the community
in retirement who have the subjective impression that their memory is failing a
little. These people probably have a normal decrease in memory which may not be
progressive, but may be aggravated by the stresses of low income, lack of meaningful work, decreasing social contacts, etc. Some memory problems seen in the
institutionalized elderly may have a similar, relatively nonorganic etiology. Lack
of hope, meaningful activity, and social contacts can lead to withdrawal and
apathy with a secondary weakening or loss of old capacities and interests.

Since some studies of drugs intended to be effective in senile dementia include
patients with "normal" or situationally aggravated cognitive deficits, the data
are difficult to interpret.

In studies involving heterogeneous institutional populations of elderly people
with memory and behavioral deficits, most of them may, in fact, have senile dementia.
However, one must watch for both the apathetic nonorganic patient and the elderly
chronic schizophrenic often placed in such facilities.

Keeping in mind the caveat of heterogeneous patient populations, drugs have long been sought which might ameliorate or even reverse the organic and social disabilities of these often tragic and helpless patients. A number of drugs are now marketed in the United States for use in this condition and a much larger number are in clinical use in Europe. The purpose of this paper is to review these drugs and to comment on their relative place in clinical psychopharmacology.

CEREBRAL VASODILATORS

The major drugs in this group can be subdivided into two categories: Agents which are "pure" vasodilators and those which possess other mechanisms of action in addition to vasodilation. Among the compounds currently available in the U.S.A. of the former type are cyclandelate (Cyclospasmol) and isoxsuprine (Vasodilan) and in the latter; papaverine (Pavabid) and dihydrogenated ergot alkoloids (Hydergine). In Europe, other similar drugs are in common use. In the "pure" vasodilator group, butalamine (Surheme) and pentoxifylline (Trental) are representative, while naftidrofuryl (Praxilene) and nicergoline (Sermion) belong to the multiple mechanism class.

These drugs pose a conceptual problem. If they really work by dilating brain arteries or arterioles, should this effect be helpful? If blood flow is reduced by arteriosclerosis, it is difficult to envision how a drug can affect a sclerosed artery; in fact, by dilating the normal arteries a vasodilator might shunt blood away from brain areas with reduced blood supply. Current evidence suggests that brain blood flow is reduced in senile dementia but that this reduction is secondary to the decrease in active brain tissue, not a cause of the cell loss. Elaborate studies of changes in regional blood flow are being carried out in Sweden; these may both help explain the nature of the deficits seen in various senile organic states and could be used to assess the actual local effects of vasodilating drugs.[4] There is also the possibility, unproven, that vasodilators may dilate capillaries or increase the deformability of red blood cells and thus improve the tissue blood supply in this manner.[5,6]

Despite the weakness of the general concept of vasodilators as an important pharmacological basis for the treatment of senile dementia, it remains a useful paradigm for screening drugs at the animal level. Several drugs originally proposed as treatments for senile dementia were initially identified as cerebral vasodilators but are now claimed to have other pharmacodynamic properties such as improving brain metabolism. Indeed, a recent review of vasodilators by Yesavage[7] et al has shown that significantly more controlled studies claim therapeutic benefits for multiple mechanism vasodilators than for "pure" vasodilators. While no satisfactory animal model for senile dementia has been available, some recent work on neurofibrillary degeneration may yield a model superior to the vasodilator animal screen.

Recent evidence obtained by Obrist[8] would suggest that reduced cerebral blood flow is the result of and not the cause of cerebral atrophy. Moreover, it has been independently demonstrated by Corsellis[9] and by Roth et al[10] that there exists a strong positive correlation between the density and the location of neurofibrillary degeneration (NFD) with the severity of neuropsychological impairment observed in senile dementia. At present, it appears that this form of neuropathology may be primarily responsible for the cortical dysfunction in both Alzheimer's disease and senile dementia. Indeed, Tomlinson[11] has suggested that 83 percent of all cases of senile organic brain syndrome may have NFD as their primary neuropathology.

Klatzo[12] et al observed that subarachnoid injections of aluminum salts in animals produced NFD. This led Crapper, et al[13] to investigate the possibility of this element playing an etiological role in the pathogenesis of the NFD that had been observed in Alzheimer's disease by Terry[14].

The atomic absorption study conducted by Crapper et al[13] on autopsied human NFD and Al^{+3}-induced feline NFD showed that both lesions contained a high concentration of aluminum, on the order of 9 to 12 micrograms per gram. This is in contrast to normal brain tissue which has an average concentration of only 0.23 to 2.7 micrograms per gram. Indeed, they showed that intracisternal injections of $AlCl_3$ which produce tissue concentrations of Al^{+3} in excess of 12 micrograms per gram of brain, will cause a profound NFD as well as a slow development of behavioral deficits in both short-term memory and associated learning in their cats.

It is enticing to speculate on the usefulness of aluminum-induced NFD as an animal model for senile dementia. Indeed, the evidence would suggest that such a model might be utilized in the preclinical assessment of agents of putative value in geriatric psychopharmacology. However, in the absence of experimental data on this model of senile dementia, the vasodilator approach may be with us for some time to come.

Papaverine

This ancient nonanalgesic and nonaddicting opium alkaloid has been used in senile conditions for decades. The most widely used preparation is Pavabid, a primitive spansule in which layers of drug alternate with layers of shellac in slow-release micro-pellets. The usual dosage of two 150 mg tablets twice a day is remarkably free of side effects. The three available placebo controlled studies show a mild advantage for the drug over placebo, especially in the areas of ameliorating conceptual disorganization, mannerisms, and uncooperativeness.[15-17] The most recent study conducted at Boston State Hospital's Geriatric Psychopharmacology Unit in symptomatic community-resident volunteers showed a little more mood improvement on Pavabid than on placebo.[18] This study, plus two earlier ones,[19,20] suggest that Pavabid does in fact alter EEG frequencies in the direction of "normality"; however, this effect has little value if unaccompanied by real clinical improvement.

The fact that papaverine is apparently a dopamine blocking agent,[18, 21] as are the antipsychotic drugs, coupled with the data from the more positive of the studies noted above, makes one wonder if the drug is not serving as a mild neuroleptic in elderly patients.

Dihydrogenated Ergot Alkaloids

A preparation containing three dihydrogenated ergot alkaloids in equal amounts is marketed as Hydergine. This drug appears to improve glucose metabolism and oxygen utilization in brain tissue, in addition to increasing blood flow. Seven controlled studies have shown Hydergine to be superior to placebo and two have shown it to be better than papaverine, although the latter drug was used at only 300 mg per day (possibly below minimal effective dose). The problem with these studies is not the lack of difference from placebo, but that the areas of superiority vary unsystematically from study to study. The effects are sometimes seen on mood, self-care, somatic symptoms, attitude, appetite, emotional instability, anxiety, and so on. If all studies showed effects on all these target symptoms, the drug might indeed seem wondrous, but the results are spotty. Notably, the areas of clear drug-placebo difference do not include memory and cognition. Further, drug-placebo differences occur very gradually over the three-month period usually employed in these studies. The dosages used were usually either 1.5 mg b.i.d. in U.S. studies, and 1.5 mg t.i.d. in European studies.[22]

The drug has no clear side effects. However, it is usually given as a sub-lingual lozenge and the cooperation necessary to handle this type of medication may be lacking in demented patients. There appears to be, as yet, no evidence that conventional oral administration would be better or worse than sublingual.

The data on the other presumed vasodilators (cyclandelate, isoxsuprine) are less extensive. For cyclandelate, one controlled study showed improvement in long term memory and reasoning;[23] our controlled study of isoxsuprine in geriatric symptomatic volunteers was essentially negative.[24]

Our attempt to confirm a previous controlled study of naftidrofuryl which was clearly positive[25] was only partially successful.[26] However, the study indicated that our Impairment Index when applied to relatively normal elderly subjects with subjective complaints of poor memory and documented deficits in several areas of neuropsychological functioning, evinced a treatment related effect.

Anticoagulants have also been claimed to improve brain oxygenation by decreasing blood sludging.[27] The evidence is mainly anecdotal and the potential hazards of this approach lead one to avoid it for the present.

Hyperbaric Oxygen

Because of the implication of hypoxia in senile dementia, the notion that increasing arterial PO_2 by hyperbaric oxygenation would be therapeutic for these patients, led to positive findings in an initial controlled study.[28] Other investigators, notably Gershon's group, have failed to replicate the initial results on several occasions.[29,30]

STIMULANTS

Analeptics

Patients with senile dementia, or related conditions, often are withdrawn, apathetic, and inert, as well as having memory and cognitive deficits. For this reason, stimulants of various sorts have been tried for decades in an attempt to energize senile dementia patients. One notable failure in this area has been Alertonic, an alcohol-containing elixir which also includes several vitamins and 2.5 mg of pipradol, an amphetamine-like stimulant. An extensive program of controlled studies developed by Blackwell failed to demonstrate any clear efficacy for this preparation.[31] However, the idea persists that there should be a good stimulant out there somewhere which will help restore mental activity or at least increase useful activity in the elderly.

The ancient and honorable drug in this area is pentylenetetrazol (Metrazol) which has been studied in senile conditions since 1953. It reflects dramatically the state of all other geriatric drugs. There are a number of very positive uncontrolled studies reporting that chronically institutionalized impaired patients blossom under the drug and at least 14 controlled studies which are much less impressive. Only two show Metrazol to be clearly superior to placebo,[32,33] five show some modest advantage for Metrazol over placebo,[17, 34-37] and seven are pretty clearly negative.[38-44] In the studies that show improvement it is usually on clinical global ratings or on, for example, total assets on the NOSIE ward behavior scale. It is not shown on psychological test performance. Dosages vary from 100 mg. t.i.d. to 300 mg t.i.d. with no clear relationship appearing between dose used and likelihood of clinical improvement. It is interesting to note, however, that one very positive study used 100 mg given six times a day.[33] If the drug is very short-acting, this type of regimen should be superior. Side effects are often more common on Metrazol than on placebo and include nausea and gastric distress, dizziness, faintness, syncope, and jitteriness. Although Metrazol has been used prior to the advent of electroconvulsive therapy and in much higher intravenous dosages to induce grand mal seizures, only three seizures were observed in the 14 studies reviewed. One occurred on placebo; the other two were noted in a study using a regimen of 200 mg four times a day.[44]

We have recently been involved in a study comparing Metrazol (600-800 mg/day for 12 weeks) with placebo in elderly community volunteers with mild memory complaints. A preliminary analysis shows, as noted above, a modest superiority for Metrazol over placebo on our battery of neuropsychological tests.[45] Also, the type and quantity of side effects observed on Metrazol did not differ significantly from placebo.[45]

On balance, in the absence of really effective drugs, pentylenetetrazol may be worth trying occasionally in elderly patients with memory deficit and behavioral problems. There are animal data showing that the drug improves the retention of learned material, at least in mice.[46] The drug seems safe in dosages under 800 mg/day.[45] Frequent small doses might have an advantage. A trial of at least six weeks, if the drug is well tolerated, may be necessary to see if improvement is occurring.

Amphetamine-like Drugs

Methylphenidate (Ritalin) has been studied a little in elderly patients, as has magnesium pemoline (Cyclert).[47, 48] The latter drug created a burst of interest 15 years ago when it was believed, incorrectly, that it increased brain nucleic acid.[49] It is now marketed for use in hyperkinetic children but may be worth trying as a mild stimulant in elderly patients. Deanol (Deaner) is another marketed antidepressant stimulant which may well act by cholinergic activation in the brain;[50] the other drugs noted above act through adrenergic mechanisms. Gershon's group finds elderly volunteers to be underreactive to methylphenidate.[51] Unfortunately, when they finally show a response to a fairly high dose (e.g., 40 mg/day) they develop side effects, not improvement.

We think it may be appropriate to try stimulant drugs cautiously in elderly patients who are underreactive and not grossly demented. Since methylphenidate and deanol may have different mechanisms of action, both should be investigated carefully.

The larger question is whether the behavior for which one might prescribe a stimulant is really a form of depression, in which case treatment with a tricyclic antidepressant might be more rational. The patient's cardiac status may be an issue in the decision. Patients with partial heart block should be given tricyclics only with caution and regular electrocardiographic monitoring. Low doses of adrenergic stimulants, though they may cause some rise in pulse rate and blood pressure, probably have less effect on cardiac conditions.

NEW THERAPEUTIC CONCEPTS

Several new approaches are worth mentioning at this time:

1. There may be a class of neglected compounds in our current pharmaceopeia. If Robinson is right, and elderly individuals have elevated levels of the enzyme monoamine oxidase (MAO) in their brains,[52] the use of an MAO inhibitor such as phenelzine (the one best studied at present) may be rational. The fear of hypertensive crisis leading to strokes tends to dampen our enthusiasm for this approach, but we would hope that a carefully controlled study could be done to determine efficacy and safety in elderly patients with depression or related symptoms in order to determine the value of this treatment strategy.

2. There is some evidence that the enzyme choline acetyltransferase is reduced in the aged.[53] Feeding patients a lot of choline, the precursor of acetylcholine,

an approach which appears to be useful in tardive dyskinesia, may not work because of the reduced level of synthetic enzyme. Physostigimine, which acts by reversibly inhibiting acetylcholine esterase, needs study in senile dementia. However, even if it improves cognitive function it will not do as a treatment because of its short duration of action and the probable need to give it parenterally. A long-acting oral cholinergic drug would need to be developed. It would probably need to be combined with a quarternary, anti-muscarinic drug like methscopolamine which would block peripheral cholinergic side effects while exhibiting minimal penetration of the blood-brain barrier thus allowing our hypothetical drug to act freely on brain cholinergic centers.

3. The growing interest in polypeptide neurohormones has led to the discovery that a fraction of the large polypeptide ACTH, namely ACTH 4-10 (OI-63) (the fourth through the tenth amino acids in ACTH) has a marked effect on rat behavior, improving memory and increasing drive.[54] We have studied this drug in elderly volunteers and find a marked improvement in self-reports of mood on the POMS, an adjective check list, and some hint that it may help subjects retrieve previously learned material from their memory store.[55] Unfortunately, the drug can only be given parenterally and has a half-life in the body of about 15 seconds! Organon, the company which developed ACTH 4-10, is working on longer lasting oral analogues. We have recently completed a study on the first of these; at the dosage used the results were not impressive.[56] Recently, lysine vasopressin has been reported in the literature to have similar effects to ACTH 4-10 on memory. One study conducted in Spain, reports that insufflation of lysine vasopressin (Diapid) reversed post-traumatic amnesias.[57] An independent research team in Belgium also reported improved memory in a group of elderly volunteers.[58] While the findings of these two groups provide clinical support for data obtained in animals, these reults are too preliminary to make any judgements regarding the clinical usefulness of lysine vasopressin.

4. Piracetam (Nootropil) is an odd drug created by cyclizing gamma-amino-butyric acid (GABA), a straight chain compound. The resulting drug does not appear to act like GABA, but does protect animals against the behavioral impairments caused by hypoxia and also vertigo.[59,60] Controlled European studies have been positive and make the drug worthy of further study in this country.[61,62]

5. A compound which has received some attention due to its ability to reduce the "aging pigment" (lipofuscin) in the brains of aged guinea pigs is centrophenoxin (Lucidril).[63] The evidence, at this time, regarding its therapeutic efficacy in senile dementia is equivocal. However, it bears some structural relationship to both procaine and naftidrofuryl, compounds which have some evidence for efficacy.[7,25,64] This would suggest that further studies should be conducted.

6. Lastly, a radical treatment approach might be suggested based upon the evidence that chronic accumulation of aluminum in the brain could lead to neuro-fibrillary degeneration (NFD).[65] If, indeed, aluminum-induced NFD is the primary neuropathology of Alzheimer's disease, as well as senile dementia, then pharmacologic intervention with a chelator might be indicated. Most chelating agents exhibit approximately the same order of preference for metals.[66] Since the binding constants for lead and aluminum with calcium disodium edetate are similar, it can be hypothesized that aluminum-induced NFD might be reversed by this agent. While no clinical trials have been conducted, there is a report in the literature of a case of "dialysis dementia" (an aluminum-induced encephalopathy) which failed to respond to treatment with BAL (dimercaprol).[67] At present there are too little data to justify clinical trials; however, animal studies should be conducted to assess the value of this approach.

CONCLUSIONS

The best existing treatment for senile dementia is, unfortunately, the positive diagnosis of some other more treatment-responsive condition which masquerades as senile dementia. If true senile dementia is clearly present, the best available drug therapies are Hydergine and pentylenetetrazol, with Hydergine having better evidence for efficacy. Neither drug has clinically dramatic effects; both have slow and subtle effects over periods of several weeks.

The most interesting newer drugs include polypeptides with clear memory-improving effects in animals, and piracetam, a drug marketed in Europe but not yet available in the United States.

REFERENCES

1. Diagnostic and Statistical Manual III (Draft), Task Force on Nomenclature and Statistics. (1977) American Psychiatric Association, Washington, D.C.

2. Katzman, R. (1977) Normal Pressure Hydrocephalus. In Wells C.E. (Ed): Dementia. Philadelphia, F.A. Davis, Chap. 4.

3. Gurland, B.J. (1976) The Comparative Frequency of Depression in Various Adult Age Groups. J. Gerontol. 31: pp 283-286.

4. Hagberg, B., Ingvar, D.H. (1976) Cognitive Reduction in Presenile Dementia Related to Regional Abnormalities of the Cerebral Blood Flow. Br. J. Psychiat. 128: pp 209-222.

5. Meier-Ruge, W., Enz, A., Gygax, P., etal (1975) Experimental Pathology in Basic Research of the Aging Brain. In Gershon, S., Raskin A. (Eds): Aging. New York, Raven Press. pp 55-126.

6. Hess, H., Franke, I., Jauch, M. (1973) Improvement in the Fluidity of Blood with Medication. Fortschr. Med. 91: pp 743-748.

7. Yesavage, J.A., Tinklenberg, J.R., Berger, P.A., and Hollister, L.E. (in press) Vasodilators in Senile Dementias: A Review of the Literature. Arch. Gen. Psychiat.

8. Obrist, W.D. (1972) Cerebral Physiology of the Aged. Influence of Circulatory Disorders. In Gaitz, C.M. (Ed): Aging and the Brain. New York, Plenum. pp 117-133.

9. Corsellis, J.A.N. (1962) Mental Illness and the Aging Brain. London, Oxford Univ. Press.

10. Roth, M., Tomlinson, B.E., Blessed, G. (1966) Correlation Between Scores for Dementia and Counts of Senile Plaques in Cerebral Gray Matter of Elderly Subjects. Nature (London) 209: pp 109-110.

11. Tomlinson, B.E. (1970) Morphological Brain Changes in Non-Demented Old People. In van Praag, H.M., Kalverboer, A.F. (Eds.) Aging of the Central Nervous System,. Haarlam, the Netherlands, De Erven and Bohn, pp 38-57.

12. Klatzo, I., Wisniewski, H., Streicher, E. (1965) Experimental Production of Neurofibrillary Degeneration. I. Lights Microscopic Observations. J. Neuropath. Exp. Neurol 24: pp 187-199.

13. Crapper, D.R., Krishman, S.S., Dalton, A.J. (1973) Brain Aluminum Distribution in Alzheimer's Disease and Experimental Neurofibrillary Degeneration. Science 180: pp 511-513.

14. Terry, R.D. (1963) The Fine Structure of Neurofibrillary Tangles in Alzheimer's Disease. J. Neuropath. Exp. Neurol. 22: pp 629-642.

15. Ritter, R.H., Nail, H.R., Tatum, P., etal (1971) The Effect of Papaverine on Patients with Cerebral Arteriosclerosis. Clin. Med. 78: pp 18-22.

16. Stern, F.H. (1970) Management of Chronic Brain Syndrome Secondary to Cerebral Arteriosclerosis with Special Reference to Papaverine Hydrochloride. J. Am. Geriat. Soc. 18: pp 507-512.

17. Lu, L., Stotsky, B.A., Cole, J.O. (1971) A Controlled Study of Drugs in Long-Term Geriatric Psychiatric Patients. Arch. Gen. Psychiat. 25: pp 284-288.

18. Branconnier, R.J., Cole, J.O. (1977) Effects of Chronic Papaverine Administration on Mild Senile Organic Brain Sundrome. J. Am. Geriat. Soc. 25: pp 458-462.

19. McQuillan, L.M., Lopec, C.A., Vibal. J.R. (1974) Evaluation of EEG and Clinical Changes Associated with Pavabid Therapy in Chronic Brain Syndrome. Curr. Ther. Res. 16: pp 49-58.

20. Cole, J. O., Branconnier, R.J., Martin, G.F. (1975) Electroencephalographic and Behavioral Changes Associated with Papaverine Administration in Healthy Geriatric Subjects. J. Am. Geriat. Soc. 23: pp 295-300.

21. Gardos, G., Cole, J.O., Sniffin C. (1976) An Evaluation of Papaverine in Tardive Dyskinesia. J. Clin. Pharm. 16: pp 304-310.

22. Shader, R.I., Goldsmith, G.N. (1976) Dihydrogenated Ergot Alkaloids and Papaverine: A Status Report on Their Effects in Senile Mental Deterioration. In Klein, D., Gittleman-Klein, R. (Eds.): Progress in Psychiatric Drug Treatment. New York, Brunner-Mazel, pp 540-554.

23. Smith, W.L., Lowry, J.B., Davis, J.A. (1968) The Effects of Cyclandelate on Psychological Test Performance in Patients with Cerebral Vascular Insufficiency. Curr. Ther. Res. 10: pp 613-617.

24. Branconnier, R.J., Cole, J.O. Unpublished data.

25. Judge, T.G. Urquhart, A. (1972) Naftidrofuryl -- A Double-Blind Cross-Over Study in the Elderly. Curr Med Res Opinion 1: pp 166-172.

26. Branconnier, R.J., Cole, J.O. (in press) The Impairment Index as a Symptom-Independent Parameter of Drug Efficacy in Geriatric Psychopharmacology. J. Gerontol.

27. Walsh, A.C., Walsh, B.H. (1972) Senile and Presenile Dementia: Further Observations on the Benefits of Dicumarol-Psychotherapy Regimen. J. Am. Geriat. Soc. 20: pp 127-131.

28. Jacobs, E.A., Winter, P.M., Alvis, H.J., et al (1969) Hyperoxygenation Effect on Cognitive Function in the Aged. N. Eng. J. Med. 281: pp 753-757.

29. Raskin, A., Gershon, S., Crook, T.H., etal (1975) Tables for the Effects of Hyper- and Normobaric Oxygen on Cognitive Impairment in the Elderly. Presented at the Annual Meeting of the American College of Neuropsychopharmacology, San Juan, Puerto Rico, December 11.

30. Goldfarb, A.L., Hochstadt, N.J., Jacobson, J.H., et al (1972) Hyperbaric Oxygen Treatment of Organic Mental Syndrome in Aged Persons. J. Gerontol. 27: pp 212-217.

31. Blackwell, B. Personal Communication.

32. Lapinsohn, L.I. (1955) Metrazol or Glutamic Acid in Treating Certain Mental Disorders. Penn. Med. J. 58: pp 42-44.

33. Linden, M.E., Courtney, D., Howland, A.O. (1956) Interdisciplinary Research in the Use of Oral Pentylenetetrazol (Metrazol) in the Emotional Disorders of the Aged. Studies in Gerontologic Human Relations. V.J. Am. Geriat. Soc. 4: pp 380-399.

34. Leckman, J., Anath, J.V., Ban, T.A., et al (1971) Pentylenetetrazol in the Treatment of Geriatric patients with Disturbed Memory Function. J. Clin. Pharmacol. 11: pp 301-303.

35. Stotsky, B.A., Cole, J.O., Lu, L., et al (1972) A Controlled Study of the Efficacy of Pentylenetetrazol (Metrazol) with Hard-Core Hospitalized Psychogeriatric Patients. Am. J. Psychiat. 129: pp 47-51.

36. Mead, S., Mueller E.E., Mason, E.P., et al (1953) A Study of the Effects of Oral Administration of Metrazol [R] in Old Individuals. J. Gerontol. 8: pp 472-476.

37. Swenson, W.M., Grimes, B.P. (1953) Oral Use of Metrazol in Senile Patients. Geriatrics 8: pp 99-101.

38. Swenson, W.M., Anderson, D.E., Grimes, B.P. (1957) A Re-evaluation of the Oral Use of Metrazol in Senile Patients. J. Gerontol 12: pp 401-403.

39. Sheard, M.H., Coyne, E., Hammons, P. (1959) A Trial of Oral Pentamethylenetetrazol in Senile Patients. Quart. Rev. Psychiat. Neurol. 20: pp 34-37.

40. Gericke, O.L., Lobb, L.G. (1964) Effect of Metrazol on the Memory of the Aged. Psychiat. Studies Projects 2: pp 2-7.

41. Ananth, J.V., Deutsch, M., Ban, T.A. (1971) Senilex in the Treatment of Geriatric Patients. Curr. Ther. Res. 13: pp 316-321.

42. Williams, J.R., Csalany, L., Misevic, G. (1967) Drug Therapy with or Without Group Discussion: Effects of Various Regimens on the Behavior of Geriatric Patients in a Mental Hospital. J. Am. Geriat. Soc. 15: pp 34-40.

43. Barrabee, P., Wingate, J.H., Phillips B.D., et al (1956) Effects of L-Glutavite Compared with Metrazol and Vitamins on Aged Female Psychotic Patients. Postgrad Med. 19: pp 485-491.

44. Robinson, D.B. (1959) Evaluation of Certain Drugs in Geriatric Patients. Arch. Gen. Psychiat. 1: pp 41-46.

45. Branconnier, R.J., Cole, J.O.   Unpublished data

46. Krivanek, J., McGaugh, J.L. (1968) Effects of Pentylenetetrazol on Memory Storage in Mice. Psychopharmacologia 12: pp 303-321

47. Raskind, M., Eisdorfer, C. (1976) Psychopharmacology of the Aged. In Simpson LL (Ed) Drug Treatment of Mental Disorders. New York, Raven Press. pp 237-266.

48. Connors, C.K. (Ed) (1974) Clinical Use of Stimulant Drugs in Children. The Hague, Excerpta Medica.

49. Plotnikoff, N. (1968) Learning and Memory Enhancement by Pemoline and Magnesium Hydroxide. Recent Adv. Biol. Psychiat. 10: pp 102-120.

50. Re., O. (1974) 2-Dimethylaminoethanol (Deanol): A Brief Review of its Clinical Efficacy and Postulated Mechanisms of Action. Curr. Ther. Res. 16: pp 1238-1242.

51. Crook, T., Ferris, G., Sathananthan, G., etal (1977) The Effect of Methyl-phenidate on Test Performance in the Cognitively Impaired Elderly. Psychopharmacologia 52: pp 251-255.

52. Robinson, D.S. (1975) Changes in Monoamine Oxidase and Monoamines with Human Development and Aging. Fed. Proc. 34: pp 103-107.

53. Signorelli, A. (1976) Influence of Physostigmine Upon Consolidation of Memory in Mice. J. Compar. Physiol. Psychol. 90: pp 658-664.

54. Flood, J.F., Jarvik, M.E. (1976) Effects of ACTH Peptide Fragments on Memory Formation. The Neuropeptides. Pharmacol. Bichem. Behav. 5: pp 41-51.

55. Branconnier, R.J., Cole, J.O., Gardos, G. (1977) ACTH 4-10 in the Amelioration of Symptomatology Associated with Mild Senile Organic Brain Syndrome. Paper presented at the Annual New Clinical Drug Evaluation Unit Program, Key Biscayne, Florida, May 19-21.

56. Branconnier, R.J., Cole, J.O.   Unpublished Data.

57. Oliveros, J.C., Jandali, M.K., Timsit-Berthier, M., et al (1978) Vasopressin in Amnesia. Lancet (1) (8054) pp 42

58. Legros, J.J., Gilot, P., Seron, X., et al (1978) Influence of Vasopressin on Learning and Memory. Lancet (1) (8054) pp 41-42.

59. (1974) Piracetam, Basic Scientific and Clinical Data. UCB Pharmaceutical Division, Brussels, Belgium. pp 40-41.

60. Giurgea, C.E., Moyersoons, F., Evraerd, ACA (1967) GABA Related Hypothesis on the Mechanism of Action of the Antimotion Sickness Drugs. Arch. Intern. Pharmacodyn. Therap. 166: pp 238-251.

61. Stegink, A.J. (1972) The Clinical Use of Piracetam, a New Nootropic Drug. The Treatment of Symptoms of Senile Involution. Arzneim-Forsch (Drug Res) 22: pp 975-977.

62. Mindus, P., Cronholm, B., Levander, S., et al (1974) Effects of Piracetam on Anxiety and Mental Performance in Middle-Aged Healthy Volunteers. Paper presented at VII European Congress of Clinical Gerontology.

63. Wietec, H.F. (1966) Zum Einfluss von Centrophenoxin Auf Das Alterspigment Lipofuscin in Nervenellen. Arzeneinittel Forschung 16 (8) pp 1123

64. Jarvik, L. F. and Milne, J.F. (1975) Gerovital-H 3: A Review of the Literature in Gershon, S., Raskin, A. (Eds.) Aging. New York Raven Press pp 203-227

65. Crapper, D.R. Krishnan, S.S., Quittkat, S. (1976) Aluminum, Neurofibrillary Degeneration and Alzheimer's Disease. Brain 99: pp 67-80.

66. Albert A., (1973) Selective Toxicity, the Physico-Chemical Basis of Therapy. London. Chapman & Hall pp 350.

67. Mahurkar, S.D., Dhar, S.K., Salta, R., etal (1973) Dialysis Dementia. Lancet 1: pp 1412-1415.

PROTEIN AND AMINO ACID METABOLISM IN THE AGED

VERNON R. YOUNG and MITCHELL GERSOVITZ
Department of Nutrition and Food Science and Clinical Research Center
Massachusetts Institute of Technology, Cambridge, MA 02139

ABSTRACT

Selected aspects of amino acid and whole body protein metabolism
during aging in human subjects are discussed for their possible
nutritional significance. The picture that emerges is one of a slow
loss of total body protein with aging, due largely to a dimimution
in the size of the skeletal muscle mass. These changes are accompanied by a shift in the overall pattern of whole body protein synthesis and breakdown. Using ^{15}N-amino acids to estimate the rate
of whole body protein breakdown and measurement of urinary N^{T}-
methylhistidine excretion to determine the rate of muscle protein
breakdown, skeletal muscle mass was estimated to account for about
27% of whole body protein turnover in the young adult declining
to 20% or less in the elderly subject. Studies of obligatory
urinary nitrogen losses (or endogenous N output) also suggest that
muscle makes a lower contribution to endogenous N output in elderly
subjects than young adults.

The factorial method for estimating dietary protein needs, as
applied by the most recent FAO/WHO Expert Committee on Energy and
Protein Requirements, based, in part, on summation of obligatory
N losses, does not predict satisfactorily the amount of good quality
protein required to support nitrogen balance in elderly subjects.
From results of direct nitrogen balance studies and taking into
consideration the various biological, environmental and social
factors that tend to increase dietary protein needs we conclude that
an appropriate dietary protein allowance for elderly people would
be about 13% of the total energy intake as dietary protein and
provided from food sources with nutritional quality comparable to
those in North American and European-type diets.

INTRODUCTION

According to Diamond[1], "the external environment may play a larger
role than has been recognized in maintaining brain cells during
aging". Environmental variables of importance include infectious
disease, use of drugs, socio-economic and cultural factors and
nutrition. Deficiencies and imbalances of dietary nutrients affect

the biochemical and functional status of body tissues, including the central nervous system[2,3]. Complex changes in the biochemical status of brain cells occur with alterations in the adequacy and level of nutrient intake and these changes presumably underlie the mental and behavioural responses that follow changes in diet and in nutritional status. Thus, a maintenance of adequate nutritional status would be expected to help optimize the biochemical and functional activity of various body organs and processes and, in the context of the principal topic covered in this symposium, the central nervous and neuroendocrine systems, in particular. It is appropriate, therefore, to review briefly selected aspects of nutrient utilization and nutrient requirements in elderly people. The focus of the present paper is on observations derived from direct human studies and we emphasize the utilization of and needs for dietary protein, a subject that we have discussed recently in several reviews[4-6]. Hence, the latter provide the basis for the present paper; a more extensive analysis of nutrient utilization was judged to be beyond the scope of the major topic of this symposium.

2. AMINO ACID METABOLISM

A major function of dietary protein is to provide substrate necessary for the maintenance of tissue and organ protein synthesis in the adult. The substrate consists of the so-called essential (indispensable) amino acids and a source of nonessential (nonspecific) nitrogen, that is required for the synthesis of the nonessential (dispensible) amino acids and other nitrogen-containing metabolites including, for example, purines and pyrimidines, neurotransmitters, porphyrins, carnosine, creatine and the peptide hormones. These various compounds play important physiological roles, but presumably they account for a relatively small proportion of total daily amino acid utilization.

A general scheme of amino acid metabolism is given in fig. 1, suggesting that the utilization and requirements for amino acids may be influenced by possible age-related changes in various processes including intestinal and cellular membrane transport, tissue enzyme activity, and the metabolic status of protein metabolism in cells and organs. More extensive information is available on the influence of age on amino acid metabolism in experimental animals because a number of practical and ethical considerations limit the exploration of this aspect of nutrient metabolism in aging human subjects. However, blood plasma can be readily obtained and a few studies have

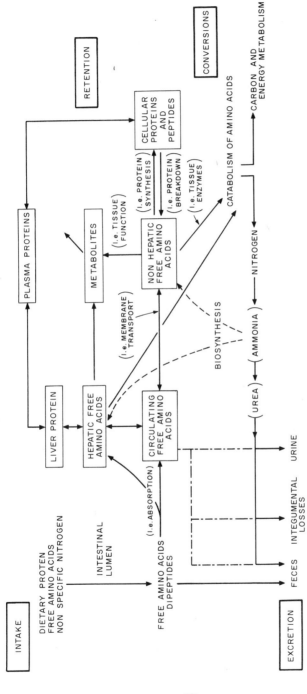

Fig. 1. A schematic outline of amino acid metabolism in the intact organism. From Young et al.[5]

289

been reported on plasma amino acid levels in older people. Although many factors regulate the concentration of amino acids in plasma[7], studies at this level in various physiological and pathological states have improved our understanding of human protein and amino acid metabolism[eg.8,9].

Our laboratory has carried out a series of studies designed to examine the relationships between plasma amino acid levels, amino acid intakes and requirements in humans of various ages (reviewed in ref. 10). Hence these studies provide an opportunity to compare plasma amino acid patterns in young adults and elderly people.

Thus, because one or more of the branched-chain amino acids (leucine, isoleucine and valine) may inhibit breakdown and stimulate synthesis of muscle protein[11,12] and because they are metabolized preferentially in the skeletal musculature[13], we examined the concentration of these amino acids in blood plasma of young adults and elderly subjects. Table 1 summarizes these data and they reveal no important differences in the concentration of branched-chain amino acids in blood plasma,during the post-absorptive phase,for the two age groups studied. However, an additional evaluation can be made by examination of the influence of a dietary change on the branched-chain amino acids in plasma in young adults and elderly subjects. Furthermore, it is also known that metabolic interactions occur among these amino acids that depend, in part, on the level of the dietary supply[14]. Therefore, table 2 shows results for the concentration of branched-chain amino acids in blood plasma under conditions of usual and reduced intakes of leucine. As can be seen from this table,a reduction in the intake of leucine in young men results in a decrease in plasma leucine and an increase in the concentration of the other two branched-cahin amino acids, isoleucine and valine. The mechanism for this effect is not known but we have suggested that the level and availability of dietary leucine regulates the uptake and utilization of the other two branched-chain amino acids[14]. As also shown in the table, elderly women show a rise in plasma isoleucine and valine concentrations when the dietary leucine intake is reduced; this change is comparable to that observed in young men. Thus, it can be tentatively concluded from these limited data that branched-chain amino acid metabolism is,at least,qualitatively similar in young adults and the elderly. However study of plasma free amino acids only provides an index of the instantaneous concentration of the amino acid in the circulation and does not reveal whether the flux and/or metabolic fate of amino acids within body tissues and organs is similar or different among the age groups.

TABLE 1

Concentrations[1] of Branched-chain Amino Acids in
Blood Plasma of Young Adult and Elderly Subjects
Consuming an Adequate Free-choice Diet[1]

Plasma Amino Acid	Young Men	Elderly Women
Leucine	14.7 ± 1.6[2]	14.1 ± 3.1
Isoleucine	8.2 ± 1.2	6.9 ± 1.5
Valine	24.9 ± 2.7	24.9 ± 3.4
Leucine:Valine Ratio	0.59 ± 0.05	0.57 ± 0.09

1. Taken from Young et al.[5]
2. Mean $\pm$ SD; results are expressed as μ moles per 100 ml.
    Samples were drawn after a 10-hr overnight fast.(Unpublished
    data of Perera, Scrimshaw, and Young). Data are from 19
    healthy young men, ages 22 ± 4 years and from 11 healthy
    elderly women, ages 69 ± 2 years.

TABLE 2

Effect of Reduced Leucine Intake on the Concentration of
Branched-chain Amino Acids in Plasma
of Young Men and Elderly Women[1,2]

Amino Acid	Young Men		Elderly Women	
	Normal	Reduced Intake	Normal	Reduced Intake
Leucine	14.2 ± 1.1[3]	11.7 ± 0.7	13.7 ± 1.5	10.4 ± 0.9
Isoleucine	7.7 ± 0.4	12.2 ± 0.3	6.8 ± 1.3	9.2 ± 1.0
Valine	24.3 ± 1.3	41.3 ± 9.8	24.9 ± 0.9	38.1 ± 0.5
Leucine: Valine	0.57 ± 0.03	0.30 ± 0.07	0.56 ± 0.08	0.27 ± 0.04

1. From Young et al.[5]
2. Four subjects comprised each group. Data are expressed as
    μmoles per 100 ml. (Unpublished data of Perera, Scrimshaw,
    and Young.) Blood samples were taken after a 10-hr overnight
    fast during a free-choice diet period (Normal) or after 7 or
    10 days with an amino acid diet providing 16 mg of leucine per
    kg of body weight per day.
3. Mean $\pm$ SD.

Studies of this phase of amino acid metabolism could be carried out with the aid of ^{13}C and ^{15}N-labeled amino acids as tracers and we are now beginning to carry out these investigations[eg.15].

Plasma amino acid levels are affected by the amount of protein and level of individual amino acids in the diet[16,17]. Therefore, additional information on the status of amino acid metabolism in elderly people can be gained by comparing the effects of alterations in essential amino acid intake on plasma amino acid concentrations in young adult and older subjects. Hence, the response of free tryptophan in blood plasma to graded decreases in the dietary intake of the amino acid in three age groups (a) school-age children with Down's Symdrome[18] (b) healthy young men[19] and (c) a group of elderly men and women[20] was studied. We found that the pattern of response was similar for all three groups, with a reduced intake resulting in a decrease in plasma tryptophan, until a new and lower concentration is achieved with further reductions in dietary tryptophan intake. Again, this study suggested that tryptophan metabolism is responsive to the adequacy of tryptophan intake and appears to respond similarly in both healthy young adults and older people. It would be worthwhile to explore in experimental animals, the relationship between diet, plasma amino acid levels and CNS function, for those amino acids, such as tryptophan or phenylalanine and tyrosine, that serve as neurotransmitter precursors.

3. BODY PROTEIN METABOLISM

   (a) Body composition and muscle mass

        Initially it is necessary to consider briefly body composition and muscle mass, because the size and activity of the body cell mass will determine the need and utilization of dietary protein and amino acids. Based on cross-sectional and longitudinal studies there is a decline in lean body mass with advancing age in human subjects[21,22] (fig.2). Although the contribution made by each of the body organs to this decline is not precisely known, dissection studies suggest that the skeletal muscles account for a significant and perhaps the major proportion of the decline in body protein content. Hence, from fig.3 it is apparent that during early growth and development the skeletal muscles account for an increasing contribution to total body weight, amounting to about 45% of body weight in the young adult. However, as the adult years progress, muscle mass continues to decline, decreasing to approximately 27% of total body weight by age about 70 years. This pattern of change in the relative size of the muscle mass with growth

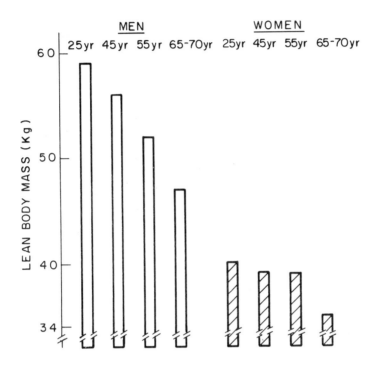

MEAN VALUES FOR LEAN BODY MASS (LBM) AT
SELECTED AGES

MEN   WOMEN

Fig. 2.   Lean body mass at various ages in adult men and women.
Drawn from data of Forbes & Reina[21].

and development and during aging contrasts to that for the liver. This
organ accounts for approximately 4.5% body weight in the newborn, 3.5%
in young adults and 2% in the elderly. From these considerations it
appears that changes in muscle mass have major significance in relation to the changes in total body protein content. Furthermore,
studies on the relationship between creatinine excretion, an index of
muscle mass[24], and body cell mass (or lean body mass) supports this
conclusion. Thus, we have observed in unpublished studies that the
lower rate of urinary creatinine excretion in elderly male and female
subjects correlates closely with their lower body cell mass, as determined from whole body potassium measurement.

   Thus, these various studies of body composition support the concept
that the reduced body cell mass in the elderly, as compared with young

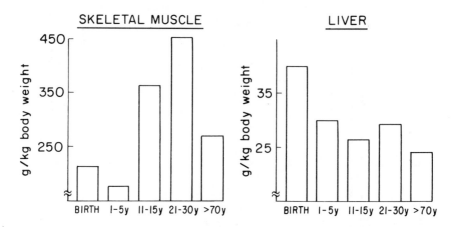

RELATIVE PROPORTION (g/kg body weight) of
MAJOR BODY ORGANS AT DIFFERENT
AGES IN MAN

Fig. 3. Contribution made by skeletal muscle and liver, each expressed as g per kg body weight, in humans at various ages.
Drawn from Korenchevsky[23].

adults, is related to a decline in the amount of protein in the
skeletal muscles. Therefore, because of the significance of the
skeletal muscles in the adaptations of body protein and energy metabolism[8,25] it is important to explore briefly some dynamic aspects of
protein metabolism and then to assess the quantitative contribution
made by skeletal muscles to overall body protein metabolism in elderly
subjects.

   (b) Whole body protein (nitrogen) turnover

     During early growth and development the rates of whole body
protein synthesis and breakdown are high and they fall as growth
diminishes and with the approachment of adulthood. A summary of some
of the published estimates of rates of total body protein synthesis
during different phases of growth and development in human subjects
is given in table 3. Although there is variation in the reported
estimates for the various age groups it is clear from the available
data that the rate of whole body protein synthesis is quite high during
early life and then declines to a much lower rate during the early
school years; in the young adult whole body protein synthesis occurs
at a rate approximating one-fifth of that in the newborn.

TABLE 3

RATES OF WHOLE BODY PROTEIN SYNTHESIS IN HUMANS
DURING GROWTH AND DEVELOPMENT

Group	No.	Age(or Wt)	Whole Body Synthesis (g protein/kg/day)	Author & Ref.
Premature Infants	3	42-68 d	10-15.5	Nicholson(26)
Premature	5	1-45 d	26.3	Pencharz et al. (27)
Infants	3	5 kg	3.3-7.7	Wu & Snyderman (30)
Infants	5	10-20 mo	6.1	Picou & Taylor-Roberts(28)
Infants	5	8.3-21 mo	6.3	Golden & Waterlow (29)
Children	8	9-16 yr	3.9	Kien et al.(31)
Young Adult	6	20-25 yr	3.0	Steffee et al. (32)
Adult	5	31-46 yr	3.5	Halliday & McKeran (33)

TABLE 4

MEAN RATES OF WHOLE BODY PROTEIN
BREAKDOWN IN YOUNG ADULT AND ELDERLY SUBJECTS[1]

Whole Body Protein Breakdown	Young Adult		Elderly	
	Male	Female	Male	Female
g/kg body wt/day	2.9	2.4	2.6	1.9
g/kg BCM/day[2]	6.7	6.1	7.5	6.6
g/g creatinine/day	115	103	169	166
g/kcal BMR x 10[3]	113*	90	117	106

1. From Uauy et al.[34].

2. BCM = Body Cell Mass

*. BMR = Basal Metabolic Rate

The effects of the advancing adult years in humans on rates of
whole body protein synthesis and breakdown have been explored less
extensively. Using the simplified model of Picou and Taylor-Roberts[28]
we have estimated rates of whole body protein synthesis and breakdown
in young adults and compared the results with those in healthy elderly
subjects, of both sexes. The results are summarized in table 4, for
rates of whole body protein breakdown;these are similar to the rates
of protein synthesis. These results suggest only a small difference in these
rates between young adult and older subjects, when the rates are

expressed per unit of body weight[34]. Golden and Waterlow[35] have concluded that the rate of whole body protein synthesis is less in elderly subjects than in younger adults.

Because body composition differences exist among young adults and elderly subjects, our studies also examined the rates of whole body protein breakdown in relation to parameters of body composition; first, creatinine, as an index of muscle mass, and second body cell mass, as determined by whole body potassium measurement. In addition, the rates were also expressed in reference to basal energy expenditure for the two age and sex groups studied. The results of these various comparisons are also given in table 4. Whole body protein breakdown (and synthesis) rates per unit of creatinine excretion were somewhat higher in the elderly than in young adults but the level of statistical significance of this difference was not high ($p < 0.1$) due to considerable variation among the subjects studied. However, this difference implies a possible change in the pattern of distribution of whole body protein turnover during aging and we explored this concept further by estimating actual rates of muscle protein breakdown in relation to whole body protein breakdown.

The rate of muscle protein breakdown in the intact organism can be assessed from a measurement of urinary N^τ-methylhistidine (3-methylhistidine) excretion[36,37]. Briefly, determination of the rate of muscle protein breakdown from 3-methylhistidine excretion involves the following considerations: (i) the major locus within the body of the amino acid is in the myofibrillar proteins, actin and myosin, of skeletal muscle; (ii) the amino acid appears in these proteins by methylation of a histidine residue after peptide bond synthesis, and (iii) upon breakdown of actin and myosin, the amino acid is released and then quantitatively excreted in the urine, without undergoing oxidation or any significant metabolic interconversion in the human subject. Thus, the daily excretion of the amino acid is related quantitatively to its rate of release from the major myofibrillar proteins in skeletal muscle, and the level of daily output reflects the breakdown rate of these proteins. Assuming that adult human muscle contains, on average, 4.2 μmoles N^τ-methylhistidine, the rate of breakdown of protein within the skeletal musculature can be computed from the measured daily urinary output of the amino acid. Furthermore, if the whole body protein breakdown rate is also known, the percentage contribution made by muscle to this parameter of whole body metabolism can be estimated. Therefore, we have measured, for this purpose, the urinary excretion of N^τ-methylhistidine in young adults and elderly subjects all consuming flesh-free diets, free of sources of the amino acid[34].

As shown in fig.4 the skeletal muscles account for about 27% of whole body protein breakdown in young adults. For the elderly, on the other hand, muscle accounts for a significantly lower proportion of whole body portein breakdown; in this case the mean values being 16% and 20% for older women and men, respectively.

The nutritional significance of this redistribution in the pattern of whole body protein breakdown is not certain but it can be explored in reference to endogenous or obligatory nitrogen losses, discussed below.

4. OBLIGATORY NITROGEN LOSSES AND FACTORIAL ESTIMATION OF PROTEIN (NITROGEN) NEEDS

Determination of nitrogen (N) losses via urine, feces and other routes, including the integument, when a protein-free diet is given, provides the data base for estimation of dietary protein allowances for adults of differing age, as discussed later. In addition, comparison of these N losses, the so-called obligatory nitrogen losses, in young adult and elderly subjects offers a further opportunity to assess the possible changes in nitrogen metabolism during advancing age in human subjects. Therefore, we[38,39] have measured the urinary N losses in elderly men and women after short-term adaptation to "protein-free" feeding. The pattern of change in urinary N excretion can be described according to a monoexponential decay and analyzed mathematically[40]. A comparison of the results obtained in our studies with young men and elderly subjects is given in table 5, from which the following observations can be made; first the obligatory urinary nitrogen output, per unit of body weight, in elderly men is essentially the same as that for young men; second when expressed per unit of creatinine excretion or per unit of body cell mass, obligatory urinary N losses are higher in elderly than in young men. These differences in N output tend to parallel those discussed above for whole body protein breakdown (and synthesis) rates, implying a relationship between whole body protein turnover and obligatory N losses. Indeed, the magnitude of obligatory urinary N losses is positively correlated with the rate of whole body protein breakdown[34]. Hence, in view of this correlation and because there is a shift in pattern of distribution of whole body protein breakdown with aging, it appears that a greater proportion of obligatory N output in elderly subjects arises from protein turnover in non-muscle tissues and organs. These differences in N metabolism

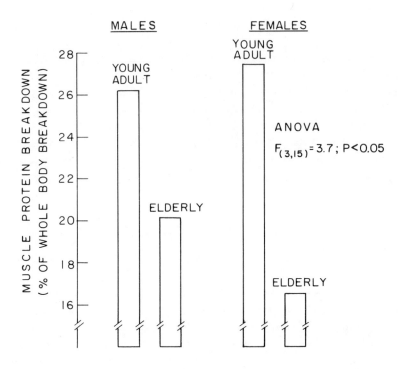

Fig. 4. Quantitative contribution by muscle to whole body protein
breakdown in young adult and elderly men and women. From
Uauy et al.[34].

TABLE 5

OBLIGATORY NITROGEN LOSSES IN YOUNG
ADULT MEN AND ELDERLY SUBJECTS

Obligatory N Loss	Young Males	Elderly	
		Males	Females
mgN per kg Body Wt	37.1	34.5	23.1[+]
mgN per kg BCM	79.7	98.1**	85.4
mgN per mg creatinine	1.54	2.2**	2.0
mgN per basal kcal	1.77	1.49*	1.41

*,** Significantly different from young males, $P<0.05$ and
     <0.005, respectively.

+   Significantly different from elderly men, $P<0.005$.

between young and old subjects might be expected to influence the efficiency of dietary portein utilization and perhaps the total protein requirement.

The most recent FAO/WHO Expert Committee on Energy and Protein Requirements[41] utilized the so-called factorial method to estimate the protein requirements of adults of various ages and to arrive at dietary protein allowances. This method of estimation is described in table 6 showing that from measurements of obligatory urinary, fecal and other N losses an estimate of total N losses is made. To convert this estimation to a requirement for dietary nitrogen (or protein) a factor in included to account for efficiency of dietary N utilization when intake approximates the mean dietary requirement. In order for the needs of nearly all members of the population to be covered an additional factor is included to account for variation in N metabolism among apparently similar subjects. Using this approach a factorial prediction of the safe practical intake for high quality, reference protein (such as egg or cow's milk) for elderly subjects is obtained. Predictions for young adults are compared in table 7 with those for elderly subjects and, by this method, the protein allowances for elderly men and women appear to be quite similar to those for young adults. However, a number of critical assumptions are made in arriving at the predictions shown in table 7. First, it is assumed that the efficiency of dietary N utilization at requirement levels of protein intake is the same in the young adults and elderly subject . Second, the extent of variability in nitrogen requirements among apparent similarly healthy elderly subjects is assumed to be the same as in young adults. Third, in converting the allowance for egg or milk protein to a diet of lower protein quality, it has to be assumed the relative nutritional value of different food protein sources is unaffected by age of the adult subject. Unfortunately, there are insufficient data to assess adequately the validity of these various assumptions and we have concluded, previously, that direct N balance studies designed to determine the physiological requirements for nitrogen in elderly subjects are essential in order to provide reliable estimates of the protein needs of a population group.

In a recent study in healthy elderly men and women, we examined the N balance response to graded intakes of good quality protein given with the submaintenance to maintenance range of protein intake[42]. This method is preferred as a basis for assessing the level of high quality protein intake that would be sufficient to maintain body N equilibrium in older subjects. Our results, based on studies in both

TABLE 6

FACTORIAL ESTIMATION OF PROTEIN REQUIREMENTS
AND ALLOWANCES FOR ADULT HUMANS[1]

---

1. Total obligatory N losses (O_N) = Obligatory urinary N +
   Obligatory fecal N + Skin N and miscellaneous N
2. Nitrogen requirement for maintenance (R_N), adjusting for
   efficienty of N utilization = O_N x 1.3
3. Safe practical allowance (for milk or egg protein),
   adjusting for individual variability (SPA) = R_N x 1.3
4. SPA predicted to be sufficient to cover needs of 97.5% of
   population

---

1. Based on method proposed by FAO/WHO[41]

TABLE 7

PREDICTION OF PROTEIN (NITROGEN) REQUIREMENTS AND OF THE SAFE
LEVEL OF INTAKE OF HIGH QUALITY PROTEIN FOR VARIOUS ADULT GROUPS

Group	Mean total obligatory N loss (mg/kg/day)	Adjusted mean N requirement[1] (mg/kg/day)	Safe level of intake[2]	
			N (mg/kg/day)	Protein[3] (g/kg/day)
Men	54	70	91	0.57
Women	49	64	83	0.52
Elderly Women	39	51	67	0.42
Elderly Men	51.7	67.2	87.4	0.55

1. Obligatory N losses are increased by 30% to account for
   efficiency of N utilization.
2. Values are adjusted requirement plus 30% to allow for
   individual variability.
3. As egg or milk protein.

elderly men and women are depicted in fig. 5, indicating that the N
requirement with egg (and presumably with milk protein) for more than
50% of elderly women is greater than 120 mg N/kg (or 0.8 g protein/kg)
and for nearly all elderly men the need lies somewhere in the range
of 0.7-0.8 g/kg/day. This estimate is considerably greater than the
level of 0.55 or even 0.42 g/kg/day that was predicted by the factorial
method to be sufficient for essentially all members of the population
(See table 7.).The reason for this large discrepancy is not clear,
but it is due to an underestimation of one or both factors (the
efficiency and variability factors) used in adjusting mean values of
total obligatory N losses to arrive at the population requirement.

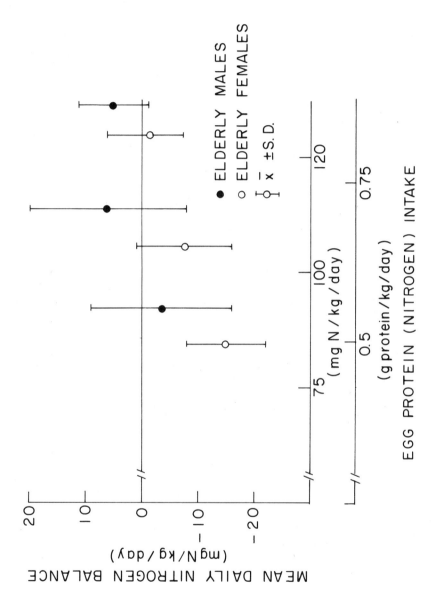

Fig. 5. Nitrogen balance response in elderly men and women receiving graded intakes of egg protein. From Uauy et al.[42].

Finally, it is necessary to consider the practical implications of these limited studies on the protein requirements of elderly subjects. Thus, it should be emphasized that our studies and discussion have focused upon observations and findings in healthy or medically privileged elderly individuals. As Exton-Smith[43] has so clearly indicated, there are numerous factors that modify the nutrient needs of individuals and population groups and/or alter the risk of nutritonal inadequacy. For protein nutrition, table 8 lists some of the factors that are applicable to elderly individuals in a population; infection, trauma and disease all increase the protein and nutrient needs of individuals, both during the acute and recovery phases. Furthermore, stress of psychological origin may also alter nutrient utilization and tend to increase protein needs[44]. Although the quantitative effects of these and other factors on the N requirement of individuals or of groups of individuals are not known, they cannot be ignored in developing safe dietary allowances for food planning, particularly because of their significance for many members of the elderly population. This makes the formulation of an appropriate, or safe, dietary protein allowance in the elderly population a difficult task.

We[44] have concluded previously that until more data become available, the safest procedure to follow in planning diets for the elderly, based

TABLE 8

SOME AGENT, HOST AND ENVIRONMENTAL FACTORS
THAT INFLUENCE DIETARY PROTEIN REQUIREMENTS
AND PROTEIN NUTRITIONAL STATUS IN THE ELDERLY

Agent (Dietary) Factors:
    1. Amino Acid Composition of Protein
    2. Energy Intake
    3. Food Processing and Preparation
Host Factors:
    1. Pathological States:
       Infection
       Trauma
       Cancer and Chronic Illness
       Malabsorptive and Gastrointestinal
         Disorders
    2. Psychological Problems:
       Loneliness, Apathy
       Mental Deterioration
    3. Drugs?
    4. Alcoholism
Environmental Factors:
    1. Socioeconomic:
       Poverty
       Food Fads, Poor Dietary Habits
    2. Biological:
       Physical Hygiene
    3. Physical:
       Unsuitable Housing

on the North American or European-type of diet, would be to adhere to the first international standard for protein of 1 g protein/kg body weight/day. If this is accepted and taking the 1974 allowances for energy as proposed by the U.S. Food and Nutrition Board[45], the recommendation translates into a diet supplying about 13% of the total energy intake as dietary protein. On this same basis the current dieatry protein recommendations of the U.S. Food and Nutrition Board for young adults and elderly males are about 7% and 9%, respectively. There is, of course, limited experimental validation for this proposal except that it is based on more recent data than those used in 1974 by the Food and Nutrition Board. Furthèrmore, it is consistent with good dietary practices and with epidemiological evidence indicating the absence of major problems associated with protein deficiency disease in elderly populations when diets provide this concentration and quality of food protein.

ACKNOWLEDGEMENTS

We thank Drs. N.S. Scrimshaw and R. Uauy for their great help in the unpublished studies referred to in this paper. The authors studies have been supported by NIH grants MA15856, AM 16654 and AG 0475.

REFERENCES

1. Diamond MC (1978) Am.Sci. 66:66.

2. Scrimshaw NS & Gordon JE (eds)(1968) Malnutrition, Learning and Behaviour, MIT Press.

3. Nowak TS & Munro HN (1977) in Nutrition and the Brain (eds. RJ Wurtman & JJ Wurtman) Raven Press, New York, pp. 193-260.

4. Young VR, Perera WD, Winterer JC & Scrimshaw NS (1976) in Nutrition and Aging, Winick M, ed, J. Wiley & Sons, New York, pp. 77-118.

5. Young VR, Uauy R, Winterer JC & Scrimshaw NS (1976) in Nutrition, Longevity and Aging. M. Rockstein & ML Sussman, eds. Academic Press, New York, pp. 67-102.

6. Uauy R, Scrimshaw NS & Young VR (1978) In: Proc. Symp. on Nutrition of the Aged, Nutr. Soc. Canada, June 1977 (in press).

7. Munro HN (1974) In: Aromatic Amino Acids in the Brain. CIBA Foundation Symposium 22, Elsevier, Excerpta Medica, North Holland, Amsterdam, pp. 1-24.

8. Cahill GF,Jr (1970) New Engl. J. Med. 282:668.

9. Felig P (1973) Metab. Clin. Exptl. 22:178.

10. Young VR & Scrimshaw NS (1978) In: Protein Resources and Technology: Status and Research Needs. Milner N, Scrimshaw NS & Wang DIC, eds. AVI Publ. Co., Inc. Westport, Conn. pp. 136-173.

11. Goldberg AL, Howell EM, Li JB, Martel SD & Prouty SF (1974) Fed. Proc. 33:1112.

12. Buse MG, Herlong HF & Weigand DA (1976) Endocrinol. 98:1166.

13. Khatra B, Chawla R, Sewell C & Rudman D (1977) J. Clin. Investig. 59:558.

14. Hambraeus L, Bilmazes C, Dippel C, Scrimshaw HS & Young VR (1976) J. Nutr. 106:230.

15. Conway JC, Bier D, Burke JF & Young VR (1978) Fed. Proc. 37:435 (abstr.)

16. Young VR & Scrimshaw NS (1972) In: International Encyclopedia of Food and Nutrition. EJ Bigwood, ed. Pergamon Press, Oxford & New York, pp. 541-568.

17. McLaughlan JM (1974) In: Improvement in Protein Nutriture. National Academy of Sciences, Washington DC pp. 89-108.

18. Tontisirin K, Young VR & Scrimshaw NS (1972) Am.J.Clin.Nutr.25:976.

19. Young VR, Hussein MA, Murray E & Scrimshaw NS (1971) J. Nutr. 101:45.

20. Tontisirin K, Young VR, Miller M & Scrimshaw NS (1973) J. Nutr. 103:1220.

21. Forbes GB & Reina JC (1970) Metabolism Clin. Exptl. 19:653.

22. Rossman I (1977) In: Handbook of the Biology of Aging. Finch CE & Hayflick L. Van Nostrand Reinhold Co., New York pp. 189-221.

23. Korenchevsky V (1961) Physiological & Pathological Ageing Hafner Publ. Co., New York.

24. Graystone JE (1968) In: Human Growth, DB Cheek, ed. Lea & Febiger, Phila, PA pp. 182-197.

25. Daniel PM, Pratt OE & Spargo E (1977) Proc. Roy. Soc. Lond. B 196:347.

26. Nicholson JF (1970) Pediat. Res. 4:389.

27. Pencharz PB, Steffee SP, Cochran W, Scrimshaw NS, Rand WM & Young VR (1977) Clin. Sci. Mol. Med. 52:455.

28. Picou D & Taylor-Roberts R (1969) Clin. Sic. 36:283.

29. Golden MHN, Waterlow JC & Picou D (1977) Clin. Sci. Mol. Med. 53:473.

30. Wu H & Snyderman SE (1959) J. Gen. Physiol. 34:339.

31. Kien CL, Young VR, Rohrbaugh DK & Burke JF (1978) Metab. 27:27.

32. Steffee SP, Goldsmith RS, Pencharz PB, Scrimshaw NS & Young VR (1976) Metab. 25:281.

33. Halliday D & McKeran RO (1975) Clin. Sci. Mol. Med. 49:581.

34. Uauy R, Winterer JC, Bilmazes C, Haverberg LN, Scrimshaw NS, Munro HN & Young VR (1978) J. Gerontol. (in press).

35. Golden MHN & Waterlow JC (1977) Clin. Sci. Mol. Med. 53:277.

36. Bilmazes C, Uauy R, Haverberg LN, Munro HN & Young VR (1978) Metabolism 27 (in press).

37. Young VR & Munro HN (1978) Fed. Proc. 37 (in press).

38. Scrimshaw NS, Perera WDA & Young VR (1976) J. Nutr. 106:665.

39. Uauy R, Scrimshaw NS, Rand WM & Young VR (1978) J. Nutr. 108:97.

40. Rand WM, Scrimshaw NS & Young VR (1976) Am. J. Clin. Nutr. 29:639.

41. FAO/WHO (1973) Energy and Protein Requirements Report of a Joint FAO/WHO Ad Hoc Expert Committee. World Health Organization Rept. Ser. No. 522 WHO Geneva.

42. Uauy R, Scrimshaw NS & Young VR (1978) Am. J. Clin.Nutr.(in press).

43. Exton-Smith AN (1973) In: Nutritional Problems in a Changing World (eds. D. Hollingsworth & M. Russell) pp. 221-231. J. Wiley & Sons, New York.

44. Young VR & Scrimshaw NS (1975) Urban Health 4:37.

45. National Research Council, Food and Nutrition Board (1974) Recommended Dietary Allowances 8th Edn. National Academy of Sci., Washington, DC.

INDEX